environment of care®
risk assessment

3rd *edition*

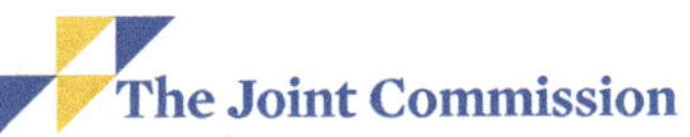

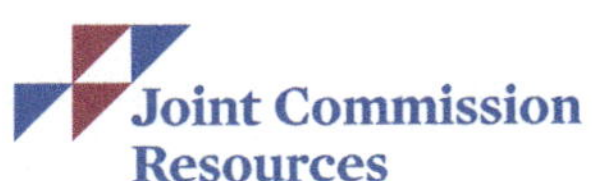

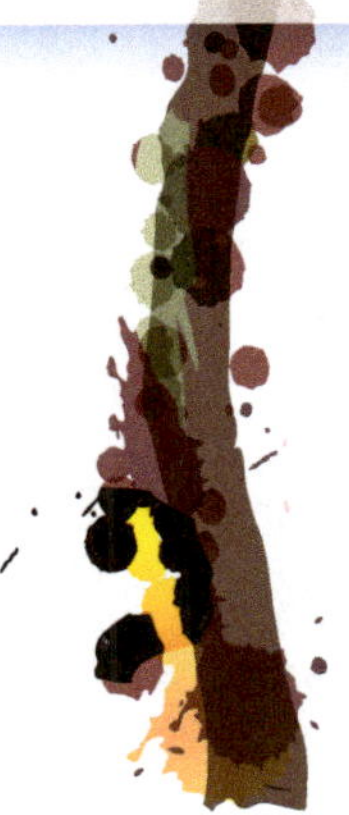

Senior Editor: Kathleen DeMase
Project Manager: Lisa King
Associate Director, Publications: Helen M. Fry, MA
Associate Director, Production and Meeting Support: Johanna Harris
Executive Director, Global Publishing: Catherine Chopp Hinckley, MA, PhD
Joint Commission/Joint Commission Resources Reviewers: Lynne Bergero, MHSA; Barbara Braun, PhD, CPH; Andrea D. Browne, PhD, DABR; Caroline Heskett, MPH; John Maurer, SASHE, CHFM, CHSP; Herman McKenzie, MBA, CHSP; Ken Monroe, PE, MBA, CHC, PMP; James G. Parker; Kathy Tolomeo, CHEM, CHSP; Lisa Waldowski, DNP, PNP, CIC; James Woodson, PE, CHFM

Joint Commission Resources Mission

The mission of Joint Commission Resources (JCR) is to continuously improve the safety and quality of health care in the United States and in the international community through the provision of education, publications, consultation, and evaluation services.

Joint Commission Resources educational programs and publications support, but are separate from, the accreditation activities of The Joint Commission. Attendees at Joint Commission Resources educational programs and purchasers of Joint Commission Resources publications receive no special consideration or treatment in, or confidential information about, the accreditation process.

The inclusion of an organization name, product, or service in a Joint Commission Resources publication should not be construed as an endorsement of such organization, product, or service, nor is failure to include an organization name, product, or service to be construed as disapproval.

This publication is designed to provide accurate and authoritative information in regard to the subject matter covered. Every attempt has been made to ensure accuracy at the time of publication; however, please note that laws, regulations, and standards are subject to change. Please also note that some of the examples in this publication are specific to the laws and regulations of the locality of the facility. The information and examples in this publication are provided with the understanding that the publisher is not engaged in providing medical, legal, or other professional advice. If any such assistance is desired, the services of a competent professional person should be sought.

ISBN: 978-1-63585-001-7 (soft cover)
ISBN: 978-1-63585-002-4 (e-book)

For more information about Joint Commission Resources, please visit http://www.jcrinc.com.

Contents

Introduction

Risk—a simple concept defined as the potential to cause harm—is an ongoing concern for health care organizations. Health care organizations are in the business of serving people; however, there is more to the care, treatment, and services of individuals than the clinical aspects. The physical environment of a health care facility—also known as the environment of care (EC)—is equally important because maintaining the environment creates a safe and secure atmosphere for staff to carry out their job functions, including providing quality care, treatment, and services to individuals. To manage risk, an organization must first identify and assess the risk.

About EC Risk Assessment

In order to ensure a safe and secure environment, organizations must assess the risks to their environment of care. Risk assessment—in the simplest terms—is a systematic method that accomplishes the following:

- Determines the potential negative consequences (risks) of an action or situation
- Evaluates the extent of those risks
- Decides whether to accept, mediate, or avoid those risks

As defined and applied throughout this book, *EC risk assessment* is a proactive examination of functions and processes in the physical environment used to assess actual and potential risks. Results from the assessment are then prioritized to identify improvement opportunities. The related concept of *risk management* involves the systematic application of policies, procedures, and practices to identify, analyze, evaluate, address, monitor, and communicate risk.

The Joint Commission requires organizations in all health care settings to conduct and document risk assessments to manage risks in the following seven functional areas of the environment of care:

1. Safety
2. Security
3. Hazardous materials and waste
4. Fire safety and life safety
5. Medical equipment
6. Utilities
7. Preconstruction

Then, organizations must establish a course of action that is both defensible and rational, implement the course of action, and analyze if the desired affect was achieved. Various health care settings manage their physical environment in different ways, and this book supports any staff who participates in EC risk-assessment activities. (*See* the matrix of applicability in Chapter 1 beginning on page 8.)

Risk assessments can vary widely in form and application, from a quick examination and judgment of a situation to a formalized set of policies and procedures that are carefully outlined and documented.

Environment of Care® Risk Assessment, Third Edition, introduces and discusses the various risk-assessment processes within the environment of care. This book is designed to help health care organizations develop and implement a comprehensive EC management program that includes risk assessment. To this end, the book provides suggestions on how to design and implement a proactive risk-assessment process and conduct effective risk assessments that address the various components of the environment of care, as well as tools to support the risk-assessment process.

In addition, this book discusses the importance of including staff from across the organization to participate in risk-assessment efforts (*see* the illustration on page ix). EC management programs see more success when a cross section of staff share their insight and expertise when evaluating potential and identified risks in the physical environment.

The Joint Commission is not prescriptive about how risk assessments are performed, allowing organizations to develop and use assessment methods that best suit their circumstances and needs. By taking a proactive approach and applying a multidisciplinary team to assessing risks in the environment of care, organizations will ensure compliance with Joint Commission standards and can achieve a safer environment for all people in their facility while improving the quality of care they provide.

About This Edition

This edition includes expanded or new chapters that cover a variety of topics including the Statement of Conditions™ (SOC), environmental tours, imaging staff, workplace bullying and violence, fire safety, hazardous materials and waste, construction, and maintaining a safe environment. It also addresses the Survey Analysis for Evaluating Risk™ (SAFER™) Matrix and changes to Intracycle Monitoring (ICM). Information has been updated throughout to reflect current standards and requirements, and the US Centers for Medicare & Medicaid Services' (CMS) adoption of the 2012 *Life Safety Code®*,* including details on the following:

- Integration of the 2012 *Life Safety Code* into Joint Commission standards and requirements
- Safety risks outside the building
- Safety data sheets and labeling requirements
- Alternative equipment maintenance (AEM) for medical equipment and utilities
- Data security
- E-cigarettes
- Emergency exercises
- Construction strategies that support risk management

---

* *Life Safety Code®* is a registered trademark of the National Fire Protection Association, Quincy, MA.

Contents of This Book

Chapter 1 provides a general overview of risk assessment, its importance to an organization, and suggestions for implementing a proactive risk-assessment process.

Chapter 2 discusses different tools and processes The Joint Commission uses that organizations can adapt as risk-assessment tools.

Chapters 3 through 9 offer information on risk assessments specific to different aspects of the environment of care, in the following order:

3. Safety
4. Hazardous materials and waste
5. Security
6. Fire and life safety
7. Medical equipment
8. Utilities
9. Emergency management

Chapter 10 discusses specific risks that arise during a demolition, construction, or renovation project.

In addition, a glossary has been added to this third edition.

Terms Used in This Book

Terms used in this book are not intended to exclude any health care setting accredited by The Joint Commission. Every attempt has been made to ensure the descriptions and the included tools are applicable to all program settings. In addition, the use of the term *patient* in this book is not intended to exclude any individuals receiving care, treatment, or services in other program settings; this book endeavors to serve readers by providing solid strategies and useful tools to ensure all individuals—whether working, visiting or receiving care—remain safe.

Features

This edition includes the following features that are meant to single out ideas, topics, tools, and examples to help the reader better understand the complexities of risk assessment in the environment of care.

Consider This

This feature provides a spotlight for information both critical and/or supplemental to the topics discussed in each chapter.

EC Risk Assessment—A Multidisciplinary Approach

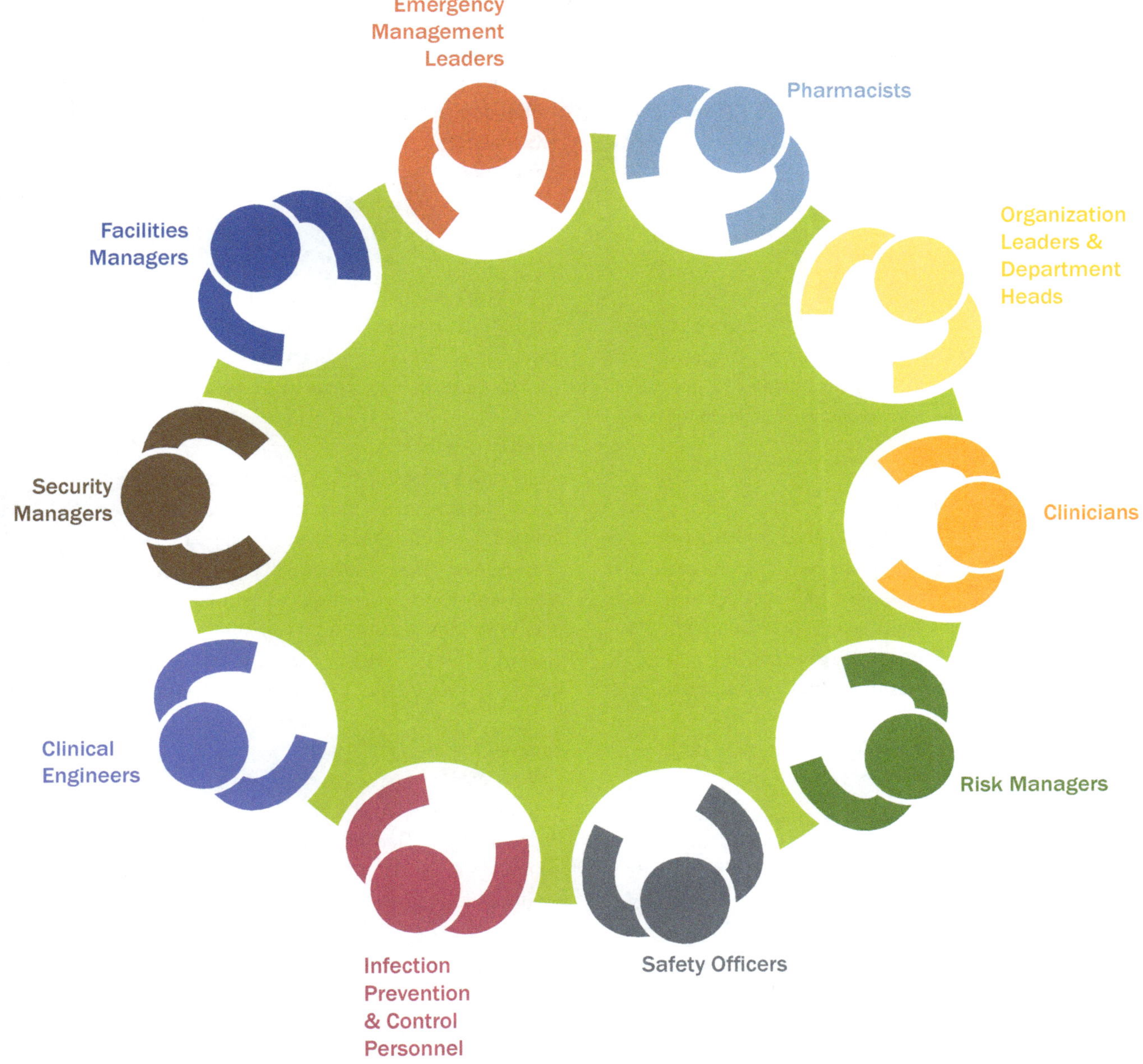

Environment of care (EC) risk-assessment activities can easily be thought of as the exclusive responsibility of facilities staff—safety officers, facilities managers, security managers, and emergency management leaders. However, to be most effective, The Joint Commission recommends conducting risk assessments with a multidisciplinary team that includes staff from a variety of areas across an organization. This cross section of staff provides valuable insight when identifying issues and contributing resources to assess and remedy any identified threats. This book is intended for anyone within an organization who can and should partici-pate in an EC risk assessment, including the disciplines identified in this illustration.

For Example. . .

Real-world examples are a fundamental tool when learning how to consider what should be assessed or why something should be assessed. These examples provide a quick snapshot of risk-assessment scenarios.

Have a Look

These infographics provide quick information in a succinct image.

Risk Assessment in the Field

While the *For example. . .* feature provides quick examples to understand concepts being discussed, this feature provides robust case studies of risk assessment in the real world. In addition to real-world solutions, real-world tools also may be included.

Risk-Assessment Toolbox

This section, at the end of each chapter, provides a complete list of the tools referenced in the chapter. In some cases, this list includes multiple versions of the same tool (for example, Tool Checklist portrait and Tool Checklist landscape) or the file contains multiple worksheets (for example, Excel files). Readers will be able to access these blank tools and sample policies in one of two ways:

1. Open the file from the flash drive (print version only)
2. Click on the tool link (electronic version only)

Once accessed, tools can be customized to the reader's needs for his or her organization.

Standards to Know

This feature, at the beginning of most chapters, lists the standards most relevant to the chapter topic as well as any standards referenced in the chapter. This is not an all-inclusive list of applicable standards, but provides readers with the most pertinent ones to reference.

Terms to Know

This list provided at the beginning of each chapter includes key terms relevant to the topic areas discussed in the chapter. Definitions for these terms are found in the glossary.

Tools

To remain in compliance with Joint Commission standards, risk-assessment efforts must be documented. Oftentimes, tools—such as the ones included in this book—can serve as that documentation or support other risk-assessment documentation. This book includes two types of tools for readers:

1. Examples—which are marked as "Tools in Use"
2. Blank—which are marked as "Tools of the Trade"

All tools are available for readers to use and adapt to their program setting and can be accessed on the flash drive (print only) or by clicking the tool link in the Risk-Assessment Toolbox (e-book only) at the end of each chapter.

Tools in Use

As the title suggests, "Tools in Use" are examples of tools—including checklists, dashboards, worksheets, and policies—that are critical to assessing the environment of care. Seeing these tools in use helps readers see the value these tools can have in their organization. Blank files of checklists, dashboards, and worksheets are available for use, while full policies are available for review and can be adapted for the reader's organizational needs.

Tools of the Trade

Checklists, worksheets, and templates make up the variety of tools presented in this book. This feature provides a snapshot of the blank tools available for download. The more than 50 tools available are fully customizable to ensure the reader can apply them to his or her organization.

Acknowledgments

This third edition of *Environment of Care® Risk Assessment* would not have been possible without our writer, Erik Martin, and our subject matter expert, Kathy Tolomeo, CHEM, CHSP. Their commitment to ensure that this book provides readers with the most up-to-date and accurate information, in a user-friendly format, has been invaluable.

In addition, we are grateful for the real-world scenarios and tools provided by the following organizations:

- Charleston Area Medical Center, Charleston, WV
- Edward Hospital & Health Services, Naperville, IL
- Gateway Foundation, Chicago, IL
- Kaiser Permanente, Oakland, CA
- Mercy Health Partners, Cincinnati, OH
- Northwestern Memorial Hospital, Chicago, IL
- Tampa General Hospital, Tampa, FL
- University of Texas MD Anderson Cancer Center, Houston, TX
- University of Toledo Medical Center, Toledo, OH
- University of Wisconsin Hospitals and Clinics, Madison, WI
- White Plains Hospital, White Plains, NY

The contributions from these organizations provide unique perspective and tools readers can apply to their own organization. Finally, we are deeply indebted to our Joint Commission and Joint Commission Resources reviewers for their time and expert knowledge (*see* copyright page for a list of these individuals.)

chapter 1

Risk-Assessment Basics

Risk—in a health care organization—occurs daily. When one aspect of the multiple processes and procedures in place to ensure the quality of the care, treatment, and services for individuals fails, the potential for harm exists. When the environment of care (EC)—that is, the physical environment—is compromised, the safety and security of any individuals in a health care facility are at risk. To understand what risk is and the importance of assessing risk in the environment of care, the sections in this chapter will explore the following seven basic questions:

1. **Why.** Why assess risks?
2. **Which.** Which Joint Commission requirements apply?
3. **When.** When should risk assessment occur?
4. **What.** What types of EC risk assessments are required?
5. **Where.** Where are the risks?
6. **Who.** Who identifies the issues needing a risk assessment?
7. **How.** How can an organization conduct a risk assessment?

Why Assess Risks?

The health care environment is fraught with risks—affecting buildings, equipment, and people (*see* the illustration on page 2). To manage these risks, Joint Commission standards require organizations to use risk assessments to identify threats in the physical environment and implement improvement measures to minimize or eliminate the identified threats. An effective method to ensure a health care organization is managing its required risk assessments is to integrate them into their EC management plans (*see* page 11 for more information on EC management plans).

Conducting risk assessments ensures that health care organizations identify potential safety and security risks and, based on what is identified, determine what actions are necessary to improve safety and security within the organization. In addition, risk assessments can provide the following benefits:

- Improve organizationwide safety and security
- Improve efficiency
- Identify training and education opportunities
- Identify performance improvement opportunities
- Justify a need
- Evaluate the effect of changes
- Inform long-term goals
- Comply with regulations and standards

TERMS *to know*

adverse event

risk assessment

sentinel event

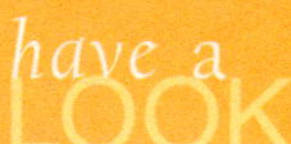

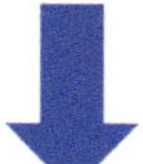

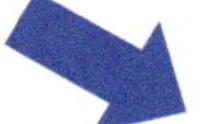

Regardless of an organization's setting, environment of care risks affect everyone—patients, residents, individuals served, staff, and visitors. These items, conditions, and events are a small sampling of risks that can be found in a health care facility.

The following sections explore the importance of conducting risk assessments in greater detail.

Improve Organizationwide Safety and Security

Safety and security are often mentioned in the same breath, but each presents distinct risks. Safety risks usually are related to *unintentional* incidents that occur in everyday tasks (covering worker safety), in the physical structure, or due to uncontrollable factors (such as weather). Security risks are related to incidents that are often *intentional* and result in harm or loss to people and property (shootings, violence, patient suicides, bomb threats, patient wandering or elope- ments, infant or pediatric abductions, drug thefts). Therefore, it is important to conduct risk assessments to identify, mitigate, and resolve threats to patient and staff safety and security—to help improve safety and security across the entire organization.

Every risk assessment affects patient and staff safety or security in some way. How a risk assessment improves patient and staff safety or security depends on the type of risk assessment and whether it can directly or indirectly protect patients and staff. Examples of such risk assess- ments include the following:

- *Organizationwide employee safety risk assessment.* Used to identify and protect staff members from risks associated with their work environments
- *Process-based safety risk assessment.* Used to review a process—such as storing sharps at the bedside—to look for potential ways to eliminate a possible patient or workplace injury
- *Security risk assessment.* Used to identify areas of potential security risk—such as dark parking lots, thick shrubbery around building exits, or areas not covered by security cameras—that could lead to a security incident with a patient or staff member if not addressed

◉ *Medical equipment risk assessment.* Used to evaluate and reveal pieces of equipment that are prone to failure and could result in patient harm if not addressed

Improve Efficiency

Just because organizations have processes in place does not mean that those processes are efficient. An organization will often engage in activities using a particular method simply because it has "always" used it or because it adopted the method from another organization. By conducting risk assessments, organizations can identify processes that are inefficient and ineffective and determine potential ways to improve efficiency, accuracy, and appropriateness.

Identify Training and Education Opportunities

Risk assessments can be valuable training tools because they identify hazards, build awareness about potentially negative situations, and point toward resolutions of those situations. For example, a security risk assessment can be used to discuss potential security concerns within organizations or within security-sensitive areas. Using the assessment as a teaching tool, the organization can build awareness about those concerns and any programs in place to reduce security risks.

Organizations also can use formalized risk assessments to guide development of their education programs by identifying areas where further education is needed to achieve safe delivery of care. For example, a risk assessment that looks at potential suicide risks for psychiatric patients may identify the need for further staff training on suicide and the environmental risks associated with suicide. Such an assessment could identify gaps in staff knowledge and areas that need improvement.

Identify Performance Improvement Opportunities

The Joint Commission requires organizations to conduct performance improvement activities. Risk assessments can pinpoint specific areas to be improved—for example, hand-hygiene compliance or staff reaction time during a fire emergency. Leadership can and should use risk assessments to prioritize performance improvement initiatives for the organization. Issues that are high risk, problem prone, and high volume should be given priority. An identified risk that has a wide scope and significant potential for harm may be targeted for improvement before a risk that has limited scope or less impactful consequences. Or a risk that directly affects patient safety on a daily basis may be given priority over an environmental risk that may or may not occur.

Justify a Need

Often the need for new equipment, staff, or space will go unmet because of budget or time constraints. The affected department or unit may need to justify its need, explaining to leadership what is needed and the consequences of not providing it. Risk assessments can serve this purpose by focusing attention on a need and the consequences of not meeting the need, and providing a clear solution.

for example...

The facilities manager in a large community hospital notices during a visual inspection that the floor deck of the air-handling unit is rusting out. He identifies the need to replace the current air-handling unit in his annual evaluation presented to senior leadership. However, after numerous requests, he receives no support because of lack of funding.

When a new chief executive officer (CEO) arrives, the facilities manager once again makes the case for a new air-handling unit. This time, he tests the air quality in the ICUs and two oncology units, where vulnerable patients are housed. He compiles the results in a dashboard. The air-quality test results are color coded in red, which indicates they are outside of acceptable ranges. This visual tool—essentially a risk assessment—helps the facilities manager demonstrate the need for a new air-handling unit to the CEO.

Evaluate the Effect of Changes

Every organization will periodically change its processes, procedures, and policies to reflect new standards, or in response to a performance improvement project or other driver. Performing risk assessments potentially can determine whether the change is managing the risk it is designed to manage, as well as expose any new risks that may emerge as a result of the change.

Complying with OSHA

The US Occupational Safety and Health Administration (OSHA) is a federal agency that aims to ensure employee safety and health in the United States by working with employers and employees to create better working environments. Its mission is to prevent work-related injuries, illnesses, and deaths. OSHA has a series of regulations that organizations must follow to ensure employee safety and health. Failure to comply with OSHA's regulations may result in violations citations from the agency.

Types of OSHA Violations[1]

Citations for failure to comply with OSHA's regulations vary based on the likelihood the hazardous condition will result in serious physical harm or death, as well as the employer's intent to actively seek a solution for or willfully disregard the hazardous condition.

Other-than-serious violations

OSHA classifies these violations as having a direct relationship to job safety and health but are not serious in nature. Violations under this classification are not considered life threatening, and the risk of serious physical harm is minimal.

Serious violations

Workplace hazards that have a high probability of causing an accident or illness resulting in death or serious physical harm are classified as "serious" violations. In these situations, the violation is cited when an employer knew or should have known of the hazard and its resulting consequences.

Willful violations

Employers that intentionally disregard OSHA regulations or show a plain indifference to employee safety and health will be cited for willful violation.

Repeat violations

Such citations occur when a violation of any standard, regulation, rule, or order where, upon reinspection, a substantially similar violation is found. In these cases, the original citation becomes a final order and a penalty may be ordered.

Failure to abate prior violations

When an employer fails to correct a prior violation a failure to abate prior violations is cited. The penalty will be applied when the violation continues beyond the prescribed abatement date.

Additional violations

In addition to the previously listed violations, OSHA may cite employers for the following actions:
- Falsifying records, reports, or applications
- Violating posting requirements
- Assaulting a compliance officer or otherwise impeding a compliance officer's performance of duties

Penalties for OSHA Violations[2]

To account for inflation, Congress passed the Federal Civil Penalties Inflation Adjustment Act Improvements Act in November 2015, directing federal agencies to adjust their civil penalties. This legislation allowed agencies a one-time catch-up increase to allow for years of nonadjustment. OSHA last adjusted its penalties in 1990, thus an increase of 78% was made effective August 1, 2016. Going forward the agency will adjust penalties for inflation based on the Consumer Price Index. Civil penalties, as well as any criminal penalties, for each type of violation, include the following:*

Other-than-serious violations. Proposed penalty of up to $12,675 per violation. Both types of violations may be adjusted depending on factors such as compliance efforts, previous inspection history, and business size.

Serious violations. Mandatory penalty of up to $12,675 per violation. Similar to other-than-serious violations, this type of violation may be adjusted downward depending on factors such as severity of the violation, compliance efforts, previous inspection history, and business size.

Willful violations. Penalty of up to $126,749 per violation, with the minimum penalty being $9,054 per violation. These violations may be adjusted depending on the size of the business and previous inspection history, but typically no credit is given for good faith.

Employers convicted of a willful violation that resulted in the death of an employee may be punishable by a court-imposed fine of up to $250,000 for an individual or $500,000 for a corporation or imprisonment for up to six months, or both. Convictions on additional violations may increase the term of imprisonment.

Repeat violations. Penalty of up to $126,749 per violation.

Failure to abate. Penalty of up to $12,675 for each day the violation continues beyond the abatement date.

---

* Penalties are based on amounts adjusted for inflation as of January 2017.

References
1. Safety News Alert. Types of OSHA Violations. Accessed Feb 20, 2018. http://www.safetynewsalert.com/types-of-osha-violations.
2. Occupational Safety and Health Administration. Press Release: US Department of Labor Announces New Rules to Adjust Civil Penalty Amounts. Jun 30, 2016. Accessed Feb 20, 2018. https://www.osha.gov/news/newsreleases/national/06302016.

for
example...

A new hand-hygiene policy in a health care facility results in the installation of touch-free faucets in patient care rooms. After the faucets are in use, the infection preventionist performs a risk assessment discovering that the new faucets are harboring bacteria. It is determined that environmental services has been cleaning the new faucets the same way as the old faucets, because they were not given the different instructions from the manufacturer of the new faucets.

Inform Long-Term Goals

Long-term—or "big-picture"—goals and strategic plans are based on data. One source of those data is risk assessments. The information gleaned from risk assessments can help leadership make decisions about expanding or eliminating services or construction or renovation projects and which investments support the health care organization's overall mission and serve to meet its patient safety goals.

Comply with Regulations and Standards

If organizations do not perform risk assessments adequately, their inaction may lead to serious consequences, including US Occupational Safety and Health Administration (OSHA) violations (*see* page 4 for more information about OSHA violations), a change in Joint Commission accreditation status, adverse events and/or sentinel events, or legal problems.

for
example...

A psychiatric patient commits suicide in his room one night at a large medical center. The organization is stunned by the event because it has many processes and interventions in place to prevent such events.

Examples of the facility's processes and interventions to minimize a patient's risk of hanging include the following:

- Providing special linens, including shorter towels—this limits a patient's ability to create a hanging risk by tying them together.
- Accounting daily for all linens—this also limits a patient's ability to create a hanging risk by ensuring that the patient has not been given extra linens or is "saving" linens.
- Installing the following in patient rooms and on the floor to eliminate hanging risk:
  - Modified doorknobs
  - Nurse call pull cords
  - Breakaway shower rods

In this case, the facilities engineer who maintains the psychiatric floor went on vacation, and the organization assigned a new engineer to that floor on a temporary basis. However, the new engineer did not receive training on the potential suicide risks associated with psychiatric patients and the environmental interventions and processes put in place to mitigate those risks. The psychiatric department called engineering to report that a shower rod broke in one of the patient's rooms and needed to be replaced. The temporary engineer did not know that only breakaway shower rods are installed on the psych unit. Consequently, a normal shower rod was installed in the patient's room, and, that night, the patient hanged himself.

In addition to the horrific nature of the sentinel event itself, this lapse in risk management could result in Preliminary Denial of Accreditation from The Joint Commission and potentially make the organization vulnerable to a lawsuit.

Which Joint Commission Requirements Apply?

The Joint Commission requires organizations to conduct a variety of risk assessments and offers recommendations for specific assessments. Joint Commission EC standards require that organizations have a process for assessing risks specifically in the physical environment and related areas. Organizations also should consider risks that could be organizationwide, department specific, and/or issue specific. For example, Leadership (LD) standards require an organization to conduct not less than one proactive risk assessment on a high-risk process a minimum of every 18 months. Infection Prevention and Control (IC) standards require organizations to identify and plan for risks for acquiring and transmitting infections. Additional EC standards require preconstruction risk assessments for air quality, infection control, utilities, noise, vibration, and other hazards associated with a demolition, construction, or renovation project. These are only a few examples of risk-assessment requirements, and not an exhaustive list. Page 9 provides an applicability matrix that includes a list of key Joint Commission standards anyone accountable for risk assessments for the physical environment, emergency management, and life safety must know. Other risk-related standards will be noted throughout the book and listed in the Standards to Know feature at the beginning of most chapters.

Documentation

The Joint Commission requires documentation for many of the previously mentioned risk assessments. (Elements of performance [EPs] that require documentation are identified with a ⓓ icon in the *Comprehensive Accreditation Manual* and online in E-dition®.) The form that documentation takes may vary, but the general rule is "not documented, not done." In other words, documentation is proof that a risk assessment was actually performed. Risk-assessment documentation also can be used to illustrate an organization's work on a particular issue.

If in doubt, document. This is a good rule to observe because documentation has benefits beyond complying with standards. Documenting is extremely useful during the risk-assessment process because it helps establish the steps involved in the risk assessment and records the results in a consistent manner. In addition, documentation aids in maintaining consistency throughout the risk-assessment process so that every time a particular type of risk assessment is conducted—such as a job hazards analysis (JHA) or a medical equipment inventory—it is completed the same way or a variation can be planned.

Risk assessments can be documented in a variety of ways. They can be completed using established forms or spreadsheets that organizations create, like one often used in the hazard vulnerability analysis (HVA) process (see Chapter 9 for more information on HVA). Or the assessment can be documented by simply drawing a line down the middle of a piece of paper and listing the pros of a project or process on one side and the cons on the other. The method chosen will depend on the situation and organization.

Although The Joint Commission does not always require a specific form of documentation, it does require organizations to follow their own policies. So, if an organization's policies require documentation, The Joint Commission will require the organization to document activities in accordance with their policies. Consequently, organizations should make sure that their developed documentation systems are used appropriately and consistently (*see* page 11 for information about EC management plans).

When Should Risk Assessment Occur?

Risk assessments are most effective when an organization clearly defines and documents the type and frequency of its required risk assessments. While The Joint Commission has some guidance on how frequently risk assessments should be conducted, ultimately the organization must determine the frequency.

Requirements of The Joint Commission

Joint Commission standards—in general—do not specifically outline risk-assessment time lines that organizations must comply with, although EC management plans must undergo an annual evaluation (every 12 months) to ensure they are still relevant, applicable, and effective. The Joint Commission tasks organizations to determine what types of risk assessments they will conduct and how often those risk assessments will be conducted. In many cases, the standards indicate that manufacturers' recommendations and state and federal requirements direct organizations to determine how often to conduct risk assessments. *See* the *Comprehensive Accreditation Manual* or E-dition for specific Joint Commission monitoring and risk-assessment requirements. (For a documentation schedule for Joint Commission–required activities to help monitor the physical environment, *see* page 10.)

Continuous Monitoring

To be effective, risk assessment cannot be conducted just to check another box on the compliance list—done once and then forgotten. Risk assessments should be used as continuous and active learning and improvement tools. Organizations must take the information gleaned from a risk assessment and respond to the risk points. This response may involve changing a process, introducing a new process, or planning for reassessment to determine the effectiveness

text continued on page 13

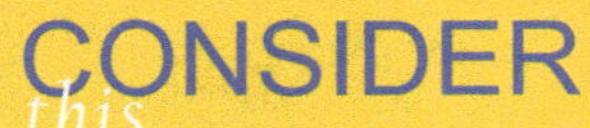

Applicability Matrix of Joint Commission Standards Related to EC Risk Assessment

This matrix provides a quick guide to review the key Joint Commission EC-related risk-assessment standards. The standards listed represent the foundational risk-assessment compliance requirements in each core area of the environment of care, including safety, hazardous materials and waste, security, fire and life safety, medical equipment, utilities, emergency management, and construction, as represented in the following standards chapters:

* Environment of Care (EC)
* Emergency Management (EM)
* Life Safety (LS)

This matrix—and this book—focuses on EC-related risk assessments, but a quick review of this list will reveal that most of these standards require organizations to *manage* risk, not *assess* risk. It's important to understand The Joint Commission interprets risk management as requiring risk assessment. The words, in some ways, are interchangeable.

Keep in mind that it is a standard's elements of performance (EPs) that outline the specific action(s), process(es), or structure(s) that must be implemented to achieve the goal of the standard—they are what the surveyor will assess during an onsite survey. Refer to the program-specific *Comprehensive Accreditation Manual* or its online E-dition® version for the applicable EPs as well as any updates to these standards.

The following list is intended to focus attention on the core areas of the environment of care. Additional standards are closely related to mitigating and managing the risks identified during an EC risk assessment. Many of these related requirements are noted throughout the book and are referenced in the Standards to Know feature that opens most chapters. For example, Infection Prevention and Control (IC) Standard IC.01.03.01 requires organizations to identify risks related to infection, which is tightly tied to environmental issues, and National Patient Safety Goal (NPSG) 15, specifically NPSG.15.01.01.01, has an EP that requires a risk assessment of the environmental features that affect the risk of patient suicide.

Standard	Program Setting							
	AHC	BHC	CAH	HAP	LAB	NCC	OBS	OME
EC.01.01.01 The [organization] plans activities to/that minimize risks in the environment of care.	×	×	×	×	×	×		
EC.02.01.01 The [organization] manages safety and security risks.	×	×	×	×	×	×	×	×
EC.02.02.01 The [organization] manages risks related to hazardous materials [and waste].	×	×	×	×	×	×	×	×
EC.02.03.01 The [organization] manages fire risks.	×	×	×	×	×	×	×	×
EC.02.04.01 The [organization] manages [medical/ laboratory] equipment risks.	×		×	×	×	×	×	
EC.02.05.01 The [organization] manages risks associated with its utility systems.	×	×	×	×	×	×	×	×
EC.02.06.05 The [organization] manages its [space/ environment] during demolition, renovation, or new construction [to reduce risk to those in the organization/laboratory].	×	×	×	×	×		×	
EM.01.01.01 The [organization] engages in planning activities prior to developing its [written] Emergency [Management/Operations] Plan.	×	×	×	×	×	×		×
LS.01.01.01 The [organization] designs and manages the physical environment to comply with the *Life Safety Code®*.*	×	×	×	×		×		×

AHC, Ambulatory Health Care; BHC, Behavioral Health Care; CAH, Critical Access Hospitals; HAP, Hospitals; LAB, Laboratory and Point-of-Care Testing; NCC, Nursing Care Centers; OBS, Office-Based Surgery Practices; OME, Home Care.

---

* *Life Safety Code®* is a registered trademark of the National Fire Protection Association, Quincy, MA.

Note: *Brackets are used to identify language that may differ across program settings although the requirements are aligned.*

EC Documentation Schedule

The Joint Commission requires that certain activities be performed to help manage the environment of care and life safety. This excerpted schedule displays how frequently the listed activities must be performed. Use this tool to help keep track of and document the on-time performance of these activities, including fire-related safety, medical equipment and utilities systems maintenance, and emergency power systems.

Note: *The complete schedule may be adapted and is available for internal use on the flash drive (print only) or by clicking the tool link in the Risk-Assessment Toolbox (e-book only) on page 24.*

Published in *Environment of Care Risk Assessment*, Joint Commission Resources, 2018.   **File Name:** 01 01 EC Doc Schedule

EC DOCUMENTATION SCHEDULE

ORGANIZATION: ___________________________________   DEPARTMENT/UNIT: ___________________________________

REQUIREMENT	FREQUENCY	JAN	FEB	MAR	APR	MAY	JUN	JUL	AUG	SEP	OCT	NOV	DEC	NOTES
FIRE DRILLS														
Ambulatory Occupancy	Quarterly													
Business Occupancy 1	12 Months													
Business Occupancy 2	12 Months													
Business Occupancy 3	12 Months													
Health Care Occupancy	Quarterly Each Shift													
Residential Occupancy	Quarterly (for 24-Hour Care)													
FIRE SAFETY EQUIPMENT AND BUILDING FEATURES														
Fire Alarm Systems*														
AHU Shutdown	12 Months													
Alarm Signal Transmission to Off-Site Responders	12 Months													
A/V Devices	12 Months													
Door Releasing Devices	12 Months													
Duct Detectors	12 Months													
Heat Detectors	12 Months													
Manual Fire Alarm Boxes	12 Months													
Sliding and Rolling Fire Doors	12 Months													
Smoke Detectors	Months													

Brief Overview of EC Management Plans

Environment of Care (EC) standards compliance is a complex undertaking that requires clearly outlined plans to ensure compliance is achieved and maintained—this is the role of EC management plans (called EC operations plans in home care settings). These written documents are required by Joint Commission EC standards and serve as a framework for management. EC management plans are considered high-level business plans and, as such, are *not* detailed descriptions of policies and procedures.

Essentially, EC management plans have a dual purpose:
- Provide a framework for how to approach the environment of care
- Explain how that approach complies with Joint Commission EC standards.

However, management plans provide many more functions for health care organizations beyond their core functions. Health care organizations can use management plans for any of the following:
- Identify and manage risks
- Guide performance improvement efforts
- Provide leadership and new EC staff with a high-level overview of EC activities
- Serve as references during mock tracers, on-site surveys, and during ongoing EC education and training programs

Management plans are required to cover specific areas of the physical environment. The areas can be combined into one EC management plan or broken out as individual plans in the following areas:
- Safety
- Security
- Life safety
- Hazardous materials and waste (not required for behavioral health care organizations)
- Medical equipment management (not required for home care organizations; laboratory refers to this as laboratory equipment)
- Utility management

Elements of EC Management Plans

Regardless of the area of focus, all management plans should include a mission statement and other features such as the following:
- **Objectives.** Broad-based statements that discuss the purpose of the plan and what the organization plans to accomplish in this EC area
- **Scope.** List or describe all the organization's sites contained in the plan, including possibly hours of operation and services offered
- **Performance.** Describe how an organization will measure the performance of the plan in reducing risk and ensuring the safety of all individuals
- **EP compliance.** Outline brief descriptions of how each element of performance (EP) for each EC standard will be met
  (**Note:** *Surveyors will hold health care organizations accountable for what identified compliance activities are included in their policies.*)

continued

- **Responsibilities.** Identify the responsibilities of individuals and groups for compliance and other activities
- **Time frames.** State time frames for performing specific compliance activities
- **Emergency response.** Provide a summary of how the organization will respond to particular emergency situations
- **Inspection, testing, and maintenance.** Describe the approach to these activities in relation to the EC standards
- **Policies and procedures.** Cite and cross-reference applicable policies and procedures
- **Supplemental information.** Reference critically related information (for example, municipal codes)
- **Risk assessment.** Explain how assessments will be used to manage risks in the EC areas
- **Staff development.** Explain the training and orientation process for staff, including contract staff
- **Annual evaluation.** Describe the process for evaluating the plan annually, including who will be conducting it

To ensure comprehensive EC management plans, relevant standards and EPs in other chapters should be cross-referenced as applicable. Chapters that may be applicable include the following:
- Emergency Management (EM)
- Human Resources (HR) (this chapter is titled "Human Resources Management" (HRM) in the *Comprehensive Accreditation Manual for Behavioral Health Care* or E-dition)
- Infection Prevention and Control (IC)
- Information Management (IM)
- Leadership (LD)
- Life Safety (LS)
- Performance Improvement (PI)

In addition, EC management plans must take into consideration the various department and staff they directly affect. Ensuring compliance with the most stringent regulations, including local, state, federal, should be highlighted in the management plans when they vary from Joint Commission standards.

Like so many aspects of maintaining the physical environment, creating and revising EC management plans provides an excellent opportunity to foster collaboration across the organization. Involving key stakeholders in this process can build well-rounded, truly comprehensive management plans.

This multidisciplinary approach also will work well when it is time to review the management plans. In accordance with the standards, EC management plans must undergo an annual evaluation (every 12 months) to ensure they are still relevant, applicable, and effective. This annual evaluation may not result in changes every time, but it provides an opportunity to reflect on the current state of the physical environment in the organization and revise as necessary. (*See* page 13 for a sample safety management plan.)

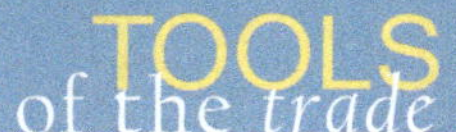

Safety Management Plan

This excerpt from a sample safety management plan can be used as a template to create a management plan for any of the identified areas of the environment of care. This sample also can be used to compare to existing management plans within an organization to determine if there are areas that can be improved.

Note: *The complete safety management plan may be adapted and is available for internal use on the flash drive (print only) or by clicking the tool link in the Risk-Assessment Toolbox (e-book only) on page 24.*

Published in *Environment of Care Risk Assessment,* Joint Commission Resources, 2018.　　　　　　**File Name:** 01 02 Safety Manage Plan

SAFETY MANAGEMENT PLAN

This sample Safety Management Plan can be used to develop an environment of care (EC) management plan for any area of the physical environment.

POLICY TITLE:	Safety Management Plan	**POLICY NUMBER:**	90.003.015
ORGANIZATION:	County Health Care	**EFFECTIVE DATE:**	11/11/17
APPROVED BY:	EC and Safety Committees	**REVISED DATE(S):**	11/10/02; 11/14/07; 11/16/12

I.　MISSION STATEMENT

---

of a changed process or the volatility of a process. The response also could be a deliberate decision to take no immediate action, but to monitor the situation after a predetermined amount of time.

New risks arise every day in the health care environment, and potential hazards associated with health care delivery can emerge and change quickly. Organizations should plan to assess and respond to risks continually and to define the nature and frequency of reassessments.

What Types of EC Risk Assessments Are Required?

The following sections offer a brief description of the various risk assessments that will be explored in greater detail throughout this book. Many are contained within the EC chapter of the *Comprehensive Accreditation Manual* and online in E-dition, while other assessments fall under different standards chapters in the manual. This list is a brief introduction to some of the more common assessments; more information will be contained in Chapters 3 through 10.

Safety Risk Assessment

Safety risk assessments (*see* Chapter 3) address safety concerns associated with the physical environment (such as falls on a wet floor) and the behavior of people being served (such as workplace violence). They include environmental tours and worker safety analyses, as well as risk assessments resulting from the ongoing monitoring of the environment, root cause analyses (RCAs), and annual proactive risk assessments of high-risk processes.

Hazardous Materials and Waste Risk Assessment

Through a hazardous materials and waste risk assessment (*see* Chapter 4), organizations identify materials that require special handling and implement processes to minimize the risks of their unsafe use and improper storage and disposal. These assessments typically take the form of inventories of all potentially hazardous chemicals within the organization.

Security Risk Assessment

Organizations perform a security risk assessment (*see* Chapter 5) to identify any security risks that may be present in the environment, as well as risks to patient, staff, and visitor security throughout the organization. Examples of security risks include elopement from a dementia unit in a nursing care center, infant abduction from the obstetrics ward, and violence toward a visiting nurse in a home care residence.

Fire Safety and Life Safety Risk Assessment

Several different assessments are required to ensure that fire and life safety risks (*see* Chapter 6) are minimized. The Statement of Conditions™ (SOC) helps organizations identify and plan for effective fire response, specifically through compliance with the National Fire Protection Association's (NFPA) *Life Safety Code*®.* Only those health care organizations that are classified as health care, ambulatory, or residential occupancies are eligible to complete an SOC (*see* Chapter 2 for additional information on determining occupancy type). When deficiencies in *Life Safety Code* compliance are found using the SOC, organizations must implement interim life safety measures (ILSM) to temporarily compensate for the identified fire safety risks.

Medical Equipment Risk Assessment

The Joint Commission requires most organizations to manage the risks associated with medical equipment (*see* Chapter 7). To do this, organizations must establish a risk-assessment process to identify, evaluate, and create an inventory of equipment. This inventory must address equipment function and the physical risks associated with the equipment's use. Organizations also must have plans to address risks associated with failure of medical equipment, including the timely replacement of equipment when that equipment is life sustaining.

Utility Risk Assessment

Similar to medical equipment risk assessment, organizations must in engage a risk-assessment process to ensure the operational reliability of utility systems (*see* Chapter 8) and identify and respond to risks. Utility systems are defined as those that provide support to the environment of care, including electrical distribution and emergency power; vertical and horizontal transport; heating, ventilating, and air conditioning (HVAC); plumbing, boiler, and steam; piped gases; vacuum systems; and communications, including data exchange systems.[1] Organizations also must have contingency plans in place that address risks associated with utility failures, such as an interruption in any utility service due to construction, natural disaster, or other cause.

Emergency Management Risk Assessment

One of the primary risk assessments used in emergency management (*see* Chapter 9) is an HVA. This assessment helps organizations identify potential threats that may affect the environment, mitigate potential risks, and develop effective and comprehensive Emergency Operations Plans. An HVA may address such threats as natural disasters, chemical spills, terrorist acts, and influenza pandemics.

Preconstruction Risk Assessment

Before any general maintenance, demolition, construction, or renovation project, organizations must perform a precon-struction risk assessment (PCRA) (*see* Chapter 10). This assessment must occur prior to work being performed to identify hazards that could potentially compromise care, treatment, and services in occupied areas of the organiza-tions' buildings. The scope and nature of the construction activities determine the extent of risk assessment, but should address all risk areas, including utility requirements, noise, vibration, and other hazards (for example, safety, hazardous materials). In addition, the PCRA must include a specific infection control risk assessment (ICRA) to manage construction-related infection risks, such as air and water quality and mold mitigation.

Where Are the Risks?

Numerous means are available to identify potential risks in organizations (*see* page 15). The Joint Commission recommends that organizations use internal and external sources to identify such issues for risk assessment.

Some areas and patient populations in health care orga-nizations are more prone to risk and should be a primary consideration when identifying issues for possible risk assessments. And there are other issues or EC–related practices, policies, or situations that would benefit from a closer look via a risk assessment. Specific points in a process that are susceptible to risk generally result from a high degree of dependence on communication (which may or may not occur), nonstandardized processes, and/or failure or absence of backup.

---

* *Life Safety Code*® is a registered trademark of the National Fire Protection Association, Quincy, MA.

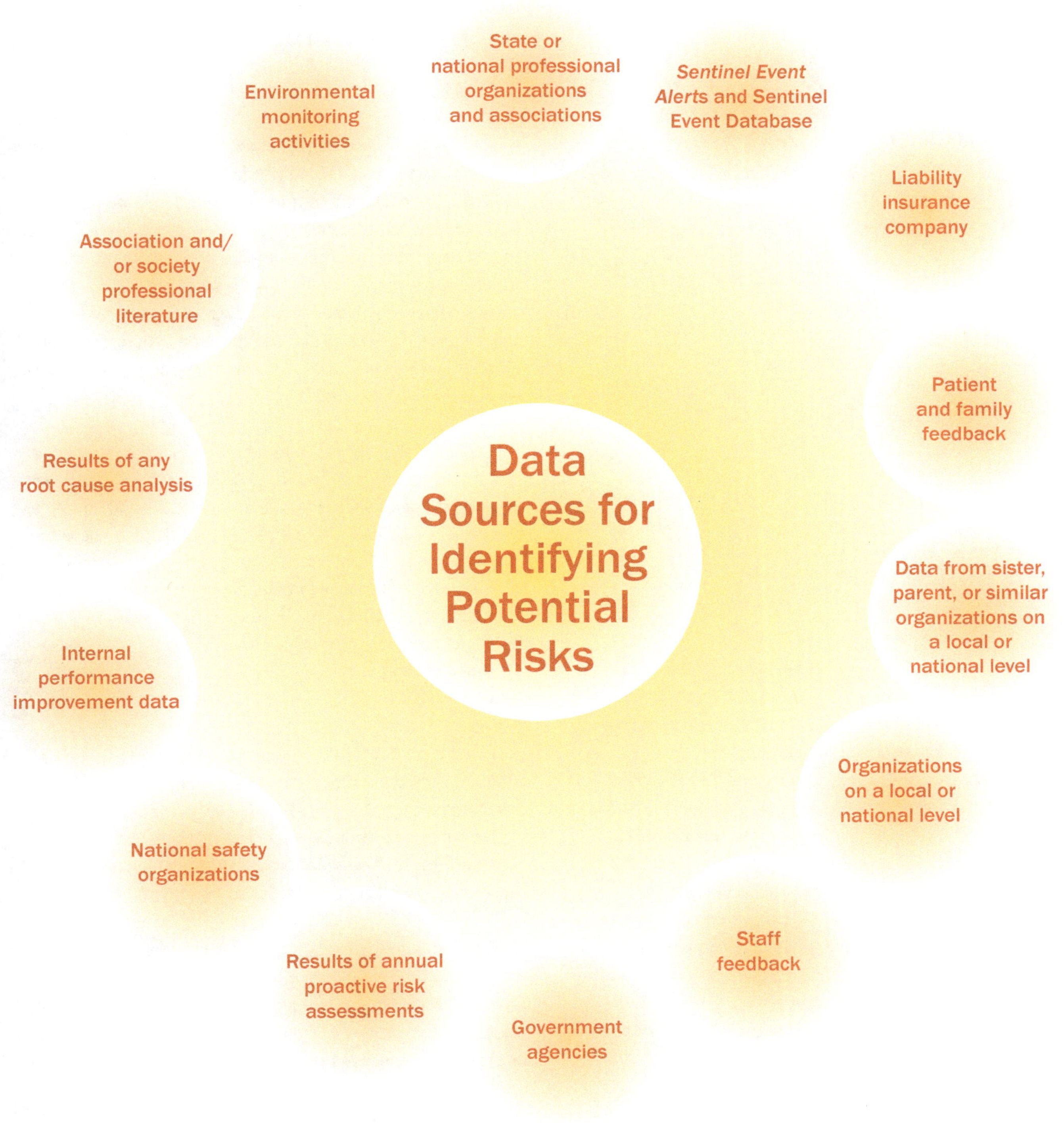

These potential data sources are only a sampling of what can be used to determine risks in the physical environment.

for

example...

Due to its frantic pace, frequent patient turnover, acute level of care, and constant access, the emergency department may be a prime location for risk in the areas of security, safety, and emergency management.

On the other hand, because of the large quantities of chemicals and drugs stored there, the pharmacy may be at greater risk for issues associated with hazardous materials and waste, as well as security.

The ICU and operating rooms are dramatically affected by utility failures and thus may present higher risks that should be considered.

Within specific patient populations, such as psychiatric patients, risk may be considered higher because of the nature of illnesses or conditions and the likelihood of suicidal tendencies.

Who Identifies the Issues Needing a Risk Assessment?

In a complex health care organization, the responsibility for deciding which issues should be targeted by an EC risk assessment can fall in a number of different places. Ultimately, the organization leadership should identify the individual or individuals who will assume responsibility for managing risk in the environment of care, including overseeing risk assessments as required by Standard EC.01.01.01. This person(s) may come from a variety of different backgrounds, including facilities management, public safety (security), nursing, or risk management. As part of coordinating risk management, the person(s) identified will work closely with EC staff and organization leadership to identify which issues should be addressed by risk assessments.

How Can an Organization Conduct a Risk Assessment?

Although The Joint Commission recommends and requires many different risk assessments, the standards do not address all the possible risks found in health care organizations. It is almost guaranteed that staff will encounter issues or problems in which a proactive risk-assessment process may be necessary, yet a requirement does not specifically exist for it in Joint Commission standards.

It is beneficial in these types of situations to have a standardized approach to assessing risk proactively. This approach should be applicable to organizationwide, department-specific, and issue-specific assessments and should be used to evaluate the gray areas in the health care environment—that is, issues for which there is no definitive right or wrong answer. The following sections describe several types of assessment processes that can be used to address many kinds of risks. (*See* page 17 for an illustration of the basic risk-assessment process.)

There is no single prescribed format required to conduct a risk assessment, and there are numerous risk-assessment or performance improvement methodologies and strategies that an organization may choose to employ. The following three methods of assessment are examples of different risk-assessment processes that can be used effectively to address many types of EC risks:

1. Simple proactive risk assessment
2. Failure mode and effects analysis
3. Dashboard tool

Simple Proactive Risk Assessment

Although a proactive risk assessment will vary for each health care organization, the following is a basic approach organizations can consider using. (For an illustration of the basic risk-assessment process and a proactive risk-assessment worksheet, *see* pages 17 and 18, respectively.)

Before embarking on this process, an organization may want to pull together a multidisciplinary team of individuals who are familiar with the many aspects of the issue to obtain the most comprehensive definition. Stakeholders representing a variety of perspectives can help ensure an unbiased analysis of the issue (*see* page 20 for additional information about assembling a team).

Steps Involved in Simple Assessments

Step 1: Identify the issue. After identifying an issue posing potential risk, clearly define it to focus the EC risk assessment. Be specific and straightforward and phrase information as a yes/no question whenever possible. Refrain from

text continued on page 20

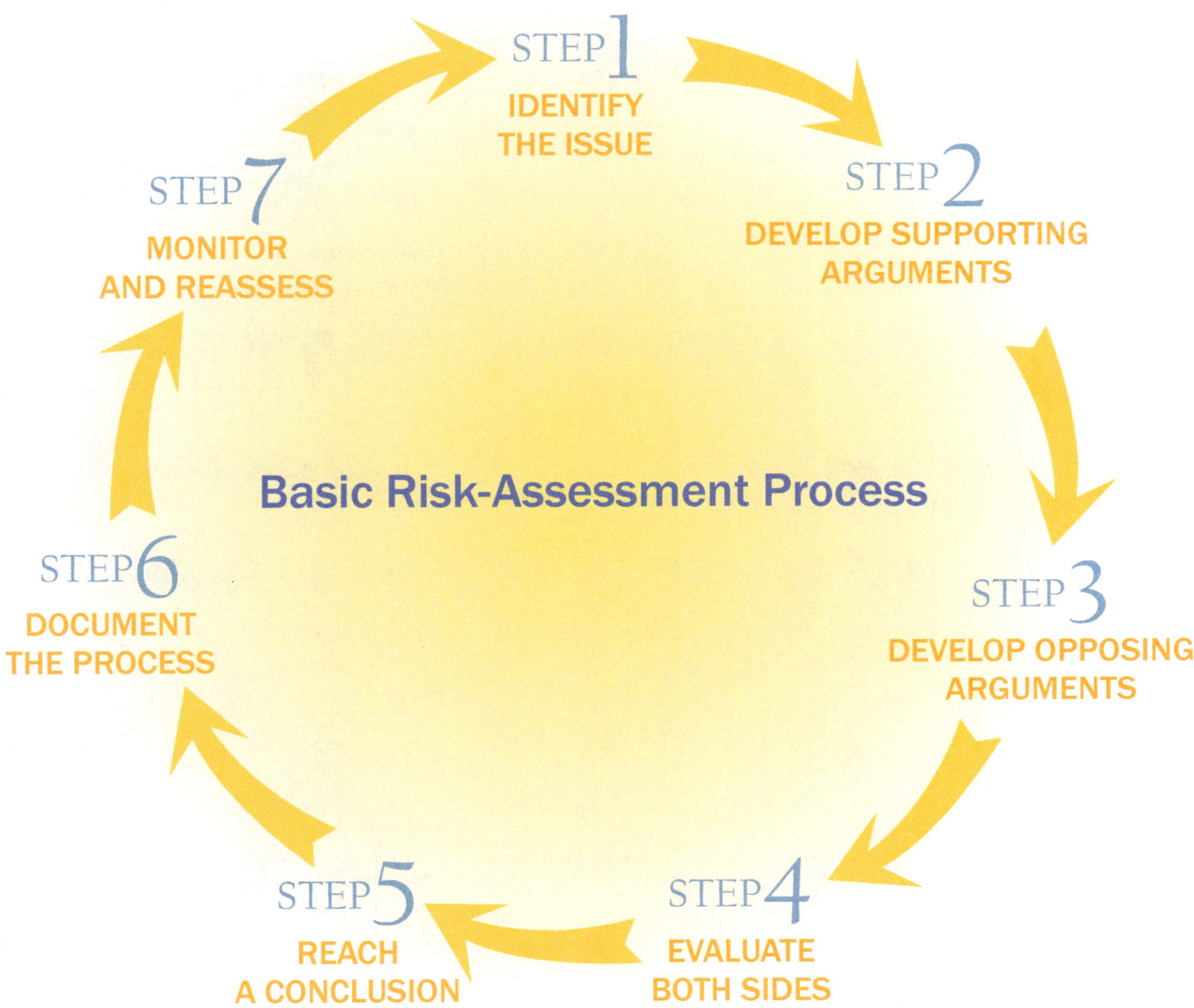

Risk assessments can be simple or multilayered processes. This illustration identifies the seven basic steps of the risk-assessment process.

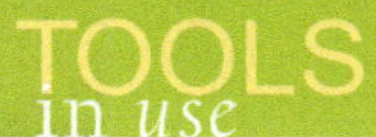

Proactive Risk-Assessment Worksheet

This excerpted worksheet can be used when an organization is confronted with a problem and is unsure of the needed plan of action to resolve the issue. Using this form, provides the organization the opportunity to study/identify the reasons to do or not to do—to take an action or not to take the action. This process assists organizations in the discussion and determination of when an issue is a risk and in the determination of the appropriate plan of action based on the situation.

Note: *This worksheet may be adapted and is available for internal use on the flash drive (print only) or by clicking on the tool link in the Risk-Assessment Toolbox (e-book only) on page 24.*

Published in *Environment of Care Risk Assessment*, Joint Commission Resources, 2018.

PROACTIVE RISK-ASSESSMENT WORKSHEET

ORGANIZATION: County Psychiatric Hospital   DEPARTMENT/UNIT: Inpatient Psychiatry

DATE OF ASSESSMENT: 1/16/2018   PARTICIPANT(S): Facilities Manager, Nursing Staff, Administration

DESCRIBE THE ISSUE

Inpatient unit nurse reported that bathroom door in a patient sleeping room could pose a ligature risk.

THOSE INVOLVED IN THE DISCUSSION

Nurse executive, facilities manager, maintenance staff, nursing staff

ARGUMENTS

SUPPORTING ARGUMENTS (WHY SHOULD THE ISSUE REMAIN THE SAME?)	OPPOSING ARGUMENTS (WHY SHOULD THE ISSUE BE CHANGED?)
No patient in the facility has ever successfully attempted suicide.	Ligature risks must be addressed for compliance with Joint Commission standards as well as law and regulation.
Mitigation strategies could be expensive if new fixtures are purchased	Risk to patients/human and financial cost of a patient suicide exceed costs of mitigation
Limited data available on some mitigation strategies	Some proven strategies do exist

ANY APPLICABLE RISK REPORTS OR PERFORMANCE IMPROVEMENT DATA?

Report of potential ligature risk from nursing Engineering department follow-up confirmed potential risk	

ANY APPLICABLE SENTINEL EVENT ALERTS?

Sentinel Event Alert No. 56 https://www.jointcommission.org/assets/1/18/SEA_56_Suicide.pdf	

ANY ADDITIONAL APPLICABLE CODES, REGULATIONS, AND/OR GUIDELINES?

• Joint Commission Environment of Care (EC) Standard EC.02.06.01, Element of Performance 1	

© 2018 The Joint Commission. May be adapted for internal use.   Page **1** of **2**

Proactive Risk-Assessment Worksheet *continued*

Published in *Environment of Care Risk Assessment*, Joint Commission Resources, 2018.

- US Centers for Medicare & Medicaid Services (CMS) Survey and Certification Memo 18-06-Hospitals: Clarification of Ligature Risk Policy

MITIGATION (POTENTIAL STRATEGIES TO REDUCE RISK)

Options include:

- Lock bathroom door, require staff assistance for patient to access
- Install alarm on door to prevent inappropriate use
- Install door with an angled upper edge or breakaway magnetic hinges

Approved for implementation? ☐ Yes ☐ No

CONCLUSION

- Unit will immediately begin locking bathroom doors in rooms housing patients assessed to be at risk of suicide.
- Unit will require staff assistance to access bathroom.
- Within 8 months, facilities management will install breakaway magnetic hinges on all bathroom doors in the unit.

COMMUNICATION PLAN

- Draft written policy on door locking and distribute to all employees
- Add to staff meeting agenda
- Post signage at nursing stations as reminders
- Inform staff of plans to install new hinges

TIME FRAME FOR REASSESSMENT (IF APPLICABLE)	DATE(S) FOR REASSESSMENT
Reassess after 8 months to ensure all hinges were replaced	On or before September 18, 2018

PERSON(S) RESPONSIBLE FOR FOLLOW-UP (IF APPLICABLE)

Facilities manager/nurse executive or designee

ROUTE TO RISK MANAGER/QUALITY IMPROVEMENT/ENVIRONMENT OF CARE COMMITTEE: _______________________________

DATE: _______________________ NAME: _______________________________

Page 2 of 2

Assembling a Team

In some cases, it may be appropriate to assemble a multidisciplinary team to conduct the risk-assessment process. This invites multiple perspectives on an issue and can ensure the most comprehensive assessment.

Selection of team members is critical. Team members should bring to the table a diverse mix of knowledge bases and should be knowledgeable about and committed to performance improvement, as well as safety. The team should include individuals with fundamental knowledge of the particular process involved. These are the subject matter or process experts. The team also should include representatives from areas that may be affected directly by changes in the process. These individuals will be the ones most impacted by changes and will have the most at stake during the redesign.

The team also might include an individual with some distance from the process—perhaps one who is not at all familiar with the process but who possesses excellent analytical skills. Functioning perhaps as an advisor or facilitator, this person can provide a fresh perspective, unencumbered by the classic "that's how we've always done it" mentality. At least one individual with decision-making authority (a leader) and individuals critical to the implementation of anticipated process changes are needed as well.

combining several issues, even if they are related, as it can complicate the assessment, cause confusion, and result in faulty conclusions. Alternately, an issue that is too broad will quickly become too vague to be useful.

Identified issue: "Can we store items under the sink in patient care areas?"

Step 2: **Develop arguments that support the proposed process or issue.** After the issue is identified clearly, develop arguments that support the proposed process or issue. It may be helpful to create a columned list of questions, with a response column for advantages. Answers should reflect the specific needs of the affected patient population.

Arguments in favor of under-sink storage might include the following:
- *Easy access*
- *Relieving crowding in other storage areas*

Step 3: **Develop arguments against the proposed process or issue.** These arguments may be perceived concerns or situations that may pose potential risks or affect

a situation negatively. It may be helpful to use the same questions in Step 2, with a response column for disadvantages.

Arguments against under-sink storage might include the following:
- *Potential damage to items from leaking faucets*
- *Infection risk from damp paper items*
- *Potential for mold growth*

Step 4: **Objectively evaluate both arguments.** It is crucial that the organization conduct an impartial comparison of the advantages and disadvantages associated with the issue. Pros and cons must be thoroughly examined by all stakeholders—which requires pulling together the right individuals who can access the relevant information. Some elements to consider in this evaluation include patient population, state and local laws and regulations, and incident reports and history.

Evaluation: The pros and cons of storing items under the sink are evaluated by representatives from infection prevention and control, facilities management, nursing, and administration, considering the criteria previously listed.

Step 5: **Reach a conclusion.** The evaluation should result in a decision to accept the risk and make no changes, or to take steps to avoid or mitigate the risk. When the conclusion is determined, it is advisable to submit the risk assessment to a multidisciplinary committee, such as the safety committee or a performance improvement committee, to secure organizational consensus regarding this conclusion.

Conclusion: Concerned about arguments against under-sink storage, but wanting to find a middle ground, the evaluation team reaches a consensus to allow storage of only non–patient care items, such as flower vases, under sinks in patient care areas.

Step 6: **Document the process.** Documentation could include the risk-assessment worksheet, a written discussion of the issue in the minutes of the safety committee (or other committee) meeting, or a formal report. At this point, any relevant policies should be updated to reflect the conclusions.

The team provides the safety committee with a copy of the risk-assessment worksheet. The risk assessment is documented in the minutes of the safety committee meeting, and the storage policy is amended to reflect the decision to allow non–patient care items to be stored under the sink in patient care areas. Staff are informed of the new policy during regular meetings.

Step 7: **Monitor and reassess the conclusion to ensure that it is the best decision.** A monitoring strategy should be decided on from the beginning and be included in the risk-assessment document that is submitted to the safety committee or performance improvement committee. The strategy should include a specific date to reassess the conclusion drawn by the risk assessment. If the reassessment determines that an unintended effect or incorrect conclusion was reached, the issue is submitted to the multidisciplinary committee for reassessment. However, if the evaluation confirms the conclusion, then the confirmation is documented and the benefits of further monitoring are decided.

After three months, the team revisits the under-sink storage issue as part of its monitoring plan. It is found that both patient care items and non–patient care items are being stored together under some sinks—a situation not allowed by the risk-assessment conclusion. It is decided that the effect was unintended, and the risk-assessment team reopens the issue for review.

This seven-step risk-assessment process is demonstrated in the real-world scenario beginning on page 32.

Failure Mode and Effects Analysis

When conducting risk assessments on complex issues, organizations may need to use more than just a simple proactive risk assessment. Failure mode and effects analysis (FMEA) is a tool that can help an organization examine a high-risk process. This team-based, systematic technique is used to prevent problems before they occur. FMEA not only provides a look at what problems could occur but also examines how severe the effects of the problems could be. It assumes that no matter how knowledgeable or careful people are, failures will occur in some situations and may even be likely to occur. The focus is on what could allow the failure to occur, rather than who.

Ideally, FMEA is used to help prevent failures from occurring. However, if a particular failure cannot be prevented, FMEA then focuses on protections that prevent the failure from reaching the patient, or, in the worst case, mitigate the failure's effects if it reaches the patient.

The FMEA Process

The FMEA technique is based on studied engineering principles and approaches to designing systems and processes. It has been used successfully in a number of industries, including the airline, automotive, and aerospace industries. Varying by the source consulted, FMEA can involve as few as 4 or as many as 10 steps.

Questions Involved in FMEA

When conducting an FMEA on a complex process, teams should answer the following questions:
1. What are the steps in the process?
   - If it is an existing process, how does it currently occur and how should it occur?
   - If it is a new process, how should it occur?
2. How are the steps interrelated?
   - For example, are they sequential or do they occur simultaneously?
   - How is the process related to other health care processes?

3. What tools should be used to diagram the process?
4. What is the manner in which this process could fail?
   - When answering this question, team members should consider how people, materials, equipment, processes and procedures, and the environment affect the process.
5. What are the potential effects of the identified failures?
   - Effects of failures might be direct or indirect, long term or short term, or likely or unlikely to occur. The severity of effects can vary considerably, from minor annoyances to death or permanent loss of function. In this part of the process, team members should think through all the possible effects of a failure and list them for reference.
6. What could be the root causes of prioritized failure modes?
   - What would have to go wrong for a failure like this to happen?
   - What underlying weaknesses in the system might allow this to happen?
   - What safeguards (for example, double checks) are present in the process?
   - Are any missing?
   - If the process already contains safeguards, why might they not work to prevent the failure every time?
   - If this failure occurred, why would the problem not be identified before it affected a patient?

After the team has identified root causes and determined any intolerable potential effects of the process, the team devises and implements actions to eliminate the possibility of error, stop an error before it reaches patients, or minimize the consequences of an error. Then the team reviews and revises, as necessary, the action or actions being taken or planned to minimize the probability or effect of failure.

Dashboard Tool

Another effective method used to identify potential issues that require a risk assessment is a dashboard. Inspired by a car's instrument panel, a dashboard is a management tool that provides a real-time snapshot of performance, helping users to see quickly the status of current work and areas that require attention. The Joint Commission does not require organizations to create and maintain dashboards to help with compliance. However, a dashboard report can be a beneficial tool—especially for organizations struggling with how to keep track of various compliance risks. A dashboard serves the following purposes:

- To collect data (as required by Standard EC.04.01.01)
- To analyze data (as required by Standard EC.04.01.03)
- To provide regular reports that can be reviewed and acted on by an EC committee (as required by Standard EC.04.01.05)

At its most basic level, a dashboard is a report that outlines an organization's progress toward a goal and points toward the necessary next steps. Continuing the analogy, although a mechanic (or process owner) needs to know what's happening under the hood with each individual system, the driver (or senior leadership) monitors only the gauges and indicator lights on the dashboard. A car dashboard displays key performance indicators (KPIs) such as the speed, fuel gauge, and so forth. Careful monitoring of these KPIs ensures successful motoring. Similar KPIs in environmental areas can be monitored to ensure successful risk mitigation. For example, in the physical environment, KPIs include barrier integrity, egress reliability, and air-exchange and air-pressure differentials.

Organizations can create a dashboard internally, using word processing or spreadsheet software. The example dashboard tool beginning on page 25 is supported by two worksheets that can be adapted so that organizations can monitor the current, real-time activity of their environmental risk assessments. The example uses Standard EC.02.05.01—which historically has been a challenging standard for all organizations—and includes the following three tabs:

1. *Standard Analysis Worksheet.* Capturing the compliance status of the EPs that are included in the desired dashboard in this tab, this worksheet is flexible. It can be used to review and/or monitor just the risk-assessment standards (as in the example), the entire EC and LS chapters, or the top 10 Joint Commission compliance issues. Or it can focus on the organization's specific Requirements for Improvement (RFIs). This worksheet works well for EPs that require a simple yes/no response.
2. *In-Depth Data Worksheet.* For more complex EPs that require data analysis, use this tab to capture data on multiple-issue, data-driven EPs that require detailed analysis before determining compliance status. The results from this worksheet are fed into the Standard Analysis Worksheet to prepare data for the dashboard. In the example, data from several units/floors have

been captured before identifying overall organization compliance.

Key Performance Indicator Summary Dashboard. This tab allows EC professionals to prepare an overview for leaders of the key performance indicators (KPIs) for the standards included in the analysis.

Performing the Compliance Assessment

An active compliance assessment of the EPs included in the dashboard is usually done by the process owner who is familiar with the EP requirements. Compliance can be assessed during EC rounds, tours, or tracers, or via other observation or document review.

Whereas a standard defines the performance expectations and/or structures or processes that must be in place, the standard's EPs detail those expectations and/or structures or processes. Evaluating compliance with each EP determines an organization's overall compliance with a standard. After compliance with each EP is noted in the worksheet, EC professionals can determine their organization's overall compliance with the standard—which is the information that feeds the Key Performance Indicator Summary Dashboard.

Compliance starts with accountability and transparency, from the process owner to the facility manager to senior leadership. A robust dashboard reporting process can be used to introduce accountability for ensuring compliance with the EC risk-assessment requirements. Organizations may find that empowering staff to manage corrective actions identified as KPIs in their dashboards (as informed by a Standard Analysis or In-Depth Data Worksheet) strengthens both the culture of safety and the support of the corrective actions.

Building the Dashboard

EC professionals can monitor current, real-time activity in their environment by building or adapting a dashboard with the following steps.[2]

Step 1: Identify the scope of the monitoring project. As previously indicated, the scope of the monitoring project can include anything from a single standard to the top 10 Joint Commission compliance issues to the entire EC or LS chapter, or an organization may choose to monitor standards related to its most recent RFIs. Regardless of the chosen scope, the monitoring project should be tailored to meet the compliance or risk-assessment needs of the organization.

Step 2: Build the Standard Analysis Worksheet(s). For each standard within the scope of the monitoring project, create an individual worksheet. The standards can be included in a single file, with individual tabs for each standard, or each standard could be in a standalone file. When populating each worksheet, make sure to include the standard number and language, each element of performance (EP), and compliance results. For multiple-issue EPs, list the individual factors that require a compliance assessment, such as each utility system that requires a written procedure for responding to a disruption. Note on the Standard Analysis Worksheet which EPs require an additional In-Depth Data Worksheet(s) to capture the data used to determine compliance status. Starter files are available on the flash drive (print only) or directly through the link in the Risk-Assessment Toolbox (e-book only) on page 24.

Step 3: Build the In-Depth Data Worksheet(s). Each In-Depth Data Worksheet will be different because each EP requires unique assessment. Organizations should include what is being analyzing, the frequency of analysis, and other appropriate factors. In some cases, a single EP might require more than one In-Depth Data Worksheet (for example, air-pressure relationships, air-exchange rates, and filtration efficiencies from EC.02.05.01, EP 15).

Step 4: Update the Standard Analysis Worksheet. The Standard Analysis Worksheet should include the summary data for all EPs in the standard, including those that needed an In-Depth Data Worksheet. After compliance with each EP in a standard is evaluated, overall compliance with that standard can be determined.

Step 5: Populate the Key Performance Indicator Summary Dashboard. This portion of the dashboard is built with the overall compliance information identified in the Standard Analysis Worksheets. The dashboard should list each standard included in the monitoring project for leadership's review. Consider using line graphs or pie charts to provide an at-a-glance summary of the compliance status of each EP or standard, and clearly label each entry.

Step 6: Monitor compliance and stay accountable. Specific noncompliant EPs identified in the Standard Analysis and In-Depth Data worksheets should be assigned for correction to the process owner. With the worksheets, process owners will have the tools they need to improve how they monitor the environment and the information they need to approach improvements. With the dashboard, leaders can efficiently monitor key indicators of compliance and be prepared to implement needed improvements.

References

1. The Joint Commission. *2017 Comprehensive Accreditation Manual for Hospitals*. Oak Brook, IL: Joint Commission Resources, 2016.
2. The Joint Commission. EC dashboard keeps compliance front and center. *Environment of Care News*. 2015;18(2): 1, 3–6, 9.

RISK-ASSESSMENT TOOLBOX

1. [Download] EC Documentation Schedule
2. [Download] Safety Management Plan
3. [Download] Proactive Risk-Assessment Worksheet
4. [Download] Dashboard Worksheets
5. [Download] Seven-Step Risk-Assessment Worksheet

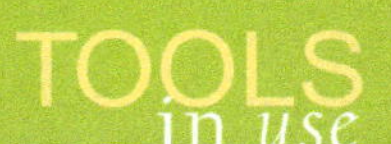

Example Dashboard Worksheets

Monitoring real-time activity of certain processes and systems is a valuable asset that allows organizations to better understand what potential environmental risks need to be addressed. These worksheets show a mock organization's monitoring of activities related to Standard EC.02.05.01.

Note: *These worksheets may be adapted and are available for internal use on the flash drive (print only) or by clicking on the tool link in the Risk-Assessment Toolbox (e-book only) on page 24.*

Standard Analysis Worksheet

Standard Analysis Worksheet

Published in *Environment of Care Risk Assessment*, Joint Commission Resources, 2018.

EP	Deficiency	In-Depth Data Required (Y/N)	Description	1st Quarter		2nd Quarter		3rd Quarter		4th Quarter		Overall Compliance
			EC.02.05.01 The hospital manages risks associated with its utility systems.	Compliant	Noncompliant	Compliant	Noncompliant	Compliant	Noncompliant	Compliant	Noncompliant	
1	SLD		The hospital designs and installs utility systems that meet patient care and operational need.	87.50%	12.50%	87.50%	12.50%	93.00%	7.00%	96.50%	3.50%	91.13%
2	SLD		Written inventory of operating components of utility systems	100.00%	0.00%	79.50%	20.50%	84.50%	15.50%	100.00%	0.00%	91.00%
3	SLD		Written documentation of identification of high-risk operating components on inventory	100.00%	0.00%	100.00%	0.00%	84.50%	15.50%	100.00%	0.00%	96.13%
4	SLD		Written documenation of the activities and frequencies for inspecting, testing, and maintaining all operating components of utility systems on inventory	100.00%	0.00%	100.00%	0.00%	84.50%	15.50%	98.30%	1.70%	95.70%
5	SLD		Written documentation of activities and frequencies for inspecting, testing and maintaining equipment in accordance with manufacturers' recommendations	100.00%	0.00%	100.00%	0.00%	84.50%	15.50%	98.30%	1.70%	95.70%
6	SLD		Written criteria by a qualified individual to support alternative methods	100.00%	0.00%	100.00%	0.00%	84.50%	15.50%	98.30%	1.70%	95.70%
7	SLD		Written documentation of identification of operating components with alternative equipment maintenance program	100.00%	0.00%	100.00%	0.00%	84.50%	15.50%	98.30%	1.70%	95.70%
8	SLD		Utility system controls are labeled for partial or complete emergency shutdowns.	93.54%	6.46%	83.50%	16.50%	90.00%	10.00%	95.00%	5.00%	90.51%
9	SLD	N	Written procedures for responding to utility system disruptions	88.88%	11.12%	100.00%	0.00%	100.00%	0.00%	90.00%	10.00%	94.72%
			Electricity	Yes		Yes		Yes		Yes		
			Natural Gas	Yes		Yes		Yes		Yes		
			Medical Air	Yes		Yes		Yes		Yes		
			Vacuum	Yes		Yes		Yes		Yes		
			HVAC (Heating, Ventilation, Air Conditioning)	Yes		Yes		Yes		Yes		
			Water	Yes		Yes		Yes		Yes		
			Sanitation	No		No		No		Yes		
			Communication Systems	Yes		Yes		Yes		Yes		
			Information Technology	Yes		Yes		Yes		Yes		
			Elevator							No		
10	SLD		Procedures address shutting off the malfunctioning system and notifying staff in affected areas.	100.00%	0.00%	100.00%	0.00%	94.50%	5.50%	94.50%	5.50%	97.25%
11	SLD		Procedures address performing emergency clinical interventions during utility system disruptions.	95.00%	5.00%	100.00%	0.00%	100.00%	0.00%	100.00%	0.00%	98.75%
13	SLD		Hospital responds to utility system disruptions as described in its procedures.	92.30%	7.70%	83.33%	16.67%	93.50%	6.50%	95.45%	4.55%	91.15%

© 2018 The Joint Commission. May be adapted for internal use.

continued

Example Dashboard Worksheets *continued*

Standard Analysis Worksheet

Standard Analysis Worksheet

Published in ***Environment of Care Risk Assessment***, Joint Commission Resources, 2018.

14	CLD		Minimizes pathogenic biological agents in cooling towers, domestic hot- and cold-water systems, and other aerolizing water systems.	95.60%	4.40%	86.67%	13.33%	87.00%	13.00%	95.00%	5.00%	**91.07%**
15	**CLD**	**Y**	**Critical Care Areas: appropriate pressure relationships, air-exchange rates, filtration, temperature and humidity**	**76.54%**	**23.46%**	**74.56%**	**25.44%**	**64.26%**	**35.74%**	**77.20%**	**22.80%**	**73.14%**
	KPI Analysis		**Air Pressure Relationship**	59.57%	40.43%	46.81%	53.19%	34.04%	65.96%	57.45%	42.55%	**49.47%**
			Air-Exchange Rates	79.30%	20.70%	88.60%	11.40%	80.25%	19.75%	85.90%	14.10%	**83.51%**
			Filtration Efficiecies	90.74%	9.26%	88.26%	11.74%	78.50%	21.50%	88.26%	11.74%	**86.44%**
16	SLD		Non–Critical Care Areas: appropriate pressure relationships, air-exchange rates, filtration, temperature and humidity	93.20%	6.80%	85.90%	14.10%	78.00%	22.00%	98.50%	1.50%	**88.90%**
17	SLD		Utility systems have maps of distribution.	100.00%	0.00%	100.00%	0.00%	93.00%	7.00%	100.00%	0.00%	**98.25%**
18	SLD		Medical gas storage rooms and transfer and manifold rooms comply with NFPA 99–2012; 9.3.7.	97.00%	3.00%	100.00%	0.00%	87.50%	12.50%	100.00%	0.00%	**96.13%**
19	SLD		EPSS equipment and environment are maintained per manufacturers' recommendations, including ambient temperature, ventilation supply and exhaust, and water jacket temperature.	84.00%	16.00%	93.00%	7.00%	93.00%	7.00%	89.60%	10.40%	**89.90%**
				103.26%	**9.24%**	**100.29%**	**12.21%**	**93.75%**	**18.75%**	**104.19%**	**8.32%**	

Element of Performance	Compliance Percentage	Noncompliance Percentage
1	91.13%	8.88%
2	91.00%	9.00%
3	96.13%	3.88%
4	95.70%	4.30%
5	95.70%	4.30%
6	95.70%	4.30%
7	95.70%	4.30%
8	90.51%	9.49%
9	94.72%	5.28%
10	97.25%	2.75%
11	98.75%	1.25%
13	91.15%	8.86%
14	91.07%	8.93%
15	73.14%	26.86%
16	88.90%	11.10%
17	98.25%	1.75%
18	96.13%	3.88%
19	89.90%	10.10%

EC.02.05.01 Element of Performance Compliance Rate

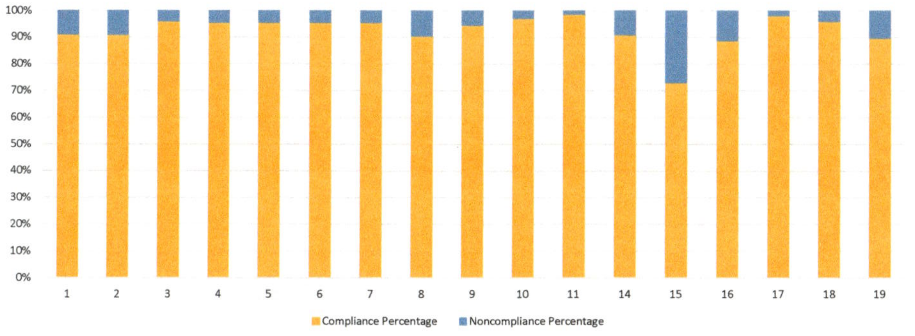

Example Dashboard Worksheets *continued*

In-Depth Data Worksheet

In-Depth Data Worksheet

Published in *Environment of Care Risk Assessment*, Joint Commission Resources, 2018.

EC.02.05.01, EP 15 Air Pressure Relationships–Daily Verification of Appropriate Air Pressure for In-Use Rooms												
Measurement	1st Quarter		2nd Quarter		3rd Quarter		4th Quarter		Total		
	Compliant	Noncompliant	Compliant	Noncompliant	Compliant	Noncompliant	Compliant	Noncompliant	Compliant	Noncompliant	Overall Compliance
AHU 1											
OR 1 (2)	174	6	157	23	148	34	157	25	636	88	87.85%
OR 2 (2)	170	10	164	16	153	29	155	27	642	82	88.67%
OR 3 (2)	149	16	176	12	92	17	92	0	509	45	91.88%
OR 4 (2)	147	11	123	12	120	14	156	0	546	37	93.65%
PACU (2)	152	7	147	9	143	13	129	27	571	56	91.07%
Clean Core 1 (4)	312	48	337	27	301	59	303	57	1253	191	86.77%
AHU 2											
OR 5 (2)	152	0	154	0	156	0	156	2	618	2	99.68%
OR 6 (2)	152	0	154	0	156	0	156	2	618	2	99.68%
OR 7 (2)	152	0	154	2	156	1	156	0	618	3	99.52%
OR 8 (2)	152	0	154	1	156	2	156	0	618	3	99.52%
OR 9 (2)	152	3	154	2	156	0	156	1	618	6	99.04%
Ciculation Corridor 1 (2)	152	0	154	4	156	1	156	0	618	5	99.20%
Circulation Corridor 2 (2)	152	0	154	0	156	3	156	0	618	3	99.52%
OR Sterile Storage (3)	270	2	273	0	276	0	273	3	1092	5	99.54%
AHU 3											
Clean Core 2 (4)	360	0	360	4	368	0	368	0	1456	4	99.73%
Clean Core 3 (4)	360	0	364	0	362	6	368	0	1454	6	99.59%
Clean Core 4 (4)	227	1	228	3	232	2	234	0	921	6	99.35%
IR 1 (2)	180	0	176	0	179	1	175	0	710	1	99.86%
IR 2 (2)	151	1	152	2	155	1	155	1	613	5	99.19%
IR Sterile Storage (1)	90	0	91	0	92	0	92	0	365	0	100.00%
AHU 4											
Endo 1 (2)	166	0	172	1	181	3	183	1	702	5	99.29%
Endo 2 (2)	152	1	148	6	156	0	153	3	609	10	98.38%
Endo 3 (2)	152	0	154	0	154	2	156	0	616	2	99.68%
Endo 4 (2)	152	0	154	0	154	2	151	5	611	7	98.87%
Endo Sterile Storage (2)	180	0	182	0	184	1	184	0	730	1	99.86%
Endo Decontamination (2)	180	0	182	0	183	1	180	4	725	5	99.32%
Vascular 1 (2)	158	0	161	0	140	0	143	0	602	0	100.00%
Vascular 2 (2)	152	0	154	0	156	0	156	0	618	0	100.00%
Vascular Sterile Storage (1)	180	0	182	0	184	0	184	0	730	0	100.00%
AHU 5											
L&D OR 1 (2)	178	2	179	3	182	2	182	2	721	9	98.77%
L&D OR 2 (2)	180	0	181	1	182	2	184	0	727	3	99.59%
L&D OR 3 (2)	149	0	161	0	175	0	173	0	658	0	100.00%
L&D Sterile Storage (1)	90	0	91	0	92	0	92	0	365	0	100.00%
ICU Isolation 1 (2)	178	6	173	5	184	3	184	1	719	15	97.96%
ICU Isolation 2 (2)	176	4	182	0	184	1	184	0	726	5	99.32%
NICU Isolation 1 (2)	179	1	176	3	184	2	184	0	723	6	99.18%
NICU Isolation 2 (2)	177	9	182	5	184	4	184	1	727	19	97.45%
AHU 6											
Medical Isolation A (2)	152	0	154	0	156	1	156	0	618	1	99.84%
Medical Isolation B (2)	180	0	182	0	182	2	184	0	728	2	99.73%
Post-Op Isolation C (2)	176	0	182	1	180	0	178	0	716	1	99.86%
Post-Op Isolation D (2)	180	0	182	0	184	0	184	1	730	1	99.86%
Pharmacy	180	0	168	14	167	17	179	2	694	33	95.46%
AHU 7											
Laboratory A	160	1	133	9	150	6	164	0	607	16	97.43%
Laboratory B	176	0	182	0	180	0	178	0	716	0	100.00%
Laboratory C	158	0	161	0	140	0	143	0	602	0	100.00%
Central Sterile - Clean (5)	450	3	455	5	460	1	460	2	1825	11	99.40%
Central Sterile - Dirty (6)	348	102	536	10	526	32	549	3	1959	147	93.02%
	59.57%	40.43%	46.81%	53.19%	34.04%	65.96%	57.45%	42.55%	17.02%	82.98%	

© 2018 The Joint Commission. May be adapted for internal use.

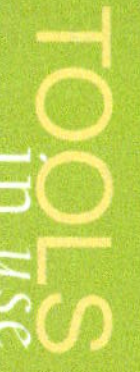

continued

In-Depth Data Worksheet

Published in *Environment of Care Risk Assessment*, Joint Commission Resources, 2018.

Air Pressure Relationships–Daily Verification of Appropriate Air Pressure for In-Use Rooms

Summary of All Areas		
Measurement	Compliance Percentage	Noncompliance Percentage
OR 1 (2)	87.85%	12.15%
OR 2 (2)	88.67%	11.33%
OR 3 (2)	91.88%	8.12%
OR 4 (2)	93.65%	6.35%
PACU (2)	91.07%	8.93%
Clean Core 1 (4)	86.77%	13.23%
OR 5 (2)	99.68%	0.32%
OR 6 (2)	99.68%	0.32%
OR 7 (2)	99.52%	0.48%
OR 8 (2)	99.52%	0.48%
OR 9 (2)	99.04%	0.96%
Ciculation Corridor 1 (2)	99.20%	0.80%
Circulation Corridor 2 (2)	99.52%	0.48%
OR Sterile Storage (3)	99.54%	0.46%
Clean Core 2 (4)	99.73%	0.27%
Clean Core 3 (4)	99.59%	0.41%
Clean Core 4 (4)	99.35%	0.65%
IR 1 (2)	99.86%	0.14%
IR 2 (2)	99.19%	0.81%
IR Sterile Storage (1)	100.00%	0.00%
Endo 1 (2)	99.29%	0.71%
Endo 2 (2)	98.38%	1.62%
Endo 3 (2)	99.68%	0.32%
Endo 4 (2)	98.87%	1.13%
Endo Sterile Storage (2)	99.86%	0.14%
Endo Decontamination (2)	99.32%	0.68%
Vascular 1 (2)	100.00%	0.00%
Vascular 2 (2)	100.00%	0.00%
Vascular Sterile Storage (1)	100.00%	0.00%
L&D OR 1 (2)	98.77%	1.23%
L&D OR 2 (2)	99.59%	0.41%
L&D OR 3 (2)	100.00%	0.00%
L&D Sterile Storage (1)	100.00%	0.00%
ICU Isolation 1 (2)	97.96%	2.04%
ICU Isolation 2 (2)	99.32%	0.68%
NICU Isolation 1 (2)	99.18%	0.82%
NICU Isolation 2 (2)	97.45%	2.55%
Medical Isolation A (2)	99.84%	0.16%
Medical Isolation B (2)	99.73%	0.27%
Post-Op Isolation C (2)	99.86%	0.14%
Post-Op Isolation D (2)	99.86%	0.14%
Pharmacy	95.46%	4.54%
Laboratory A	97.43%	2.57%
Laboratory B	100.00%	0.00%
Laboratory C	100.00%	0.00%
Central Sterile - Clean (5)	99.40%	0.60%
Central Sterile - Dirty (6)	93.02%	6.98%

Summary of Least Compliant Areas		
Measurement	Compliance Percentage	Noncompliance Percentage
OR 1	87.85%	12.15%
OR 2	88.67%	11.33%
OR 3	91.88%	8.12%
OR 4	93.65%	6.35%
PACU	91.07%	8.93%
Clean Core 1	86.77%	13.23%
Pharmacy	95.46%	4.54%
Central Sterile - Dirty (6)	93.02%	6.98%

EC.02.05.01 EP 15 Areas of Noncompliance

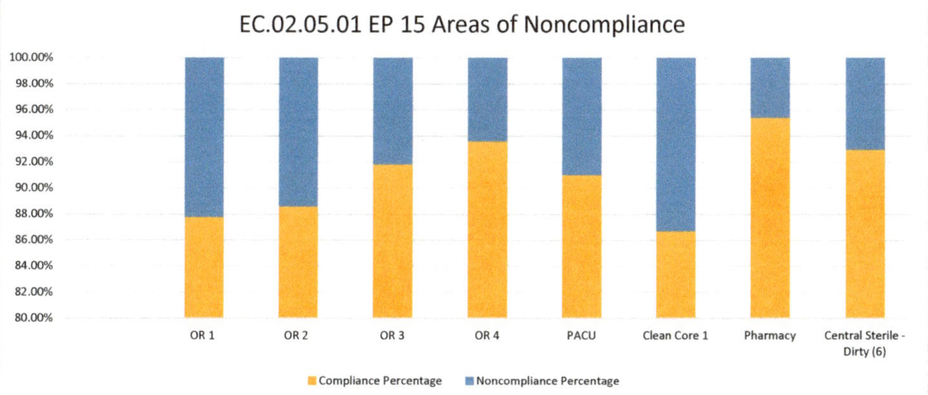

OR 1, OR2, OR 3, OR 4, PACU, and Clean Core 1: 1989 system that has a very extensive PM system due to the age of the equipment; 129 OR cases in the past year have been re-scheduled, moved or postponed due to a malfunctioning system and approximately $53K in repairs.
Pharmacy: Staff error due to not having the system on when required or propping door open. Manager follow-up and staff education and accountability.
Central Sterile Supply: Multiple issues—department error by not monitoring one pressure relationship from the dirty side into a staff work area, an electrical mechanical door holder that was removed from a door entering the area from the corridor, and staff propping the door once the electrical mechanical door holder was removed, and corrective maintenance needs. Corrective action taken immediatly and documented; manager follow-up and staff education and accountability.

Key Performance Indicator Dashboard

Published in *Environment of Care Risk Assessment*, Joint Commission Resources, 2018.

Environment of Care & Life Safety Key Performance Indicators		1st Quarter		2nd Quarter		3rd Quarter		4th Quarter		Overall
Standard	Description	Compliant	Noncompliant	Compliant	Noncompliant	Compliant	Noncompliant	Compliant	Noncompliant	Compliance
EC.02.05.01	The hospital manages risks associated with its utility systems.	94.50%	5.50%	96.70%	3.30%	96.20%	3.80%	97.80%	2.20%	96.30%
LS.02.01.20	The hospital maintains the integrity of the means of egress.	98.70%	1.30%	96.23%	3.77%	95.36%	4.64%	99.48%	0.52%	97.44%
EC.02.06.01	The hospital establishes and maintains a safe, functional environment.	93.68%	6.32%	96.61%	3.39%	91.50%	8.50%	94.39%	5.61%	94.05%
EC.02.03.05	The hospital maintains fire safety equipment and fire safety building features.	100.00%	0.00%	98.75%	1.25%	97.59%	2.41%	99.32%	0.68%	98.92%
LS.02.01.10	Building and fire protection features are designed and maintained to minimize the effects of fire, smoke, and heat.	96.40%	3.60%	98.72%	1.28%	95.33%	4.67%	98.72%	1.28%	97.29%
LS.02.01.30	The hospital provides and maintains building features to protect individuals from the hazards of fire and smoke.	96.19%	3.81%	93.65%	6.35%	89.05%	10.95%	95.99%	4.01%	93.72%
LS.02.01.35	The hospital provides and maintains systems for extinguishing fires.	93.68%	6.32%	96.61%	3.39%	91.50%	8.50%	94.39%	5.61%	94.05%
EC.02.02.01	The hospital manages risks related to hazardous materials and waste.	98.77%	1.23%	98.77%	1.23%	96.53%	3.47%	95.04%	4.96%	97.28%
EC.02.05.09	The hospital inspects, tests, and maintains medical gas and vacuum systems.	100.00%	0.00%	99.35%	0.65%	100.00%	0.00%	98.93%	1.07%	99.57%
EC.02.05.07	The hospital inspects, tests, and maintains emergency power systems.	99.53%	0.47%	98.12%	1.88%	100.00%	0.00%	98.12%	1.88%	98.94%

* Bolded standards are examples of noncompliance for an organization with a goal of 95% or greater.

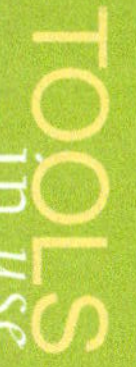

continued

Example Dashboard Worksheets *continued*

Key Performance Indicator Worksheet

Key Performance Indicator Dashboard

Environment of Care
Overall Compliance

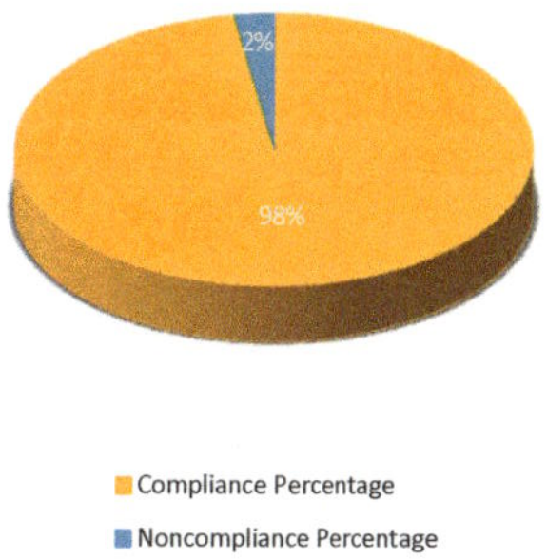

Life Safety
Overall Compliance

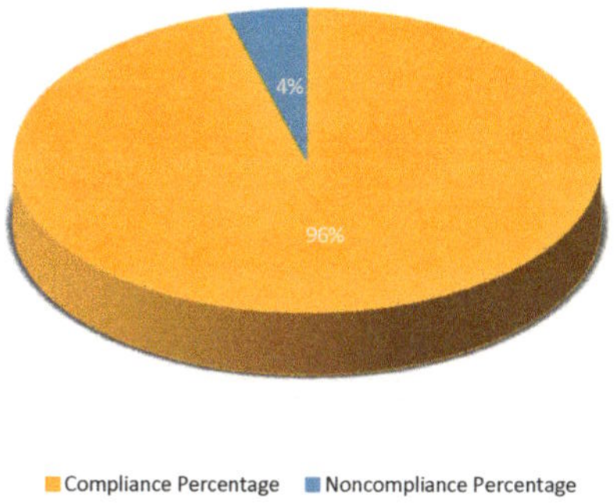

Standard	Compliance Percentage	Noncompliance Percentage
EC.02.05.01 Utility Mgmt	96.30%	3.70%
LS.02.01.20 Egress	97.44%	2.56%
EC.02.06.01 Safe & Functional Environment	94.05%	5.96%
EC.02.03.05 Fire Safety Equipment	98.92%	1.09%
LS.02.01.10 Fire Safety Design	97.29%	2.71%
LS.02.01.30 Fire Safety Maintenance	93.72%	6.28%
LS.02.01.35 Extinguishment	94.05%	5.96%
EC.02.02.01 Hazmat	97.28%	2.72%
EC.02.05.09 Medical Gas & Vacuum	99.57%	0.43%
EC.02.05.07 Emergency Power	98.94%	1.06%
Environment of Care	97.51%	2.49%
Life Safety	95.63%	4.38%

Example Dashboard Worksheets *continued*

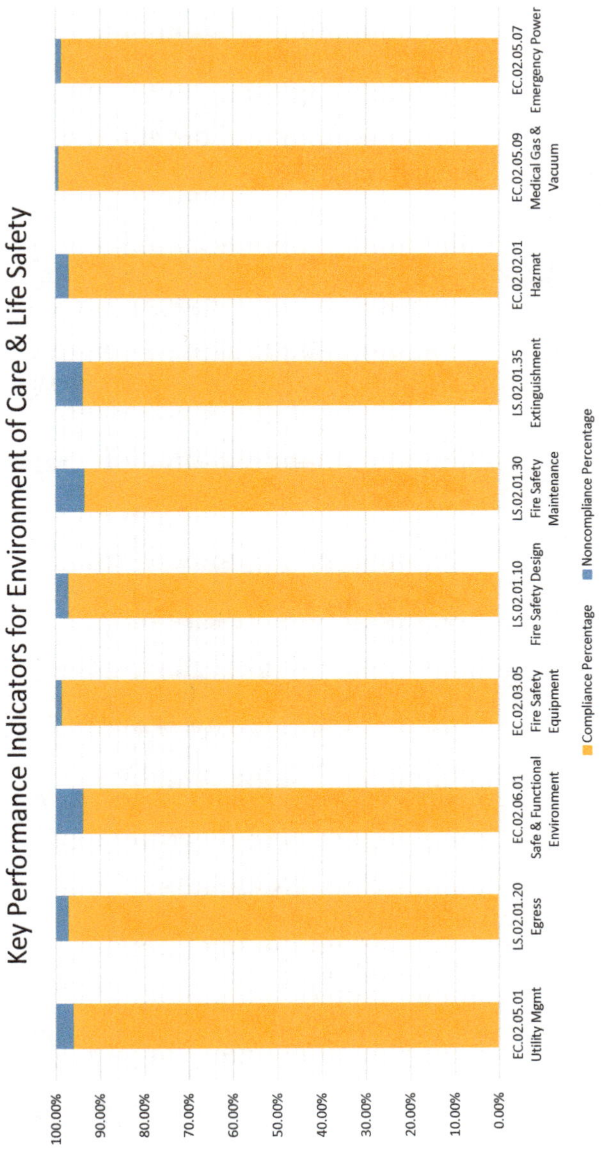

Key Performance Indicator Worksheet

Storage of Endoscope Supplies

As this chapter outlines, risk assessments are conducted for numerous reasons and may take a variety of forms. In some cases, risk assessment can simply be a matter of spending an hour considering the issue in a straightforward, structured way; while in other cases, a more in-depth assessment must be conducted that can take days or weeks to complete.

When staff at UW Health—an academic health system associated with the University of Wisconsin Hospitals and Clinics—became concerned about the storage of endoscope supplies, they employed a seven-step risk-assessment process that they adapted and modified from an assessment process created by The Joint Commission. This assessment is best used when making a decision between two processes. Generally, the assessment will be between a current process and a new alternative; however, it can be used when deciding between two new processes.

About the Project

Staff at one of UW Health's ambulatory facilities identified a potential risk related to its storage of endoscope supplies. At this location, endoscope supplies that contain sharps were stored in unlocked cabinets in limited-access procedure rooms. Staff were unsure whether this posed a risk to patient or visitor safety. They decided to conduct a risk assessment to determine whether these particular endoscope supplies should be kept in a locked storage cabinet. "This risk assessment has proven to be quite a valuable tool," says Jackie Smith-Helmenstine, senior quality analyst, regulation and accreditation coordinator for UW Health. "It helps staff come up with a quantitative score that supports decision making."

Step 1: Define the Issue

The first step is to define the issue that will be assessed for risk. This includes several areas of information. First, the participants and/or stakeholders should be identified. These might include the individuals who work in and oversee the department or area being assessed. It also should include a strong facilitator, according to Smith-Helmenstine. This person is responsible for guiding the group through the assessment process and keeping it on task.

Next, the current and alternative situations must be stated simply and clearly. In this case, the current situation was that endoscope supplies containing sharps were kept on shelves in an unlocked limited-access (restricted) procedure room. The alternative condition, or proposed change, would be to keep endoscope supplies containing sharps in a locked drawer in that same limited-access procedure room.

"It's important to keep the focus as specific as possible," says Smith-Helmenstine. "If it's too broad, it becomes very complicated very quickly. Broad issues are best handled by multiple risk assessments."

The final piece in defining the issue is the scope of the impact. Some risk assessments affect the entire organization or facility, while others affect only a single floor, department, or room. In this case, the risk was limited to two procedure rooms in one outpatient facility.

Steps 2 and 3: Assess Benefits and Risks

These steps look at a range of topics that may be affected by the process in question. Such topics include patient safety, patient satisfaction, quality of care, environment of care, budget, and work flow. Each topic is discussed individually for both the current situation and the proposed alternative, and respective benefits and risks are assigned a number value.

UW Health uses the following scoring system:
- 5 = high
- 3 = moderate
- 1 = low
- 0 = not applicable

Smith-Helmenstine says this system sharpens the distinction between the scores, forcing the team to make strong decisions and eliminating the "gray areas."

Step 2 focuses on the current situation—in this case, storing the endoscopic sharps in unlocked cabinets in the limited-access area. The team goes down the list of topics and first considers the benefits, then the risks, associated with each.

For example, what is the benefit to patient safety of keeping these sharps unlocked? Discussion revealed that patient safety was increased by unlocked sharps because staff could quickly and easily access needed supplies. The group gave this a 5, or high, score. Then what is the risk to patient safety of keeping these sharps unlocked? The team determined that because the sharps were stored in a limited-access area, the risk to patient safety from keeping them unlocked was minimal. This was scored as 1, or low.

Step 3 follows the same process as Step 2, only this time focusing on the alternative situation (that is, locking up the sharps). When assessing patient satisfaction, the team determined that locking sharps would have minimal benefit but may create moderate risk, as the procedure length and wait time increases.

Not all topics will necessarily apply to all risk assessments. In this case, the safety to the environment—that is, prevention of damage to the physical structures—was not an issue, and was scored as 0.

Step 4: Evaluate the Scores

Now it is time to add up scores for each column: current situation benefits, current situation risks, alternative situation benefits, and alternative situation risks. The resulting numbers can be evaluated to see if an overall picture emerges. The numbers can be evaluated from several perspectives. First, the current situation's overall benefit can be compared to its overall risk, and the same for the alternative situation. In this case, keeping the sharps unlocked had a benefit scored at 34, while the risk of this practice scored a 10—the benefits far outweighed the risks. The alternative, locking the sharps, had risks (34) outweighing the benefits (9).

Another way to evaluate the scores is to compare the benefit of the current situation to the benefit of the alternative, and the risk of the current situation to the risk of the alternative. Again, in this case, the benefit of keeping the sharps unlocked was much greater than locking them up, while the risk was the inverse.

For this particular risk assessment, the numbers gave a very clear picture. This may not be the case for all situations. If the scores are close, the team may wish to look at the individual topics and weigh their importance based on the particular situation. For example, work flow and budget may be the primary concerns, and those scores could be considered directly.

Step 5: Reach a Conclusion

This is the part of the assessment in which a decision is made to either continue the current practice or implement the alternative. Smith-Helmenstine emphasizes that this assessment is only one tool used to inform a decision. In this case, the team decided that the results were overwhelmingly in favor of keeping the sharps unlocked, and recommended that the practice continue.

Step 6: Document the Results

This is the part of the assessment in which the results and recommendation are reported to the appropriate committee, according to organizational policy. Sometimes, if the issue is complex or wide in scope or impact, the safety committee or other body of authority will need to review the assessment before any action is taken. In other situations, that may not be necessary. In the example described here, the scope was limited to two rooms in one building, and no changes were being recommended. Therefore, the team leadership did not require formal review or approval from the safety committee.

"It's helpful to have someone on the risk-assessment team who either has the authority to approve changes or can access someone with that authority," says Smith-Helmenstine. "This can keep the process from becoming unnecessarily complicated."

continued

Step 7: Monitor and Reassess

A monitoring strategy and time line for reassessment, including the responsible parties for each process, should be determined as part of the original assessment. In a simple risk assessment, such as this example, the monitoring can be as easy as checking back after a few months to inquire if there have been any safety events related to endoscope supplies. If the answer is "no," document your follow-up, and your risk assessment is complete.

See the completed seven-step worksheet used to evaluate the risks associated with the facility's current method of storing endoscope supplies beginning on page 35.

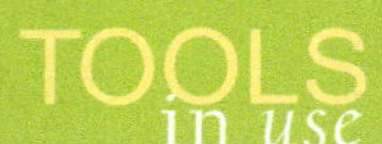

Example Seven-Step Risk Assessment

This worksheet from the University of Wisconsin Hospitals and Clinics shows the results of the seven-step risk assessment completed to evaluate the risk posed to patients and visitors by storing endoscope supplies in unlocked cabinets in limited-access procedure rooms.

Note: *This worksheet may be adapted and is available for internal use on the flash drive (print only) or by clicking the tool link in the Risk-Assessment Toolbox (e-book only) on page 24.*

Source: University of Wisconsin Hospitals and Clinics, Madison, WI. Used with permission.

Published in *Environment of Care Risk Assessment*, Joint Commission Resources, 2018.

SEVEN-STEP RISK-ASSESSMENT WORKSHEET

DATE: 5/1/2017
FACILITATORS: Jackie Smith-Helmenstine, Lisa LeClair
PARTICIPANT(S)/STAKEHOLDER(S): Anne Rikkers, Denise Leroy, Brittany Nesbit, Jackie Stubbe

Step 1a	Current Issue/Condition	Scope supplies with sharps kept unlocked in limited-access (restricted) area in procedure rooms
Step 1b	Alternative Condition/Proposed Change	Scope supplies containing sharps locked in drawer in limited-access area in procedure rooms
Step 1c	Location of Current Issue/Condition	Digestive Health Center Endoscopy

☐ Inpatient Unit ☒ Outpatient Area ☐ Housewide ☐ Emergency Department ☐ Other

STEPS 2 & 3	ASSESS BENEFITS VS. RISKS		Key	Low – 1 Moderate – 3 High – 5 Not Applicable – 0

DISCUSSION TOPICS ▼	1A CURRENT ISSUE/CONDITION			1B ALTERNATIVE CONDITION/PROPOSED CHANGE		
PERSPECTIVE ▶	BENEFIT	RISK	RATIONALE/EXAMPLES	BENEFIT	RISK	RATIONALE/EXAMPLES
Patient safety	5	1	Removing barriers to access	1	5	Adding barriers to supplies. Benefit pertaining to the scope supply sharps is minimal. Airway supplies covered by sharps.
Patient satisfaction	3	1	Procedure length is shorter when access isn't restricted.	1	3	Patient sees secure environment. Patient experiences wait time for staff to attain supplies.
Outcome (quality) of patient care	5	1	Able to get to supplies quickly. Airway supplies not covered or affected by locked sharps.	1	5	
Staff and volunteer safety	3	1		1	3	Pinched fingers, hit head, throw out back
Staff and volunteer satisfaction	5	1	Techs can function independently and readily access needed supplies.	1	5	Limited access to supplies and tools needed to care for patients
Visitor safety	1	1		1	1	
Visitor satisfaction	3	1	Visitors/family not waiting for patients.	1	3	Limiting time visitors are waiting for patients

Source: University of Wisconsin Hospitals and Clinics, Madison, WI. Used with permission.

Page **1** of 2

continued

Example Seven-Step Risk Assessment *continued*

Published in *Environment of Care Risk Assessment*, Joint Commission Resources, 2018.

Environment safety, including building and grounds	*0*	*0*			*0*	*0*	
Financial operation, budget	*3*	*1*	*Less staffing, no badge access*		*1*	*3*	*Losing keys, badge access readers, staffing requirements*
Work flow efficiency	*5*	*1*	*Allowing tech to independently retrieve supplies*		*0*	*5*	*Access to supplies limited and extends length of procedures.*
Compliance with regulatory requirements	*1*	*1*	*No contradiction in policy, no direct regulation for sharps storage*		*1*	*1*	

STEP 4	EVALUATE THE DISCUSSION TOPICS						
PERSPECTIVE ▼	**SCORE ▶**	**BENEFIT**	**RISK**	**PERSPECTIVE ▼**	**SCORE ▶**	**BENEFIT**	**RISK**
Assess impact of current issue/condition		*34*	*10*	*Assess impact of alternative condition/proposed change*		*9*	*34*

DISCUSSION POINT(S)

Current condition benefit far outweighs risk. The alternative risk far outweighs the benefit. The benefit of current condition outweighs the benefit of the alternative. The risk of the current condition is much less than the risk of the alternative. There has never been a safety issue with current practice.

STEP 5	TEAM CONCLUSION	☐ Continue Current Practice	☐ Implement Alterative Practice

STEP 6   **DOCUMENT THE RESULTS**—*not applicable; narrow scope, local area decision*

a   Date Submitted to the Health Safety Committee: ____

b   Summary Report to Health Safety Committee   *(attach report if additional space is needed)*

____

____

c   Oversight Committee Decision   ☐ Continue Current Practice   ☐ Implement Alterative Practice

d   If Implementing Alternative, Responsible Party for Implementation: _________________________

e   Projected Implementation/Completion Date: ____

f   Monitoring Strategy

____

____

STEP 7   **MONITOR AND REASSESS**

a   Findings of Monitoring Strategy

____

____

b   Reassessment   ☐ Continue 6c Decision   ☐ Develop Alterative Practice
     (repeat risk-assessment process)

____

____

Source: University of Wisconsin Hospitals and Clinics, Madison, WI. Used with permission.   Page **2** of **2**

chapter 2

Joint Commission Tools for Risk Assessment

Assessing risk in the environment of care (EC) in health care facilities comes with many challenges. These challenges do not have to be so daunting and, with the right tools, risk assessment can help organizations keep their physical environments safe and secure and maintain survey readiness.

In addition to surveying organizations for accreditation and/or certification, The Joint Commission strives to partner with organizations to ensure they are providing high-quality health care in a safe environment. This is apparent with the tools and processes The Joint Commission has cultivated to help health care organizations maintain their survey readiness over the entire three-year accreditation cycle.* These tools and processes—often considered strictly part of the survey or between-survey processes—also function as risk-assessment tools any organization can use to identify and assess risks. The Intracycle Monitoring (ICM) process, the newly developed Survey Analysis for Evaluating Risk™ (SAFER™) Matrix, and the Statement of Conditions™ (SOC) all work at some level to identify risks. The following sections will discuss each tool and its components in more detail;

---

* For laboratory organizations, the accreditation cycle is biennial.

accredited and/or certified organizations can visit their *Joint Commission Connect™* extranet site to put these tools to work.

Intracycle Monitoring

Managing risk in the environment is an ongoing process; one that is never considered "done." One valuable tool organizations can use to accomplish this is the ICM process. The Joint Commission has implemented ICM to help organizations monitor, improve, and maintain performance, all of which lead to minimized risks.

ICM is designed as a dynamic, interactive, comprehensive work space that supports compliance between on-site surveys.

ICM Basics

Organizations access their ICM Profile on their *Joint Commission Connect* extranet site. In addition to the Focused Standards Assessment (FSA), ICM provides resources, reports, and a place to ask questions (*see* the "Focused Standards Assessment" section on page 38).

(see the "Focused Standards Assessment" section on page 38)

STANDARDS to *know*

APR.03.01.01

LS.01.01.01

TERMS to *know*

Intracycle Monitoring (ICM)

Requirement for Improvement (RFI)

Statement of Conditions™ (SOC)

Survey Analysis for Evaluating Risk™ (SAFER™) Matrix

Layout of the ICM Profile

Upon accessing its ICM Profile, an organization will encounter a dashboard that provides a wealth of educational content as well as important contact information. When the organization enters the ICM work space, eight tabs lead to tools the organization can use to monitor performance. Following is a brief discussion of some of those tabs.

Accreditation Status

This section gives an organization a high-level review of its current status by tracking its monitoring efforts. It includes survey results as well as unfinished tasks such as completing and submitting an Evidence of Standards Compliance (ESC) or an FSA.

Accreditation Program Risks

This section is a good source to consult when identifying EC risks to target for assessment. Here, The Joint Commission identifies key risk areas for each accreditation program. These are determined by survey-related data as well as experts who weigh the probability and severity of harm resulting from a particular risk; proximity to the patient, resident, or individual served; and scope of the potential impact. Standards that relate to each risk are identified.

In addition, this tab provides risk areas specific to each organization, which include standards related to any Requirements for Improvement (RFIs) from the current accreditation cycle surveys.

Focused Standards Assessment

This tab is the home for the FSA tool, and organizations can access and complete the tool through this portal. Details on the FSA are discussed beginning on this page.

Topics for Conference Call

In this area, organizations can note specific issues or standards to discuss with The Joint Commission's Standards Interpretation Group (SIG). This option is available to all organizations completing the ICM process.

This procedure provides an opportunity for both the organization and SIG staff to prepare for a discussion of those topics during a phone conference (sometimes called a TouchPoint call). During that call, the SIG staff answers the organization's questions and offers guidance for compliance.

Reports

In this section, an organization can generate reports based on the work included in the other tabs. For example, an organization can create a list of all noncompliant standards it has scored in the FSA tool.

Resources and Measures

This tab compiles all relevant Joint Commission tools, newsletters, publications, and other resources. It includes links to *Sentinel Event Alert*s, Frequently Asked Questions, and material from the US Centers for Medicare & Medicaid Services (CMS), among other valuable information.

ICM Time Line

As the name implies, ICM takes place between the triennial on-site surveys (biennial for labs). The illustration on page 40 provides a visual display of the accreditation cycle and when various activities occur, including ICM and FSA activities. It is important to note that the ICM and FSA tools are made available when an organization seeking accreditation for the first time submits its E-App (Electronic Application for Accreditation) and deposit. All organizations should complete and submit an ICM Profile by months 12 and 24 of the cycle, including which FSA option it has selected.

Focused Standards Assessment

The central component of the ICM is the FSA, or Focused Standards Assessment.

Completing the FSA, or an approved alternative, is required by The Joint Commission in accordance with its Accreditation Participation Requirement (APR) Standard APR.03.01.01.

The FSA focuses an organization's attention on standards related to that organization's identified risk areas. The FSA lists all standards that apply to an organization, based on the accreditation program and services identified in its E-App, and which should be addressed in the self-assessment. Standards associated with risk categories are labeled with an **R** icon. These include standards in the following categories:

- National Patient Safety Goals (NPSGs)
- Joint Commission–identified risk areas
- RFIs identified during the current accreditation cycle survey events

FSA Options

Organizations acknowledge their compliance with this requirement through one of four ICM Profile submission options:

- *Full.* An organization choosing this option uses the tool to conduct a self-assessment of its standards compliance. At least the minimum subset of **R** standards must be scored in order to accomplish a full submission. Data entered into the FSA tool are copied to a historical submission record—accessible only to the organization—for future reference.
- *Option 1.* An organization choosing this option uses the FSA tool to conduct a self-assessment of its standards compliance. An organization choosing this option may elect not to submit data to The Joint Commission, but it can still submit topics for discussion and engage in the SIG conference call.
- *Option 2.* An organization choosing this option uses the FSA tool to indicate that it would prefer to undergo an FSA survey, for which it is charged a fee. The results of this survey are provided to the organization in a written report of findings.
- *Option 3.* An organization choosing this option also uses the FSA tool to indicate its desire for an FSA survey, and it is charged the relevant fee. The results of this survey, however, are reported verbally to the organization, and no written documentation is provided.

Details on activities related to the FSA submission options can be found in "The Accreditation Process" (ACC) chapter of the *Comprehensive Accreditation Manual* or E-dition.

Responding to the FSA

The Joint Commission has enhanced the FSA tool to include the new SAFER process. Two new optional fields have been added:

1. Likelihood to Harm
2. Scope

These fields will be displayed only if an element of performance (EP) is scored as not compliant.

When the FSA identifies an area of noncompliance, the organization is required to respond by creating a Plan of Action (POA). This is a detailed description of how the organization plans to bring itself into compliance, including what actions will be taken and target dates of implementation. The FSA will affect an organization's accreditation decision only if the organization fails to participate in the FSA process, whether the full FSA or one of the three options, or an Immediate Threat to Health or Safety situation is identified through the FSA process and a special survey is conducted.

The SAFER™ Matrix

The Joint Commission developed the Survey Analysis for Evaluating Risk™ (SAFER™) Matrix to provide health care organizations with the information they need to prioritize resources and focus corrective action plans. Each RFI noted within a final survey report is plotted on the SAFER Matrix according to the likelihood the RFI could cause harm to patients, residents, individuals served, staff, and/or visitors and the scope at which the RFI was observed. As the risk level of an RFI increases, the placement of the standard and EP moves from the bottom left corner (lowest risk level) to the upper right corner (highest risk area).

Use the required follow-up activity table to help prioritize areas of noncompliance. These activities and time frames also can be used to ensure that identified risk areas have been addressed and resolved. Risk assessment is more than finding the areas of risk—it is also following through to mitigate or eliminate the risk entirely.

SAFER is a transformative approach for identifying and communicating risk levels associated with deficiencies cited during survey. The additional information related to risk provided by the SAFER Matrix helps organizations prioritize and focus corrective actions. Organizations can use the SAFER Matrix as a risk-assessment tool themselves to determine their own compliance or when conducting mock tracers (*see* page 48 for additional information about mock tracers). The SAFER Matrix provides one comprehensive visual representation of survey findings in which all RFIs are plotted. The SAFER Matrix replaces the previously used scoring methodology, which was based on predetermined categorizations of EPs (such as direct and indirect impact)—instead allowing surveyors to perform real-time, on-site evaluations of deficiencies. Placement of RFIs within the matrix determines the level of detail required within the organization's ESC follow-up. (For information about the recently redesigned ESC, *see* page 52.) The SAFER Matrix also assists in prioritizing follow-up actions, as these actions will be based on the severity of risk for each finding (*see* page 41 for an example of the SAFER Matrix in use).

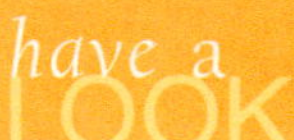

Key Milestones in the Accreditation Process

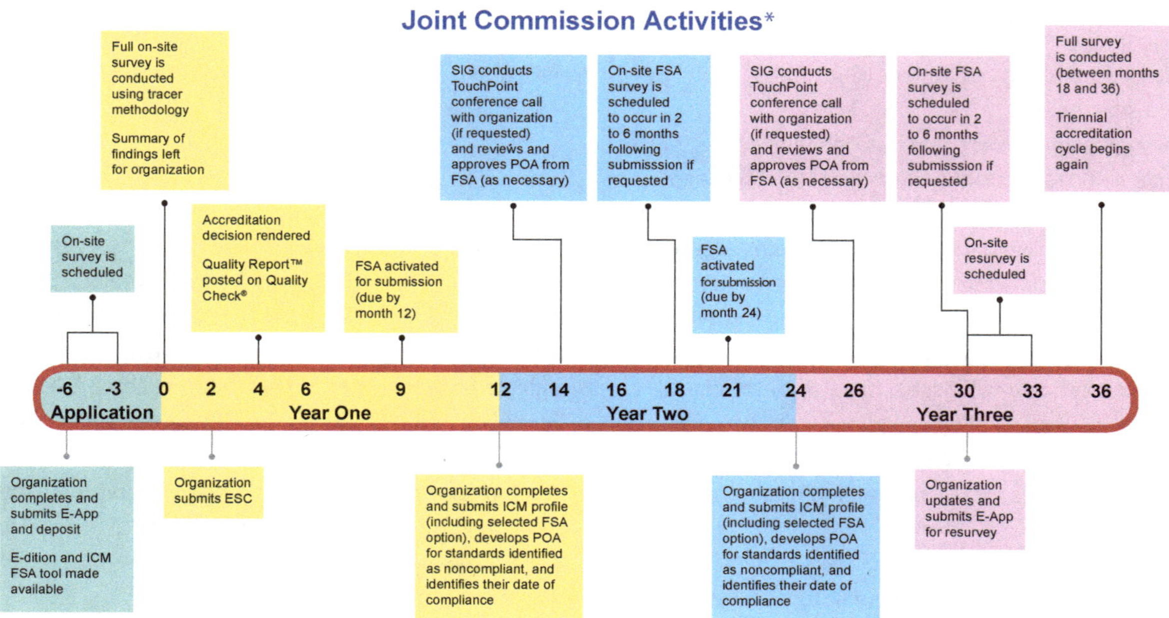

Accredited Organization Activities

This graphic outlines the various stages in the accreditation process (a triennial survey; laboratory organizations adhere to biennial surveys), including timeframes for milestone activities such as Intracycle Monitoring, Focused Standards Assessment submission, and anticipated on-site survey time.

* Activities The Joint Commission completes appear above the time line; activities conducted by an organization appear below the time line.

E-App, Electronic Application for Accreditation; ICM, Intracycle Monitoring; FSA, Focused Standards Assessment; ESC, Evidence of Standards Compliance; POA, Plan of Action; SIG, Standards Interpretation Group.

Example SAFER™ Matrix

Multidisciplinary team members can use the same SAFER Matrix tool Joint Commission surveyors now use to assess compliance within specific areas of the organization, including the physical environment. The illustration shows example placements of elements of performance (EPs) on the matrix. Placement on the matrix will vary based on the scope and likelihood to harm in the organization. After these areas have been identified, team members can prioritize the areas that are in immediate need of attention based on their likelihood to harm and the scope of the risk. Using this matrix as a risk-assessment tool also provides a visual representation that can be brought to leadership to inform them of the on-going assessment activities being conducted to ensure quality and safety, as well as to obtain project support and/or funding.

Risk assessment is more than finding the areas of risk—it is also following through to mitigate or eliminate the risk entirely. Reference the required follow-up activity table to help prioritize areas of noncompliance. These activities and time frames also can be used to ensure that identified risk areas have been addressed and resolved in a timely manner.

Note: *This matrix may be adapted and is available for internal use on the flash drive (print only) or by clicking the tool link in the Risk-Assessment Toolbox (e-book only) on page 58.*

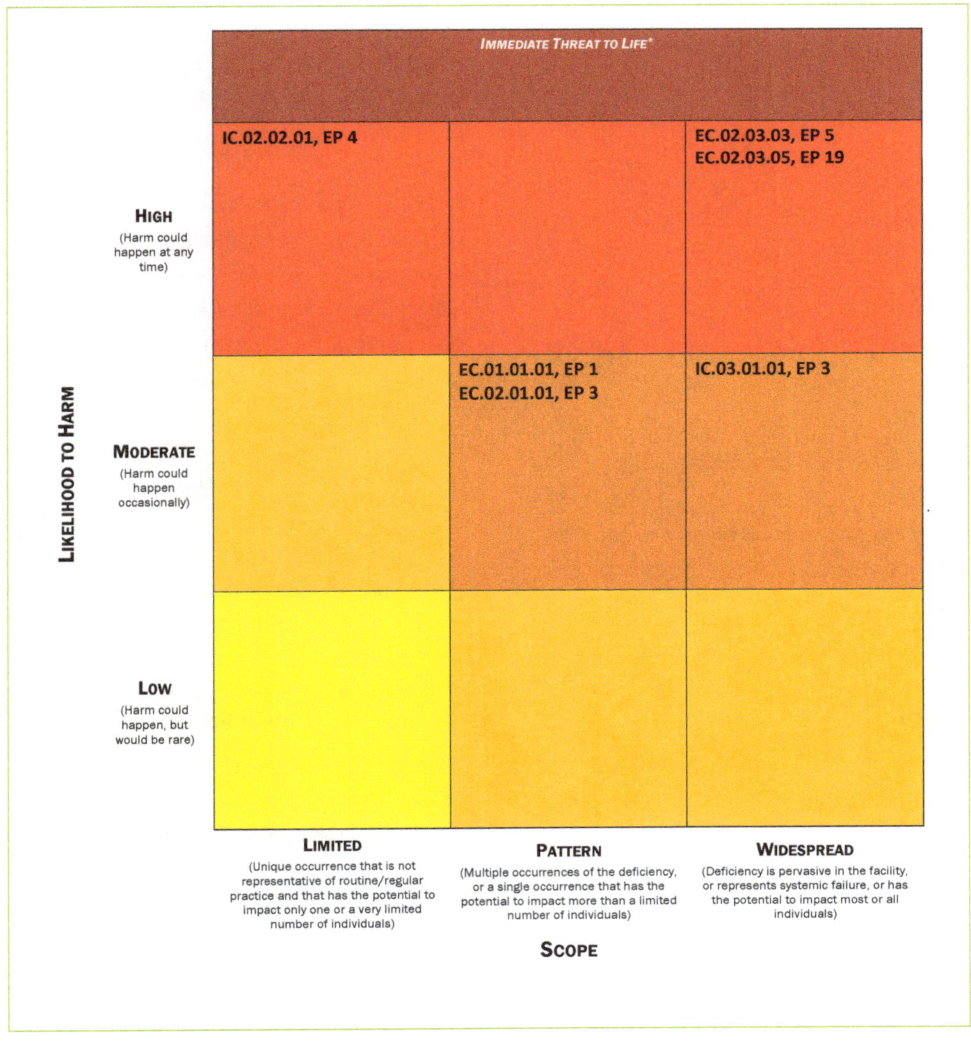

Implementation of SAFER for all accreditation and certification programs became effective in January 2017. The SAFER Matrix is now embedded within all on-site survey reports. The status of the matrix will be shared by surveyors throughout the course of the survey for multiday events. The updated, post-survey process is also in effect, resulting in the organization's ESC being due within 60 days. (Note that if a survey event results in a Preliminary Denial of Accreditation status, other follow-up events and time frames for completion/submission may apply.)

The SAFER Matrix tool, which will be made available to organizations on their *Joint Commission Connect* extranet site following their survey, allows organizations to filter RFIs within the SAFER Matrix and creates a more dynamic interaction with the survey/review information. Filters include such categories as Standard Chapter, Conditions of Participation/Conditions for Coverage, Site, and CLIA (Clinical Laboratory Improvement Amendments) Number.

In summary, SAFER will help organizations to accomplish the following:
- More easily identify RFIs with higher risk
- Identify the potential for widespread quality initiatives
- Better organize survey findings by likelihood to harm patients, residents, individuals served, visitors, and/or staff, and by scope
- Have one comprehensive visual representation of survey or self-assessment findings

In addition, SAFER will affect your organization the following ways:
- The SAFER Matrix will be included in all survey reports and drive the level of post-survey follow-up required.
- All RFIs will be addressed in a 60-day ESC Report.
- For higher–risk level RFIs (those that fall into the dark orange and red boxes on the matrix), additional detail is required concerning leadership involvement in a preventive analysis.
- Higher–risk level RFIs (those that fall into the dark orange and red boxes on the matrix) will be highlighted for surveyors to potentially review on subsequent surveys through the next full survey/review event.

The Statement of Conditions™

Complying with the Environment of Care (EC) and Life Safety (LS) standards is not a one-time endeavor but an ongoing, continuous improvement process. Health care buildings almost always are evolving through new services, equipment, renovation, and construction, and the use of the space within these facilities changes frequently. As a result, health care buildings may not be fully compliant with physical environment (EC and LS) requirements at any given moment.

To help organizations in their journeys toward compliance, The Joint Commission developed the Statement of Conditions™ (SOC). This proactive tool helps an organization conduct a critical self-assessment of its environment of care, fire safety risks, and current level of compliance with the *Life Safety Code*®[†] (*see* the "Interim Life Safety Measures" section in Chapter 6 on page 137). The SOC also helps organizations manage deficiencies identified during self-assessment. (For more information about accessing and maintaining the SOC, *see* page 43.)

Format of the SOC

Basic Building Information (BBI). This tab allows for a summary of care facilities that are defined by the *Life Safety Code* as health care, ambulatory, or residential occupancies, as applicable. Although The Joint Commission does not require health care organizations to use the SOC, it is still recommended. Sites are populated based on an organization's E-App, while buildings for each site are created and managed by the organization. Although no longer mandatory, a BBI is required to manage other parts of the SOC (*see* page 43 for a more detailed discussion of the BBI section). If an organization chooses to complete the BBI section of the SOC, it can use a portion of this section to identify the location(s) of its life safety drawings, which are required to be maintained by The Joint Commission.

Plan for Improvement (PFI). This optional section of the SOC allows organizations to manage non-survey-related EC and LS deficiencies to help maintain continuous compliance. That is, when organizations self-identify deficiencies between surveys, they can log them in the PFI section to track improvement plans and progress. By managing

---

[†] *Life Safety Code*® is a registered trademark of the National Fire Protection Association, Quincy, MA.

text continued on page 47

Accessing and Maintaining the Statement of Conditions™

All accredited Joint Commission health care organizations have a *Joint Commission Connect*™ extranet site. This extranet site is a primary point of communication between a health care organization and The Joint Commission, and provides a wealth of resources and tools—such as Focused Standards Assessment (FSA) and Intracycle Monitoring (ICM).

The Statement of Conditions™ (SOC) is another component organizations can access on their extranet site that includes the following four tabs:
1. Basic Building Information (BBI)
2. Plan for Improvement (PFI)
3. Survey-Related Plan for Improvement (SPFI)
4. Time-Limited Waiver (TLW)/Equivalency

As discussed on page 42, the SOC is a self-assessment tool organizations can use to determine its level of compliance with environment of care and fire safety risks and with the National Fire Protection Association's *Life Safety Code*®.* Although no longer required by The Joint Commission, organizations are encouraged to maintain their SOC to assist with ongoing compliance efforts.

Basic Building Information

The BBI section is used to capture the life safety features of each building that provides patient care. When an organization has multiple sites, one BBI form is completed for each site; however, a single BBI form may encompass multiple buildings if they are physically connected at that site.

This section includes the following two categories:
1. **Sites.** These are populated and removed based on the organization's E-App. The site typically is the main campus or the primary address for an organization.
2. **Buildings.** These are populated by the organization and include important information about each care facility as defined by the *Life Safety Code*, including the following:
   - Health care occupancy
   - Ambulatory occupancy
   - Residential occupancy (hotel/dormitory)
   - Business occupancy
   - Mixed occupancy (which contains a minimum of health care, ambulatory, and/or residential occupancies)

Information required for each building entry is dependent on its occupancy type. The first phase of information needed includes the building name, total square footage (rounded to the nearest 10%), building address, and occupancy type; after this information is entered, save and continue. An additional set of fields will need to be completed based on the occupancy type selected. Information required may include the following:

---

* *Life Safety Code*® is a registered trademark of the National Fire Protection Association, Quincy, MA.

continued

- Total licensed patient beds (same as the E-App)
- Building size and type (including total stories, number of exits, building construction type)
- Building age renovation
- Percent of building that is sprinklered
- Life safety features (including fire alarm system, smoke detection system, emergency power)
- Special features (including grease-producing devices, locked or secured units, laundry/trash chutes)
- Previous inspections (including US Centers for Medicare & Medicaid Services [CMS], state and local fire marshal)
- Name and qualifications of SOC preparer(s)
- Location of life safety drawings
- Additional optional notes

After this information has been entered and saved, this section of the SOC is complete.

Plan for Improvement

With the BBI section complete, it is time to address the identified *Life Safety Code* deficiencies in the PFI section. These identified deficiencies may be a result of organizational, local or state, authority having jurisdiction, and/or insurance inspections.

The PFI menu offers the following seven options:
1. **Search.** This option allows users to search for open or closed PFIs.
2. **Open.** Open PFIs for the organization are included in this option, as well as the last modified date, and a summary of open SPFIs. This selection also offers an option to export open PFIs and SPFIs to Excel, and summarizes the number of accepted and new equivalency items.
3. **Closed.** A summary of closed PFIs and an option to export them to Excel are offered by this selection.
4. **View All.** This option shows a summary of all open PFIs. Fields that can be viewed may include interim life safety measures (ILSM) requirements, site, building, PFI ID, description (of the deficiency), scheduled completion date, and status. Unique to this section is a color-coded system used to draw attention to specific PFI dates:
   - Light blue is a PFI that is within 30 days of its scheduled completion date
   - Yellow is a PFI that is within 15 days of its scheduled completion date
   - Red is a PFI that has passed its scheduled completion date
   - Orange is a PFI that is completed (closed) past the scheduled completion date
5. **Convert Excel PFI.** This option provides instructions and formatted Excel spreadsheets for organizations to import PFI(s) into their SOC. To complete this successfully, the format must be followed exactly.
6. **Create New.** This option is chosen when creating a new PFI.
7. **History/Audit Trail.** The following information is documented in this section
   - Survey event
   - Approved/rejected equivalency
   - Approved/rejected extension requests
   - Coaching calls
   - Additional SOC–related communications

Survey-Related Plan for Improvement

The SPFI section documents survey-related *Life Safety Code* deficiencies cited as a Requirement for Improvement (RFI) that cannot be corrected with the 60-day evidence of standards compliance (ESC) time frame. Menu options for this section are similar to the PFI section.

Creating a new SPFI begins by choosing "yes" when a pop-up box asks if the PFI is related to a Joint Commission RFI from an onsite survey. After the new SPFI is created, details about the deficiency (including site, building, last day of survey, cited standard and element of performance) need to be entered. A brief description summarizing the specific deficiency is the next step. If an ILSM is necessary, information documenting it and risk mitigation in place must be documented.

After the overall information is documented, a detail page will be completed that includes information about the resolution (including the proposed action, source of funding, projected cost, and projected start and scheduled completion dates). For SPFIs that require more than 60 days to complete, a time-limited waiver (TLW) must be submitted to request an extension.

Time-Limited Waiver/Equivalency

The TLW section is used when organizations need to request additional time to complete a *Life Safety Code* RFI that will take more than the 60-day ESC allotted time to complete or to request an equivalency of a *Life Safety Code* RFI deficiency that cannot be corrected without major construction.

All fields of the TLW form are required to be completed and include the following:
- Organization information
- Submitter information
- Request information
  - Request type (TLW or equivalency)
  - Survey date
  - SPFI ID
  - *Life Safety Code* chapter and section (for RFIs associated to *Life Safety Code* deficiencies only)
- ILSM/mitigation actions implementations
- Request summary (including a description of the deficiency, an explanation for the requested time, and identifying unreasonable hardships)
- Proposed corrective action

In addition to the information required in the form, organizations must provide the following documentation:
- Deemed Accreditation Organizations
  - Final Survey Report
  - Facility Request for Waiver
  - Facility Plan for Correction
  - Supporting Evidence

continued

- Non-Deemed Accreditation Organizations
  - Final Survey Report
  - Supporting Evidence

Failing to provide all mandatory documentation will result in a rejection of the TLW/equivalency. Also note that a TLW/equivalency is not guaranteed.

For additional information about accessing and maintaining the SOC, visit The Joint Commission Standards Interpretation Frequently Asked Questions: https://www.jointcommission.org/standards_information/jcfaq.aspx.

deficiencies as PFIs, the organization can demonstrate a proactive approach to identifying, mitigating, and correcting deficiencies during the survey process. The PFI process is used to address deficiencies that are complex enough to need longer time frames and/or special funding sources to correct (*see* page 44 for a more detailed discussion of the PFI section). A PFI would not be used to correct minor deficiencies, such as a burned-out exit bulb, or for EC–related testing and inspection requirements.

Survey-Related Plan for Improvement (SPFI). When EC and LS deficiencies are identified during an on-site survey (as an RFI), the organization is required—in accordance with Standard LS.01.01.01—to manage it as an SPFI within the SOC (*see* page 45 for a more detailed discussion of the SPFI section). Similar to the PFI process, SPFIs are more complex and/or need special funding to correct or equivalize. If the resolution of the deficiency can be corrected within 60 days from last day of survey in the ESC, the organization must apply for a time-limited waiver (TLW) to complete it.

Time-Limited Waiver/Equivalency (TLW) . This section is used to request either a TLW or equivalency (*see* page 45 for a more detailed discussion of the TLW section). The TLW is a request for additional time to address an EC or LS RFI that will take longer than the allowed 60 days provided in the ESC. An equivalency is a means to address a *Life Safety Code* deficiency that may not meet the prescriptive requirement of the code but does meet the intent of the code (refer to Chapter 6 for additional information on equivalencies).

Assigning an Individual(s) to Manage the SOC

Organizations accredited under the Ambulatory Health Care, Behavioral Health Care, Critical Access Hospital, Hospital, and Nursing Care Center Accreditation Programs are required to assign an individual(s) to manage the SOC when addressing survey-related deficiencies, in accordance with Standard LS.01.01.01. This applies to all buildings where care or treatment is provided and that meet the *Life Safety Code* definition of a health care, ambulatory, or residential occupancy. (It is not required for organizations classified as business occupancies.) One individual may manage the documentation of the deficiencies within the SOC, but an EC committee and leadership should oversee the management of these identified deficiencies for appropriate mitigation strategies and resolution.

Who Completes the SOC?

Although there are no strictly defined qualifications of who should complete an SOC, Joint Commission standards require organizations to appoint competent individual(s) to do the task. This individual(s) should have a strong knowledge of the environment of care and the *Life Safety Code*, as well as the buildings being evaluated. His or her qualifications should be in line with the scope and difficulty of the assessment. Things to consider when choosing who should complete the SOC include the following:

The assessment's complexity and scope. Some facilities have a greater number of physical environment requirements than others, which will make the assessment more complicated. Also, factors such as age and size of buildings will affect the assessment's complexity. For example, older buildings may have outdated systems or have undergone multiple renovations or additions that would make assessment more involved.

The assessor's knowledge. In general, as building complexity increases, an assessor's knowledge of the *Life Safety Code*, regulations, and the building becomes more important. In-house personnel can be a good choice for ongoing SOC assessment, as they often know the building the best. If a staff person or the building owner can be trained on EC and LS, he or she might be an ideal assessor. However, if appropriate staff resources are not available or the building is particularly complex, an outside consultant or a team of consultants may be contracted.

The assessor's experience. A specific background in health care safety, fire safety work, or health care construction can be invaluable in an SOC assessor. There can be trade-offs between formal education and experience. For example, if a person has 30 years of experience in assessing buildings, it could be equivalent to a background with a heavier mix of formal education. Another option is to use outside help as a backup. In-house assessors should know when they are in over their heads. If these assessors encounter a tricky problem, they may want to consider bringing in someone who understands the nuances.

Regardless of who is chosen to complete the SOC, organizations that give some forethought to the selection can help ensure a thorough assessment process that reflects the true status of safety in the organization.

text continued on page 51

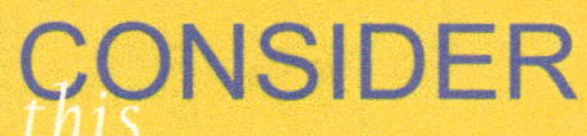

Mock Tracers in the Environment of Care

A tracer is a tool used by surveyors during on-site surveys to follow—or "trace"—a person through his or her process of care, treatment, or services. Some tracers focus on the experience of the person and how the various aspects of an organization interact to meet the individual's needs and maintain safety. Other tracers examine a specific program or system in the organization.

Like the other tools discussed in this chapter, the tracer can be used by organizations the same way it is used during a survey. "Mock tracers" mimic what occurs during an on-site survey tracer and help in the following ways:

- *Identify deficiencies.* By conducting a mock tracer, an organization can take a closer look at certain systems and processes. When deficiencies are identified, an organization can address them and develop sustainable improvements.
- *Engage staff and leadership.* Because mock tracers are conducted by staff, they provide an opportunity to reach out to leadership and other departments to demonstrate the ongoing survey readiness methods used to keep facilities safe.
- *Prepare for survey.* A mock tracer is an excellent tool to use to maintain survey readiness.
- *Reduce the anxiety of an on-site survey.* Conducting a mock tracer provides an opportunity to demonstrate to staff what can be expected during a Joint Commission on-site survey. In addition to identifying potential deficiencies, this exercise can alleviate stress on staff since they will be more knowledgeable about the survey process—including the expectations— and provide valuable insight regarding possible deficiencies and solutions.

Environment of Care Tracers

For the physical environment, The Joint Commission does not have a defined "EC tracer." Surveyors most commonly will assess an organization's degree of compliance with relevant Environment of Care (EC), Emergency Management (EM), and Life Safety (LS) standards in two ways:

- As part of patient or system tracers
- As part of the environment of care/emergency management system session during a survey

EC tracers examine an organization's systems and processes related to the physical environment, emergency management, and life safety. An EC tracer is often triggered by something a surveyor observes during another tracer. For example, a surveyor conducting an individual tracer of a patient might notice an employee mishandling hazardous waste, which would spark a follow-up tracer directly related to this important EC area. Other related areas may become involved during an EC tracer, such as infection prevention and control and clinical areas that manage medical equipment. (*See* pages 49 and 50, respectively, for a mock tracer form, an evaluation checklist, and tracer questions for the physical environment.)

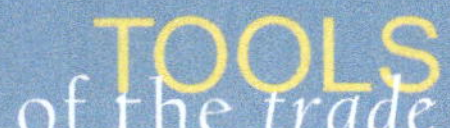

Mock Tracer Form

This worksheet can be customized by choosing tracer questions from those provided throughout this book or with questions created by the mock tracer survey team.

Note: *The complete form may be adapted and is available for internal use on the flash drive (print only) or by clicking the tool link in the Risk-Assessment Toolbox (e-book only) on page 58.*

Published in *Environment of Care Risk Assessment*, Joint Commission Resources, 2018.　　**File Name:** 02 02 Form Mock Tracer color

Mock Tracer Form

Organization		Department/Unit	
Date of Tracer		Time of Tracer		Tracer Topic	
Type of Tracer	☐ Individual　☐ System　☐ Program　☐ High-Risk ☐ Environment of Care　　☐ *Life Safety Code®**	Tracer Team	
Patient Record # (if applicable)		Documents Reviewed	

Tracer Question(s)	Relevant Standard(s)
Person(s) Asked	

Tracer Question(s) go here.　　Compliant?　　If insufficient compliance　　☐ Immediate Threat to Life

---

Mock Tracer Evaluation Checklist

This checklist itemizes the elements of an effective mock tracer and can be used to evaluate the effectiveness of mock tracers in an organization. This tool also can be used to develop a procedure checklist for an organization's mock tracer program.

Note: *The complete checklist may be adapted and is available for internal use on the flash drive (print only) or by clicking the tool link in the Risk-Assessment Toolbox (e-book only) on page 58.*

Published in *Environment of Care Risk Assessment*, Joint Commission Resources, 2018.　　**File Name:** 02 03 Checklist Mock Tracer Eval

MOCK TRACER EVALUATION CHECKLIST

This checklist itemizes elements of an effective mock tracer. Organizations can use it to evaluate mock tracers conducted in their facilities. In addition, the evaluation criteria can be used to develop a procedure checklist for mock tracers in an organization's mock tracer program. Answers to all questions should ideally be **Y** *for* **Yes** *(unless they aren't applicable). If an answer is* **N** *for* **No,** *use the "Notes" section to document needed changes. Unless otherwise noted, this checklist is applicable to all program settings.*

ORGANIZATION: ___________________________　DEPARTMENT/UNIT: ___________________________

DATE OF ASSESSMENT: ___________________　PARTICIPANT(S): ___________________________

DATE OF MOCK TRACER: _________________　MOCK TRACER TOPIC: _______________________

QUESTION	YES	NO	NA	NOTES

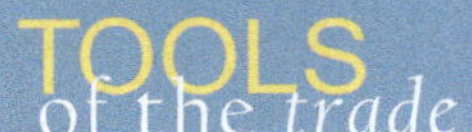

Tracer Questions for the Physical Environment

When creating an environment of care (EC) mock tracer, the mock survey team can pull from this 14-section listing of questions and adapt them as appropriate to their specific program setting.

Note: *The complete worksheet may be adapted and is available for internal use on the flash drive (print only) or by clicking the tool link in the Risk-Assessment Toolbox (e-book only) on page 58.*

Published in *Environment of Care Risk Assessment*, Joint Commission Resources, 2018.   **File Name:** 02 04 Tracer Qs for EC

TRACER QUESTIONS FOR THE PHYSICAL ENVIRONMENT

These sample questions—applicable to all Joint Commission program settings unless otherwise indicated—can be used when creating a mock tracer for the physical environment. There are 14 sections of questions to choose from, and all may be adapted as appropriate to a specific program setting. Questions can be chosen then copied into the Mock Tracer or another form.

SECTION 1. ENVIRONMENT OF CARE MANAGEMENT PLANS AND RISK MANAGEMENT TRACER QUESTIONS	USE QUESTION AS IS	ADAPT QUESTION FOR USE
1. Who is responsible for risk management activities in the organization? Is this person also responsible for intervening in cases of threat to life or health, or damage to equipment or buildings? If not, who is responsible for that?*	☐	☐
2. Please describe the process for creating the environment of care management plans.*	☐	☐
3. Who is responsible for creating the environment of care management plans? Is an interdisciplinary team involved? If so, who is on the team?*	☐	☐
4. Does your organization have environment of care management plans covering all of the environment of care functional areas, such as fire safety and utilities?*	☐	☐
5. How do your environment of care management plans focus on risk management?*	☐	☐
6. Do the environment of care management plans include objectives, performance monitors, and scope definitions? Do they cover all organization sites, including any leased sites? Do they explain briefly how relevant standards and elements of performance (EPs) are met?*	☐	☐
7. Do your environment of care management plans identify those responsible for completing specific tasks within required time frames?*	☐	☐
8. How does your organization evaluate your environment of care management plans? How often do you perform an evaluation? Who participates in the evaluation? Does your organization document the date of evaluations?*	☐	☐
9. How does your organization ensure that the evaluation process occurs in a timely way?*	☐	☐
10. Does your organization compare the evaluations of the environment of care management plans against the minutes of your improvement committee?*	☐	☐

Using the SOC Effectively

The state of an organization's SOC is key to its overall EC and LS management. The SOC is not a "once-and-done" exercise. Rather, it must reflect the current conditions in the health care facility. The SOC is meant to be a "living document" that evolves with changes in the building and environment.

Because of the electronic format of the SOC, it also can serve as an effective risk-management tool. Through the many different reports available on the tool, an organization can effectively track its SPFIs and optional PFIs, TLWs, and equivalencies and identify any trends and patterns that may be cause for concern. For example, an organization can view the status of all open SPFIs and PFIs and further sort this list by building. This can help the EC professional get a sense of the improvement initiatives occurring within the organization and where resources need to be allocated.

Basic Steps in the SOC Process

The SOC tool consists of a series of forms or actions that, as they are completed, guide the organization through the process of assessing EC and LS compliance, identifying deficiencies that result in risk, mitigating the risks, and correcting those deficiencies. A brief overview of the SOC process is included in this book; detailed instructions are available within each section of the SOC.

Identify Occupancy Type

Before an assessment of EC and LS compliance can begin, the organization must identify each care building's occupancy type. This step is important because the type of occupancy determines which *Life Safety Code* requirements are applicable (*see* page 55 for additional information about occupancy types).

Complete the BBI

The next step is to complete the BBI portion of the SOC, which consists of providing key information about each building being surveyed by The Joint Commission. This information will include occupancy type, fire protection features (for example, sprinklers, fire alarm systems), and other related information.

Each building in which care, treatment, or services are received must be identified within the BBI, regardless of ownership. If the organization is renting or leasing the space, the BBI should cover the areas it is occupying. The exception to these requirements is a building(s) that is a business occupancy. In that situation, no BBI is required, regardless of ownership or lease/rental arrangements. It is recommended that these organizations at least document the building occupancy type. The BBI is connected to the organization's Joint Commission E-App. When an organization submits or updates its E-App, the "sites" are inserted into or deleted from the BBI. When a site is within the BBI, it is the organization's responsibility to create each building in which health care services or treatment are provided for that site. Separate buildings may be required based on different occupancies or addresses.

Create PFIs

This is an optional section for organizations to use in detecting and managing deficiencies identified outside of the Joint Commission survey process (for example, the organization self-assessment, state surveys, ICM). After the organization has entered the necessary information into the BBI, it can use the information gleaned from its EC and LS assessments to create PFIs in the SOC.

If the EC and LS assessments determine that there are no deficiencies, the organization may note that in the PFI by creating a new PFI and selecting the "no deficiencies" option.

However, many organizations will find deficiencies during their EC and LS assessments. These are issues that do not comply with the standards set forth by The Joint Commission or the *Life Safety Code*. Deficiencies must be addressed to bring the organization into continuous compliance. The PFI tab in the SOC is a means for doing this.

As previously stated, minor deficiencies such as burned-out exit bulbs can be dealt with through a work order system or, possibly, by using the Building Maintenance Program (*see* page 134 in Chapter 6 for a more detailed discussion of the Building Maintenance Program). Use PFIs to manage non-survey–related deficiencies that have complex solutions needing a longer time frame to complete and that require special funding sources. A PFI is recommended within 45 days of the problem's identification.

Redesigning the Evidence of Standards Compliance Format

The Joint Commission recently redesigned its Evidence of Standards Compliance (ESC) format to help organizations focus on communicating the critical aspects of their corrective actions that resolve post-survey Requirements for Improvement (RFIs). The ESC clearly and concisely lays out expectations for successful completion, as it aligns with proven performance-improvement methodologies. Information for submission within the ESC includes assigning accountability, correcting the noncompliance, and ensuring sustained compliance for all RFIs. For those RFIs that fall within the higher-risk boxes on the Survey Analysis for Evaluating Risk™ (SAFER™) Matrix (dark orange and red matrix boxes), communicating leadership involvement and conducting a preventive analysis also are required components within the ESC submission. The following table provides a side-by-side comparison of the previous format versus the redesigned format.

Then	Now
WHO is ultimately responsible for the corrective action?	**Assigning Accountability** • Who is ultimately responsible for corrective action and sustained compliance?
NA prior to the rollout of the SAFER Matrix	**Assign Accountability—Leadership Involvement*** • Which member(s) of leadership support future compliance?
NA prior to the rollout of the SAFER Matrix	**Correcting the Noncompliance—Preventive Analysis*** • What analysis was completed to ensure not only that the noncompliant issue was corrected (surface/high-level resolution) but also that any underlying reasons for the failure were addressed?
WHAT actions were completed to correct each finding? **WHEN** were each of the actions completed?	**Correcting the Noncompliance—*The "What" and "When" Sections Combined*** • What actions were taken to correct each finding? • When were all actions completed (indicated by one final date)?
HOW will compliance be sustained?	**Ensuring Sustained Compliance** • What procedures/activities have been identified to monitor compliance? • What is the frequency of the monitoring activities? • What data will be collected from these activities? • To whom, and how often, will the data be reported?

* ESC field implemented with the rollout of the SAFER Matrix and required for higher-risk RFIs only, within the dark orange and red matrix boxes

NA, not applicable; SAFER, Survey Analysis for Evaluating Risk; RFI, Requirement for Improvement.

Life Safety Drawings

Joint Commission Standard LS.01.01.01 requires organizations to maintain accurate life safety drawings that identify the location of the life safety features of a facility. In addition to a legend that clearly identifies what is being shown in the drawing, the following life safety measures should be included:

- Sprinklered areas—fully sprinklered areas if the building includes partially sprinklered areas
- Hazardous storage areas
- Barriers—including all rated barriers, smoke barriers, and designated smoke compartments
- Suite boundaries—indicating the size of the suites, both sleeping and nonsleeping
- Chutes and shafts—including elevators, laundry, and other vertical openings
- Any approved equivalencies or waivers

If an organization is completing the Basic Building Information (BBI) section of the Statement of Conditions™, an organization can identify the location(s) of the life safety drawings in the "Additional Notes" portion of this section.

The PFI should contain details on the following:
- What specific actions the organization plans to take to correct the deficiency, including interim life safety measures (ILSM)/mitigation actions, when appropriate
- Scheduled start and completion dates
- Sources of funding for the project

Completion dates are particularly important. These should be set far enough ahead that they are reasonable but not so far ahead that the project loses urgency. It also is important to understand exactly what the form is asking and to answer accordingly. For example, in the field labeled "ILSM/Risk Mitigation Required," the organization will need to document (based on organization risk assessment) if ILSM (*Life Safety Code*–related) or mitigation actions (non-*Life Safety Code*–related) are required. If "yes" is selected, the organization will need to either select the appropriate EPs in accordance with the ILSM and/or document in the text box provided.

Manage and Track PFIs

PFIs are not intended to be created and forgotten. Although organizations have full editing rights for their PFIs, including their scheduled completion dates, the goal should be to track progress on each PFI, with the ultimate goal of "closing" it—that is, marking it as completed. When completing a PFI, the organization should document the actual completion date, reason code, and any additional comments if the PFI was not completed based on the actions documented in the resolution.

The SOC allows organizations to sort PFIs in many ways, including by all open PFI entries, by closed PFI entries, and by PFIs that are nearing their proposed completion dates. In addition, organizations may want to sort by status. An organization can look at these different categories for the organization as a whole or by different buildings or locations, provided they are set up in the BBI.

Create SPFIs

The SPFI section is mandatory and requires organizations to manage all survey-identified EC and LS RFIs within the 60 days allowable in the ESC process. The organization must document the deficiency as an SPFI and submit a TLW request within 30 days from last day of survey in order to request additional time to resolve the deficiency.

The SPFI and PFI formats are similar, but there are a few fields that differ between the two. The SPFI will require additional information regarding the survey, including last day of survey and the standard and EP scored during the survey. The description of the deficiency should be a summarization of what was cited during the survey, that is, the surveyor's description of noncompliance.

Manage and Track SPFIs

SPFIs, unlike PFIs, that do not meet the scheduled completion date will generate an unannounced survey for failing to manage the SOC. As mentioned previously, organizations may identify an individual(s) to manage the SOC, but it is the responsibility of an EC committee and organizational leadership to oversee the correction of all deficiencies as scheduled.

Another difference between SPFIs and PFIs is that The Joint Commission accepts the plan of correction documented within the SPFI and TLW. When a TLW is accepted by CMS, or by The Joint Commission for non-deemed organizations, the SPFI is accepted. When the SPFI is accepted, the organization can no longer edit any of the information within it, with the exception of documenting the completion information.

Create TLWs

When an organization needs additional time to resolve SPFIs, it must formally request and justify its request for a TLW. As noted previously, The Joint Commission requires that the organization submit a TLW request within 30 days from last day of survey. Along with submitting the required form, the organization must provide the following documentation:

1. Letter of Request for a TLW (deemed status only)—a formal letter describing the deficiency and justification of hardship
2. A Plan of Correction (deemed status only)—a formal letter describing a detailed time line and resolution of the cited deficiency
3. A copy of the Accreditation Survey Findings Report
4. Any Supporting Documentation, including, but not limited to, purchase orders, financial information, pictures, and so forth

Occupancy Types

The National Fire Protection Association's (NFPA) *Life Safety Code*®* (NFPA 101–2012) defines *occupancy* as "the purpose for which a building or other structure, of part thereof, is used or intended to be used." Several types of occupancies that are used for the provision of health care are affected by the *Life Safety Code* and, therefore, the Statement of Conditions™ (SOC). Following is a brief description of several different occupancy types, as defined by NFPA.

Health Care Occupancy

A *health care occupancy* is defined in NFPA 101, Section 3.3.188.7, as "an occupancy used to provide medical or other treatment or care simultaneously to four or more patients on an inpatient basis, where such patients are mostly incapable of self-preservation due to age, physical or mental disability, or because of security measures not under the occupant's control." *Incapable of self-preservation* means that the individual would not be able to get up and walk out of the building in case of a fire. Health care occupancies include "general hospitals, psychiatric hospitals, and specialty hospitals," as well as "nursing and convalescent homes, skilled nursing facilities, intermediate care facilities, and infirmaries in homes for the aged."

Ambulatory Health Care Occupancy

NFPA 101, Section 3.3.188.1, defines an *ambulatory health care occupancy* as "an occupancy used to provide services or treatment simultaneously to four or more patients that provides, on an outpatient basis, one or more of the following: (1) treatment for patients that renders the patients incapable of taking action for self-preservation under emergency conditions without the assistance of others; (2) anesthesia that renders the patients incapable of taking action for self-preservation under emergency conditions without the assistance of others; (3) emergency or urgent care for patients who, due to the nature of their injury or illness, are incapable of taking action for self-preservation under emergency conditions without the assistance of others."

Several points deserve special mention here. First, it is the intention of NFPA that four or more individuals must be rendered incapable of self-preservation for a facility to be classified as an ambulatory health care occupancy. Second, the word *rendered* in this context means that the individuals must be made incapable of self-preservation by the treatment provided at the facility. For example, in an outpatient surgery center, having four or more people under anesthesia and/or recovering from it at one time would result in a classification of ambulatory health care. On the other hand, individuals who arrive in wheelchairs might be considered to be incapable of self-preservation before any treatment is provided. Each organization must carefully evaluate the services and treatment it provides to determine whether the individuals served will be rendered incapable of self-preservation.

Finally, when the US Centers for Medicare & Medicaid Services (CMS) adopted the 2012 edition of the *Life Safety Code* it did so with two exceptions. Although The Joint Commission accepts the definition of the ambulatory health care occupancy as just explained, CMS requires that ambulatory surgery centers where even one person is rendered incapable of self-preservation be classified as ambulatory health care. (The Joint Commission would view

---

* *Life Safety Code*® is a registered trademark of the National Fire Protection Association, Quincy, MA.

continued

such facilities as business occupancies, but will survey such organizations as ambulatory health care occupancies if they are pursuing accreditation for deemed status purposes.)

Business Occupancy

In accordance with NFPA 101, Section 3.3.188.3, a *business occupancy* is "used for the transaction of business other than mercantile." This is a very broad definition, but as it applies to health care, it is understood to refer to a facility where no occupants stay overnight and where three or fewer individuals are rendered incapable of self-preservation at any given time.

The SOC is applicable to business occupancies only under certain circumstances. Freestanding business occupancies do not require that an SOC be completed. A Joint Commission surveyor would ensure that these occupancies are maintained in a fire-safe condition and that they do not have any blocked or locked exits, but he or she would not survey for compliance with the *Life Safety Code.*

A freestanding business occupancy is a separate building that is not physically attached to a health care or ambulatory health care occupancy. Or, it is a building attached to one of these occupancies but separated from it by a two-hour fire-resistance-rated assembly, as long as there is no required fire exit from the health care occupancy into the business occupancy. Note that there can be a door between these occupancies, as long as it is labeled "Not an Exit" on the health care side.

The only business occupancy for which an SOC must be completed is one through which a health care occupancy is required to exit in a fire emergency. In this case, the organization would have to complete the business occupancy portion of the SOC and be maintained in compliance with the business occupancy chapter of the *Life Safety Code.*

Other Occupancies That Relate to Health Care

Two other types of occupancies that are addressed by the SOC appear at first glance to have little to do with health care. Both are classified as residential occupancies. The lodging and rooming house occupancy is used for facilities that provide sleeping accommodations for 16 or fewer occupants who are capable of self-preservation. Similarly, hotel and dormitory occupancies provide sleeping accommodations for 17 or more occupants who are capable of self-preservation. Both types of residential occupancies can be used for residential treatment facilities, which are often accredited as behavioral health care facilities. As designated by the local authority having jurisdiction (AHJ), assisted living facilities also may be classified as one of these types of residential occupancies. Note that these occupancies do not apply to sleeping facilities that a health care organization might maintain for the convenience of outpatients or relatives of patients; in these cases, no SOC is required because no health care is provided in the facilities.

Mixed Occupancy

In some facilities classified as health care occupancies, areas of the building may have uses other than the housing or treatment of patients or individuals who are incapable of self-preservation. These facilities are called mixed occupancies. For example, there may be a wing that is used strictly for administrative offices or an area that is only for outpatient services that do not render individuals incapable of self-preservation. These areas may be classified as other occupancies, provided that they are separated from the health care occupancy by a minimum two-hour fire-resistance-rated assembly. There are some advantages to doing this. Health care occupancies are required to have the highest—and most costly—level of protection in accordance with the *Life Safety Code*; maintaining some areas as business occupancies may save an organization money by allowing it to comply with less stringent regulations.

When all required documentation is uploaded, the option to submit will appear at the bottom of the page.

TLWs will be reviewed by The Joint Commission and, if approved, will be submitted to CMS (deemed status only) for final approval. Organizations will need an SPFI and a Joint Commission– or CMS–approved TLW to furnish as ESC or as evidence of resolution during any type of follow-up survey.

Update the SOC

To be most effective, the SOC should be updated periodically to account for construction, renovation, building maintenance, changes in use, and other variables. It is expected to reflect the current status of the building at all times, including at the time of the organization's on-site survey.

The currency of the SOC and the status of any PFIs, SPFIs, TLWs, and equivalencies should be reviewed by an EC committee. To use the SOC to its full potential, organizations should consider looking at the SOC at least twice a year or at a higher frequency, depending on the scheduled completion dates of the PFIs and SPFIs. This allows a facilities manager to determine the size, scope, and nature of deficiencies, where to allocate resources, how to effectively address problems, and the best way to manage the compliance process.

Surveys and the SOC

Although The Joint Commission no longer reviews PFIs as part of the survey process, PFIs can still be a beneficial tool for organizations to manage deficiencies identified outside the scope of survey. If a surveyor identifies a deficiency that has already been documented by the organization as a PFI (or equivalent means), it is recommended that the organization share this information at the time of survey. Provide documentation to the surveyor as to your organization's proactive approach, documentation of any applicable ILSM or mitigation actions, and plan of correction. The surveyor will still cite the deficiency as an RFI, but if the organization is managing and minimizing the risk to the safety of its patients, residents, or individuals served this may affect how it is scored in the SAFER Matrix.

In addition, when the decision rule requires a follow-up survey to address EC and LS findings, the organization will be required to provide evidence of either (1) corrective action, (2) resolution within 60 days from last day of survey, or (3) a documented SPFI and Joint Commission– or CMS–approved TLW within the SOC. If option 3 is chosen, the organization should be prepared to share the SOC with the surveyor.

Using the SOC to Help Improve Performance

In addition to using the SOC to manage EC and LS compliance and the status of PFI and SPFI completion, organizations can use it as a tool to help identify and prioritize high-risk areas and those in need of performance improvement. By analyzing open PFIs and SPFIs, an EC manager can look for similarities and patterns that might indicate a more global need for improvement. For example, if several PFIs and SPFIs relating to an organization's fire barriers are open at the same time, it might indicate the need to take a closer look at the maintenance of fire barriers for potential performance issues. Likewise, if there are several PFIs and SPFIs in a particular building or location, it might indicate the need for renovations or improvements to that building. This kind of information can inform the performance improvement committee and leadership when making decisions about prioritization of projects and resources.

RISK-ASSESSMENT TOOLBOX

1. **SAFER Matrix and Required Follow-Up Activities**
   - [Download] **Landscape**
   - [Download] **Portrait**
2. **Mock Tracer Form**
   - [Download] **Black and White**
   - [Download] **Color**
3. [Download] **Mock Tracer Evaluation Checklist**
4. [Download] **Tracer Questions for the Physical Environment**

chapter 3

Safety

Every organization has inherent safety risks that are associated with providing services to patients, residents, and individuals served; performing daily activities; and functioning in the physical environment (*see* page 60). Safety risks also arise from circumstances beyond the health care organization's control, such as weather events. For example, during or immediately following a rainstorm there may be increased risk of slipping on wet floors.

Overview of Assessing Risks

The Joint Commission standards require organizations to manage their safety risks. Consistent and comprehensive risk assessment is key to safety management. This chapter discusses some required safety risk assessments, as well as some common safety risk assessments that organizations should consider performing.

(**Note:** *Some organizations treat safety and security as a single function. Although safety and security are related, there are several important distinctions that are discussed on page 62. This chapter will focus on safety risks and safety risk assessments; security risks and security risk assessments will be discussed in Chapter 5 beginning on page 105.*)

Participants in the Process

For most health care organizations, the individual filling the role of safety manager, facilities manager, or environment of care (EC) director typically is responsible for identifying and implementing any safety risk assessments, including those required by The Joint Commission in accordance with Standard EC.01.01.01 and those that result from a proactive look at potential safety issues. The organization's multidisciplinary improvement team—commonly known as the safety or EC committee—also should be involved in the risk-assessment process (*see* page 63 for a further discussion about the EC committee).

Frequency of Assessments

Safety risks are always present wherever health care services are provided, particularly in a health care facility; therefore, safety should always be a primary focus. Though

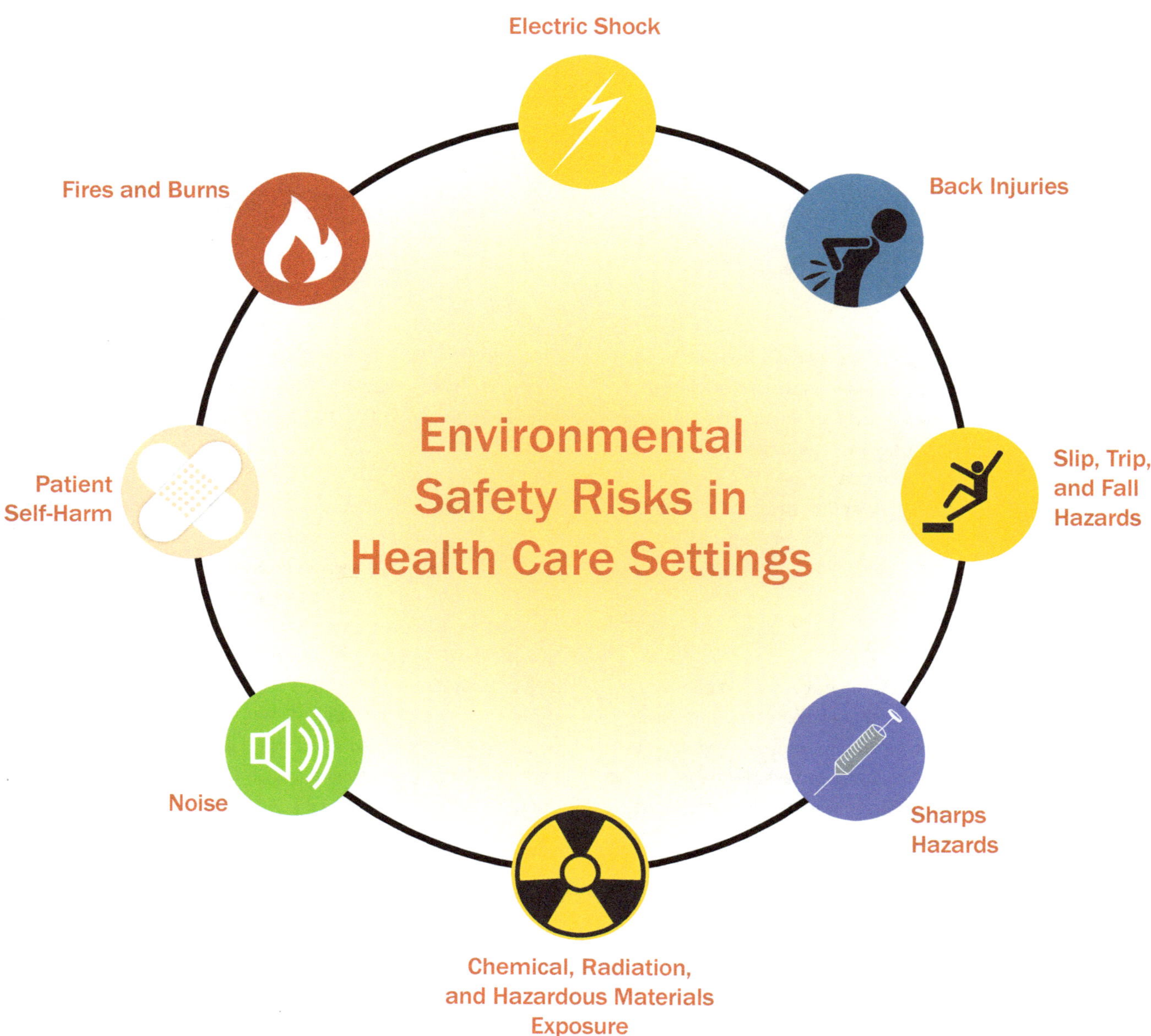

In any health care setting, there are any number of safety risks that can affect the physical environment. This illustration provides a sampling of safety risks that can impact patients, residents, individuals served, staff, and visitors in a health care organization.

safety incidents may prompt a risk assessment, organizations should not wait until a patient or staff member is harmed before assessing safety risks. Performing frequent, proactive safety risk assessments maintains a consistently high level of awareness to safety risks and addresses risks before they can result in safety events.

Although safety risks should be assessed continually on an informal basis, the time lines for performing formal safety risk assessments vary based on data collected by the organization through environmental tours, incident reports, external resources, and so on. Joint Commission standards are not prescriptive as to who should be involved in the risk assessment process, but it is recommended that it is a multidisciplinary approach for both assessment and periodic evaluations (*see* page 65 for an example EC committee reporting schedule). Recommendations for improvements may be determined by risk assessments. In addition, Joint Commission Leadership (LD) standards for hospitals and critical access hospitals require organizations to conduct a proactive risk assessment on a high-risk process, which may be safety related, a minimum of every 18 months.

Identifying Risks

To proactively determine safety risks in organizations, safety managers and EC committees should review data and get a big picture of what is occurring in their organization and where potential risks are located (*see* page 67).

In addition, safety managers should consider recently renovated or constructed areas as sources for potential risk assessments. If a department or environment is new or has undergone significant renovation or conversion, the safety manager should consider conducting a risk assessment to examine potential threats and determine mitigation efforts. This assessment should involve all individuals in the department and those who visit the department. (*See* Chapter 10 for additional information about assessing risks associated with construction.)

When potential risks are identified, the organization can use a proactive risk-assessment process to determine the extent of the risks and identify potential solutions. As described in Chapter 1, having a defined proactive risk-assessment process can help ensure that any potential risks identified are assessed appropriately, consistently, and completely.

for example...

A nurse calls a safety manager to ask if the intensive care unit (ICU) can store needles or sharps at the bedside. This sounds like a bad idea because of all the traffic in the ICU; however, no Joint Commission standards or other regulations state that nurses cannot store sharps at the bedside. In addition, there is no best-practice information on the concept, and the organization has not dealt with this issue before. So the safety manager conducts a risk assessment to ascertain the potential risks associated with storing sharps at the bedside, as well as the potential benefits to staff.

After weighing the pros and cons, the safety manager decides to allow the storage of sharps at the bedside but determines the issue will need to be closely monitored. If any incidents occur because a patient, child, or visitor gains access to these unsecured sharps, this process will change immediately. All parties agree. The safety manager assigns a representative from the ICU to attend the monthly safety committee meetings to report the status. The organization documents the process through the minutes of the safety committee.

Every month the ICU nurse manager reports to the safety committee to discuss how the process is going. By using a proactive risk-assessment process, the organization is able to confidently address a need, knowing that all the positives and negatives associated with that question have been considered.

Environmental Tours

Although most programs are no longer required by The Joint Commission to conduct environmental tours, they are still considered a best-practice process for identifying risks within the physical environment. (**Note:** *The Joint Commission still requires environmental tours for specifically identified areas of nursing care centers.* See *the* Comprehensive Accreditation Manual for Nursing Care Centers *or E-dition for additional information.*) Organizations should determine frequency and contents of the environmental tours based on identified or potential risks within the physical environment.

Safety vs. Security

Issues of safety and security are often grouped together when discussing the environment of care, but they are distinct issues. These risk areas should be evaluated for the specific hazards and threats they may pose to an organization's environment of care.

Safety incidents arise from the physical environment itself, from performance of everyday tasks in that environment, and from conditions that affect the environment (such as the weather). A safe environment protects people from harm. Safety incidents most often are accidental.

Security incidents are the result of actions by individuals, either internal to the organization (for example, staff members) or from outside (for example, visitors or community members). A secure environment protects both people and property from harm or loss. Security incidents usually are intentional. (*See* Chapter 5 for security-related risk assessment.)

These tours can help organizations identify hazardous conditions, observe safety practices and behaviors, eliminate potential hazards, and monitor staff knowledge in an effort to maintain safe environments for patients, visitors, and staff.

Most organizations use the environmental tour as a multi-functional inspection of the building, organization activities, and grounds of health care facilities. This strategy can yield maximum benefit for organizations. Many departments need to tour the facilities to collect data to support their services; combining as many functions as possible into one tour saves time and effort, as well as minimizing disruption of routine activities.

Use a Team Approach

To effectively conduct environmental tours, organizations should consider having multidisciplinary groups participate in the process. These groups can have a variety of members, including the safety manager and other health care representatives such as clinical staff and staff working in the physical environment.

Involving such a diverse group brings multiple perspectives to the tour process. People with different areas of expertise may notice things that the safety manager might overlook. For example, a member of the infection prevention and control (IC) department may recognize potential IC issues that the safety manager may not have considered. Likewise, the facilities director may notice issues of which the nursing staff may be unaware.

It also may be helpful to include individuals who are familiar with the EC needs and risks for specific populations, such as psychiatric, geriatric, or pediatric patients. Such experts may notice safety issues relevant to these populations that others may miss. For example, an expert on psychiatric patients may notice EC risks for self-harm that the safety manager initially may not see.

Train the Team for an Effective Tour

Having assembled a team with various levels of expertise, it is still important for you to train them to have a successful and effective environmental tour. Training may include, for example, the following:

- How to effectively document deficiencies
- How to report deficiencies and to whom
- How to properly educate staff
- The location of various resources, policies, and procedures
- How to document immediate corrective action

In addition, it is recommended that members of your team be familiar with other aspects of the tour outside of their areas of expertise. By cross-training your team, there is a higher likelihood that deficiencies will be identified during your tour.

As a team works together to tour and assess the environment, different disciplines will become aware of the issues affecting other disciplines. For example, an IC manager may start to notice safety violations, and the safety manager may identify IC issues. This is helpful in the event of holidays,

The EC Committee

The Environment of Care (EC) standards address and affect multiple areas in an entire organization. To address the multiple facets efficiently, any health care organization may consider creating a multidisciplinary team—sometimes known as a "safety committee," an "EC committee," or an "oversight committee." Although, the creation of this team is not required by The Joint Commission, its establishment is highly encouraged to manage the various responsibilities that are required to maintain a safe physical environment. The core of the EC committee should involve staff from the seven core EC management areas as seen in the following illustration.

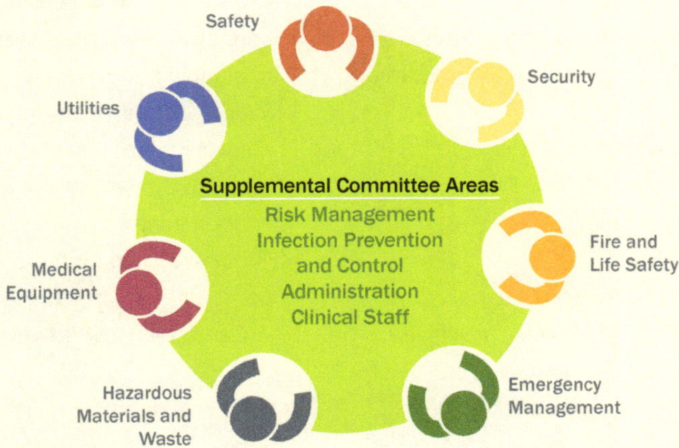

An EC committee that includes representatives from the areas of EC management ensures that the whole of the physical environment is represented. However, health care organizations are made up of staff with various areas of knowledge. Supplementing the committee with other staff outside of the EC management arena will ensure a well-rounded committee that can address the varying issues unique to each department in the organization (*see* the following illustration for potential supplemental committee members).

By structuring the committee in this manner, an organization can maintain a manageable size for the committee while still achieving optimal multidisciplinary participation. In some organizations, the safety manager* is the chairperson of the EC committee or oversight committee. This ensures that the safety manager has a direct role in all aspects of safety in the environment of care.

---

* As each organization has its unique job titles, this title is meant to be indicative of the individual within the organization charged with overseeing safety concerns.

vacations, and vacancies in positions because the team still can be effective, as all the members are familiar with the various aspects of the environment of care.

Establish a Schedule

It is important to establish a regular schedule for environmental tours. Frequency should be set by the organization, based on reliability, to ensure a safe environment. For nursing care centers, The Joint Commission still requires environmental tours to be conducted every six months for patient and resident care areas and annually for nonresident care areas. Other program settings that previously were required to conduct environmental tours—hospitals, critical access hospitals, home care, and laboratories—are now recommended to use this best-practice method to identify safety and security risks, as well as monitor compliance with the physical environment. Ambulatory health care, behavioral health care, and office-based surgery organizations were never required to conduct environmental tours, but also are encouraged to consider them.

Very few organizations can conduct a comprehensive and actionable environment tour of their entire facility in one session. To ensure that every department and location is toured, as defined by the organization, the safety manager or other designated individual should create a calendar for the year that maps out which department, including off-site locations, will be examined and when.

To help ensure a successful environmental tour process, it can be helpful to keep the schedule consistent; for example, every Wednesday from 9:00 A.M. to 11:00 A.M. This helps participants manage their own schedules so they can be consistently present.

Create a Checklist

Environmental tours are most effective when they are both thorough and efficient. To achieve this balance, organizations may want to create a preprinted checklist (*see* the EC tour checklist beginning on page 68). This checklist helps groups avoid overlooking or forgetting particular areas. Each member of the team participating in the tour should have a copy of the checklist to fill out during the tour. Different team members can be in charge of filling out different sections of

the checklist as appropriate. For example, the IC manager could be responsible for looking at and documenting IC and hand hygiene issues. The safety manager should review all checklist forms and may wish to merge all identified issues onto one form. This will prevent duplication of information and also ensure that every issue is documented.

Interview Staff

An environmental tour presents a good opportunity to question staff members about their roles in the environment of care, thus keeping them current on the requirements, as well as obtaining information regarding needs for subsequent educational programs. Talking to people who are on the front lines of providing care is a good way to determine real-world safety in the environment of care.

It may be helpful to prepare a list of standard questions to ask staff members during the environmental tour. These may be adapted to suit the particular area being toured; however, some issues are common among most areas. These include the following:

- Hazards and safety issues. Are staff members aware of the safety issues they may encounter?
  - Example: Where are sterile supplies stored, and how are they transported to patient care areas?
- Policy and procedure. Do staff members know policies that relate to their jobs, and does that knowledge translate into practice?
  - Example: How do you empty sharps containers? (Observe whether they are emptied according to established policies.)
- Workarounds. Are staff members using workarounds, or shortcuts, that save time but compromise safety?
  - Example: Observe whether any automatically latching door is being propped open during short trips.
- Processes. Do staff members know what actions to take in particular circumstances?
  - Example: How do you report defective equipment?

A culture of safety is critical to staff interviews during the environmental tour. Staff should feel comfortable expressing concerns or reporting incidents without fear of reprisal. Joint Commission LD standards require leaders to create and maintain this culture of safety.

text continued on page 68

Example EC Committee Reporting Items Schedule

This reporting schedule can help committee members track who is responsible for what documentation, as well as when required reports are due (for example, monthly, quarterly, annually).

Note: *This worksheet may be adapted and is available for internal use on the flash drive (print only) or by clicking the tool link in the Risk-Assessment Toolbox (e-book only) on page 77.*

ORGANIZATION: ___________________________   DEPARTMENT/UNIT: ___________________________

Insert an "x" for months in which a report is required.

REQUIRED REPORT	JAN	FEB	MAR	APR	MAY	JUN	JUL	AUG	SEP	OCT	NOV	DEC	RESPONSIBLE
MONTHLY													
Construction reports/updates	x	x	x	x	x	x	x	x	x	x	x	x	George Washington
EC committee report	x	x	x	x	x	x	x	x	x	x	x	x	Tom Jefferson
EC risk assessment (when applicable)													Tom Jefferson
EC rounds report/trends	x	x	x	x	x	x	x	x	x	x	x	x	Tom Jefferson
Follow-up/action log/PI log	x	x	x	x	x	x	x	x	x	x	x	x	Joan Adams
Incident reports	x	x	x	x	x	x	x	x	x	x	x	x	Jamie Madison
Inspection reports/updates	x	x	x	x	x	x	x	x	x	x	x	x	George Washington
Survey readiness committee report	x	x	x	x	x	x	x	x	x	x	x	x	Jamie Madison
Regulatory/standards reviews	x	x	x	x	x	x	x	x	x	x	x	x	Jamie Madison
Site safety report	x	x	x	x	x	x	x	x	x	x	x	x	George Washington
Testing, inspection, and maintenance documentation	x	x	x	x	x	x	x	x	x	x	x	x	George Washington
QUARTERLY													
EM	x			x			x			x			Adam Quincy
Fire safety	x			x			x			x			Van Martin
Grounds surveillance	x			x			x			x			Bill Harrison
Life safety	x			x			x			x			Van Martin
PI goals (site and system)	x			x			x			x			Joan Adams
Policy review	x			x			x			x			Tom Jefferson
Security	x			x			x			x			Jane Tyler
Clinical engineering		x			x			x			x		Jamie Madison
WSD		x			x			x			x		Jim Monroe
Gas monitoring		x			x			x			x		Jamie Madison

Page 1 of 2

continued

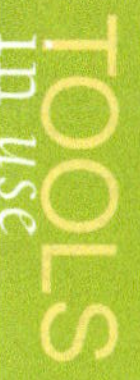

Example EC Committee Reporting Items Schedule *continued*

REQUIRED REPORT	JAN	FEB	MAR	APR	MAY	JUN	JUL	AUG	SEP	OCT	NOV	DEC	RESPONSIBLE
Infection control		x			x			x			x		Ruth Polk
Lab safety		x			x			x			x		Lincoln Pierce
OR safety		x			x			x			x		Ted Roosevelt
Radiation safety		x			x			x			x		Will Taft
Utility		x			x			x			x		Adam Quincy
Safety management			x			x			x			x	Jamie Madison
Employee incident summary			x			x			x			x	Tom Jefferson
Hazardous material(s)			x			x			x			x	Jack Andrews
Waste management			x			x			x			x	Jim Monroe
Green initiatives			x			x			x			x	Joan Adams
Product recall			x			x			x			x	Jamie Madison
Pharmacy recall			x			x			x			x	Jack Andrews
ANNUAL													
Annual effectiveness evaluations		x											Tom Jefferson
Chemical inventory		x											Jack Andrews
EM report (HVA, EOP, supply inventory)	x												Tom Jefferson
Tier 3 EC management plans	x												Jamie Madison
Injury summary												x	Joan Adams
WSD inspection			x										Jim Monroe
Reporting calendar	x												Tom Jefferson

EC, environment of care; PI, performance improvement; EM, emergency management; WSD, Waste and Sewage Department; OR, operating room; HVA, hazard vulnerability analysis; EOP, Emergency Operations Plan.

Data Sources for Identifying Safety Risks

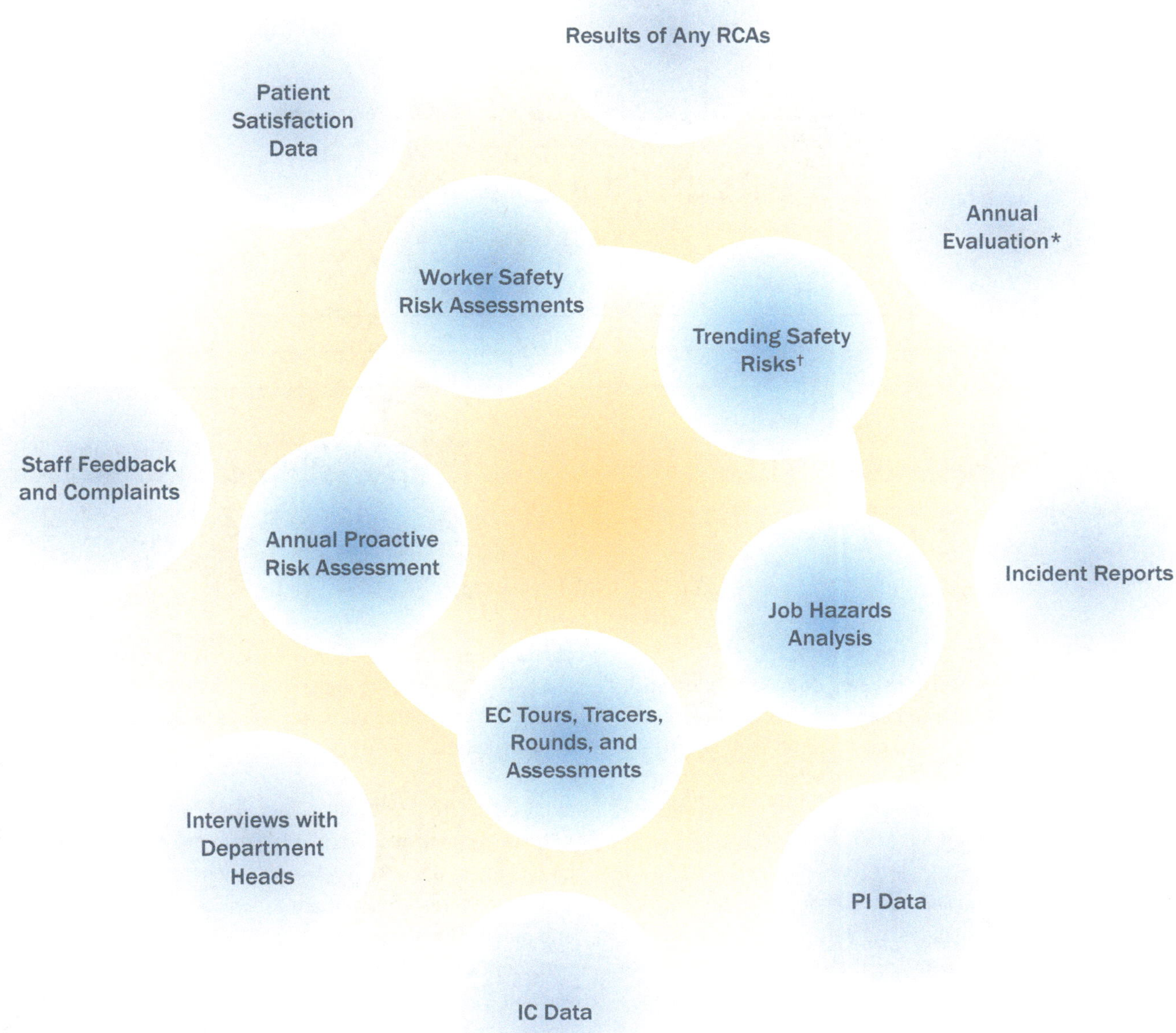

Sources that directly relate to safety and could provide data to organizations that need to proactively assess risk are shown in the inside circle. The outer circle shows other potential sources that may be useful when trying to identify safety risks. The following sections provide additional discussions on EC tours (*see* page 61), worker safety risk assessments (*see* page 70), and job hazards analysis (*see* page 70)

---

* Annual evaluation refers to the review of EC management plans that is required in accordance with Joint Commission Standard EC.04.01.01.

† Trending safety risks can be those identified by The Joint Commission or external sources.

EC, environment of care; RCAs, root cause analyses; IC, infection prevention and control; PI, performance improvement.

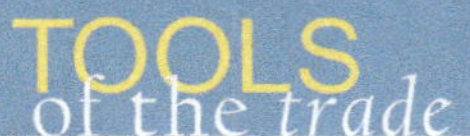

EC Tour Checklist

This checklist can be used to track compliance with requirements related to the physical environment. If the # symbol is present in the Yes and No columns, use hash marks to capture the number of observations found compliant in the Yes column or the number found noncompliant in the No column for that item. If the # symbol is not present, check the Yes column for compliant or check the No column if noncompliant.

Note: *The complete checklist may be adapted and is available for internal use on the flash drive (print only) or by clicking the tool link in the Risk-Assessment Toolbox (e-book only) on page 77.*

Published in *Environment of Care Risk Assessment*, Joint Commission Resources, 2018. **File Name:** 03 02 Checklist EC Tour

EC TOUR CHECKLIST

ORGANIZATION: ____

DEPARTMENT/UNIT: ____________________________________ BUILDING:_________________________________

DATE OF TOUR:________________ REVIEWER: ____

If the # symbol is present in the "Yes" and "No" columns, mark the number of observations found compliant in the "Yes" column or the number found noncompliant in the "No" column for that item. If the # symbol is not present, check the "Yes" column for compliant or the "No" column for noncompliant.

ITEM	OBSERVATION	YES	NO	NA	RESOLVED ON-SITE		COMMENTS
					YES	NO	

Respond to Information Collected

Organizations should be sure that data obtained during an environmental tour are appropriately analyzed and reported. Any problematic findings should be acted on, with appropriate feedback regarding problem correction. In accordance with Joint Commission standards, corrective actions are required to be documented.

During the tour, any identified condition or hazard that may pose an immediate threat to life, health, or safety should be reported to the department manager and corrected immediately. (If an immediate correction is not possible, mitigation strategies must be in place.) Other problematic findings, compliance issues, or potential risks should be documented in a report to the appropriate department manager or supervisor to review. The report should outline any hazards found in the department and/or opportunities for improvement. Individual department managers are then responsible for initiating appropriate action to address any findings.

Health care organizations should designate time frames for safety issues to be corrected, such as 15 days after inspection, 30 days, or 60 days. After the designated time frame, a follow-up tour of the department should be conducted to determine if any outstanding deficiencies still exist. All corrective action plans should be reviewed by the EC committee (*see* page 69 for a corrective action plan worksheet).

Document and Analyze Information

Although organizations are not required to conduct environmental tours, Joint Commission Standards EC.04.01.01 and EC.04.01.03 *do* require organizations to collect information and monitor the environment. Organizations may want to consider documenting environmental tours data in some type of database for analysis purposes. This documentation also is useful if a regulatory agency requests specific safety inspection information. In addition, information collected during environmental tours should be analyzed by the EC committee and used to monitor and improve the EC program.

Organizations should consider creating summary reports of the tours that provide overviews of the results and highlight any significant trends, problems, failures, user errors, concerns, and/or positive responses and feedback. These reports should be shared with organization leadership and other internal stakeholders.

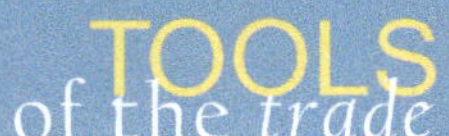

Corrective Action Plan Worksheet

This worksheet can be filled out and submitted to an environment of care (EC) committee for review.
It also can serve as a task list of what needs to be corrected within what time frame.

Note: *The complete worksheet may be adapted and is available for internal use on the flash drive (print only) or by clicking the tool link in the Risk-Assessment Toolbox (e-book only) on page 77.*

Published in *Environment of Care Risk Assessment*, Joint Commission Resources, 2018.   **File Name:** 03 03 Worksheet Correct Act Plan portrait

CORRECTIVE ACTION PLAN WORKSHEET

LOCATION/DEPARTMENT: _________________________   SPONSOR: _________________________

PROBLEM: ____

CAUSE: ____

DESIRED OUTCOME: ____

TASK	RESPONSIBLE PARTY	RESOURCES	DUE DATE	NOTES

By having a systematic process in place for environmental tours, organizations can regularly and consistently identify and respond to potential safety risks throughout the organizations—and maintain compliance with Joint Commission standards at the same time.

Tour vs. Tracer vs. Rounds vs. Assessments

Environment of Care tour. This proactive multidisciplinary comprehensive facility tour is used to evaluate the physical environment and the effectiveness of current EC–related policies and procedures in place to manage environmental safety risks. In addition, an EC tour is used to determine staff knowledge and evaluation compliance with Joint Commission standards, as well as compliance with codes, regulations, and laws. EC tours are focused on the environmental factors affecting the safety and security of everyone in a health care facility. This tour is not required by The Joint Commission, but organizations who elect to conduct them set the frequency of the tours.

Environment of Care tracer. A key survey assessment method used by Joint Commission surveyors, tracers assess a health care organization's compliance with Joint Commission standards. An EC tracer involves *tracing* an organization's systems and processes related to the environment of care, emergency management, and fire protection and life safety. (*See* page 48 in Chapter 2 for a discussion on mock tracers.)

Environment of Care rounds. EC rounds are a daily walk-through of an area in which staff look for basic EC issues that can be corrected right away, rather than waiting until a more in-depth environmental tour. Organizations can use EC rounds as a monitoring tool and catch basic EC issues right away, before they become a hazard. This type of monitoring is not required under Joint Commission standards. (*See* page 72 for an EC rounds assessment checklist.)

Environment of Care risk assessment. A proactive examination used to assess actual and potential risks, an EC risk assessment examines functions and processes in the physical environment. After it is completed, results from the assessment can be prioritized to identify improvement opportunities from serious to nonserious. This assessment is required in accordance with Joint Commission standards in each of the seven functional areas of the environment of care:

1. Safety
2. Security
3. Fire and life safety
4. Hazardous materials and waste
5. Medical equipment
6. Utilities
7. Preconstruction

Organizations can use EC tours, tracers, or rounds as data collection tools for their EC risk assessments.

Building assessment. This assessment uses established processes to assess compliance with the *Life Safety Code** and self-identified deficiencies in the built environment, as well as establishing corrective action measures. The Joint Commission requires each organization to conduct a building assessment at a time frame established by the organization; however, is recommended annually.

Worker Safety Risk Assessment

Patients are not the only individuals who face safety risks; worker safety also is an important consideration. One way to assess worker safety is to conduct a comprehensive, organizationwide worker safety assessment, which examines the EC risks to worker safety in all the different departments of an organization.

The scope of this process may seem daunting. However, it can be simplified by using a standardized form that consistently assesses environmental risks across departments. Using a form to help conduct an organizationwide safety assessment allows the safety manager to see—at a glance—the potential risks that exist within the various departments of the organization. It also ensures consistent assessments across departments and over time.

Evaluate and Score Risks

Using the form, the safety manager, individual(s) responsible for safety, or, alternately, a subcommittee of the safety committee can identify and score EC risks for each department of the organization (*see* page 72 for a worker safety

department assessment worksheet). These scores indicate the severity and immediacy of each risk. Scores can be determined by evaluating information from several sources, including the following:

- Physical tour of the department
- Review of annual incident and accident statistics
- Review of the past 12 months' safety committee minutes
- Environmental tour, round, tracer, and risk-assessment reports
- Interviews with department heads
- Interviews with a representative sampling of staff

Should any situations constituting an imminent danger be discovered during the course of an organizationwide worker safety assessment, the individual discovering the risks should report them immediately to the safety manager and appropriate department manager for prompt follow-up action.

Alternative Methods

If the safety committee does not have time to analyze all the departments—such as within a large multisite organization—the safety manager may send the forms—with instructions on how to complete them—to the departments and have them complete the forms individually. After the departments complete and return their forms, the safety manager can review them for accuracy and comprehensiveness and then give them to the safety committee for further review and recommended action.

Even if an organization chooses not to conduct an organizationwide worker safety assessment, it may be helpful to assess worker safety issues in departments at highest risk for EC issues. Such departments may include the emergency department, surgery department, intensive care unit (ICU), psychiatric unit, pharmacy, and laboratory.

The Job Hazards Analysis

Organizations may wish to examine the safety risks associated with specific job tasks. This type of assessment also can help organizations manage the safety of health care workers. Although this type of safety assessment is not specifically required by The Joint Commission, the US Occupational Safety and Health Administration (OSHA) does require such an assessment, calling it a job hazards analysis (JHA). Joint Commission Standard LD.04.01.01 requires organizations to comply with law and regulation, including OSHA.

---

* *Life Safety Code** is a registered trademark of the National Fire Protection Association, Quincy, MA.

OSHA defines a JHA as a technique focusing on job tasks to identify hazards before they occur within a job. The analysis looks at the relationships among the worker, the task, the tools, and the work environment. Ideally, after an organization identifies uncontrolled hazards associated with jobs, it takes steps to eliminate the hazards or reduce them to an acceptable level of risk.

Organization leaders, including department managers and supervisors, can use the findings of a JHA to eliminate and prevent hazards in the workplace. This can result in the following:
- Fewer worker injuries and illnesses
- Safer, more effective work methods
- Reduced workers' compensation costs
- Increased worker productivity

The analysis also can be a valuable tool for training new employees in the steps required to perform their jobs safely. In addition, any time a JHA is revised, organizations should train employees affected by the changes in the new job methods, procedures, and personal protective measures adopted.

Certain jobs within the organization may present more risks than others. The following high-risk jobs should be kept in mind during a JHA:
- Jobs with the highest injury or illness rates
- Jobs with the potential to cause severe or disabling injuries or illness, even if there is no history of previous accidents
- Jobs in which one simple human error could lead to a severe accident or injury
- Jobs that are new to an organization or have undergone changes in processes and procedures
- Jobs complex enough to require written instructions

The employee health nurse will be an important resource in creating and evaluating the JHA. This individual is on the front line of employee injuries and is responsible for documenting and reporting such injuries. This insight is valuable when identifying health hazards facing employees in various departments and jobs.

Start by Reviewing Data

As a first step in conducting a JHA, organizations may want to review their histories of injuries, accidents, losses, and occupational illnesses that needed treatment—The

Joint Commission already requires that such information be collected and monitored under EC standards. These events are indicators that the existing hazard controls (if any) may not be adequate and deserve more scrutiny. "Near misses"—events in which an accident or loss did not occur, but could have—are another indicator of possible hazardous conditions.

Break It Down into Steps

Next, organizations should consider conducting preliminary job reviews of those jobs that could be considered high risk for worker safety. Such job reviews could involve discussing with employees the hazards they know exist in their current work and surroundings and brainstorming with them for ideas to eliminate or control those hazards.

Nearly every job can be broken down into job tasks or steps. When beginning a JHA, organizations should consider watching the employees perform their jobs and listing all steps as the workers take them. The job steps should be reviewed with the employees to make sure no step is omitted. It is important to make sure the employees understand that it is the jobs that are being evaluated, not the employees' job performances.

Evaluators should record enough information to describe each job action without getting overly detailed. While recording this information, evaluators need to ensure that they are striking a balance so the job and its actions are captured accurately. Meticulously breaking down the steps of a job until it is unnecessarily long or so vague that basic steps are missing will not present a clear indication of what the job, in fact, entails and the hazards it presents.

Other valuable methods to consider when gathering information while conducting a job review may include getting input from other workers who have performed the same job, as well as photographing or recording the employee performing the job. The visual records, in particular, can be useful references when doing a more detailed analysis of the work.

Respond to Issues That Arise

If any hazards exist that pose an immediate danger to an employee's life or health, organizations should take immediate action to protect the worker. Also, any problems that can be corrected easily should be corrected as soon as possible and not be delayed until the JHA is complete.

EC Rounds Assessment Checklist

This checklist can be used for regular assessments that supplement the recommended annual environment of care risk assessment.

Note: *The complete checklist may be adapted and is available for internal use on the flash drive (print only) or by clicking the tool link in the Risk-Assessment Toolbox (e-book only) on page 77.*

Published in *Environment of Care Risk Assessment*, Joint Commission Resources, 2018. **File Name:** 03 04 Checklist EC Rounds Assess

EC ROUNDS ASSESSMENT CHECKLIST

This checklist includes questions to ask to assess a range of risks in the physical environment. It can be used for regular rounds that supplement the annual environment of care risk assessment. Answers to all questions should ideally be Y for Yes (unless they aren't applicable). If an answer is N for No, use the "Notes" section to document needed changes. Unless otherwise noted, this checklist is applicable to all program settings.

ORGANIZATION: _________________________________   DEPARTMENT/UNIT: _________________________________

DATE OF REVIEW: _________________________   REVIEWER: _________________________________

QUESTION	YES	NO	NA	NOTES
SAFETY				
Lighting				
Is there adequate lighting indoors and outdoors?				

Worker Safety Department Assessment

The worksheet featured can be used to comply with an assessment required by Environment of Care (EC) Standard EC.02.01.01 and should be completed by the individual identified by the organization to assess and score the safety risks in a department. Using the scores, organizations can determine what risks require immediate attention and what risks are most severe.

Note: *The complete assessment worksheet may be adapted and is available for internal use on the flash drive (print only) or by clicking the tool link in the Risk-Assessment Toolbox (e-book only) on page 77.*

Published in *Environment of Care Risk Assessment*, Joint Commission Resources, 2018. **File Name:** 03 05 Worker Safety Assess portrait

WORKER SAFETY DEPARTMENT ASSESSMENT WITH SCORING GUIDELINES

ORGANIZATION: _________________________________   DEPARTMENT/UNIT: _________________________________

DATE OF ASSESSMENT: _________________   REVIEWER(S): _________________________________

RISK ELEMENTS	RISK SCORE	RECOMMENDED						ADDITIONAL PPE NEEDED		NOTES
		PROCESS CHANGE		ADDITIONAL TRAINING		ADDITIONAL P&P				
	0–4	YES	NO	YES	NO	YES	NO	YES	NO	
Asbestos Exposure		☐	☐	☐	☐	☐	☐	☐	☐	

It is very important to involve employees in all phases of the JHA process, from reviewing job steps and procedures to discussing uncontrolled hazards and recommended solutions. Employees have unique understandings of their jobs, and this knowledge is invaluable for finding hazards. Involving employees will help to minimize oversights, ensure a quality analysis, and get workers to buy in to any potential solutions because they will share ownership in their safety and health program.

After an organization has conducted job reviews, it should list, rank, and set priorities for hazardous jobs. When ranking high-risk jobs, consider the level of risk they pose, the likelihood those risks will occur, and the severity of the consequences if they do occur.

Using a Form to Conduct a JHA

As with an organizationwide safety assessment, organizations may consider creating a standardized form or template to help conduct a JHA (*see* page 74 for a JHA worksheet). This form can be used when interviewing staff members about their jobs or can be completed by different departments as a starting place for discussion.

Special Risk Considerations

The following sections explore several important issues to consider when addressing safety risks.

Patient Suicide

In 2014 the US Centers for Disease Control and Prevention reported more than 42,000 deaths by suicide, making it the 10th leading cause of death in the United States.[1] Certain populations are at greater risk for suicide, such as the terminally ill, persons with mental and substance abuse disorders, youth, the elderly, and those who identify as gay, lesbian, bisexual, or transgender. Individuals can commit suicide anywhere and at any time. Unfortunately, health care organizations are not immune from this tragedy. In fact, patient suicide is consistently among the most frequently reported sentinel events to The Joint Commission.

In fact, Joint Commission National Patient Safety Goal (NPSG) NPSF.15.01.01 is designed to help organizations reduce the risk of patient suicide. The goal is applicable to behavioral health care organizations, psychiatric hospitals, and general hospitals treating individuals for emotional or behavioral disorders. It requires these organizations to

conduct a thorough and complete suicide risk assessment to organizations to reassess these patients when appropriate. The focus of the goal, and a critical component of reducing the risk of suicide in health care organizations, is first and foremost the identification of patients at risk. Based on an assessment of risk, several preventive strategies may then come into play, including environmental considerations.

The environment plays a key role in an organization's efforts to prevent suicide. Deficiencies in the physical environment are often implicated in suicide sentinel events reviewed by The Joint Commission. Patients considered high risk for suicide should be cared for in environments that minimize suicide risks yet are as natural, humane, and therapeutic as practical. A balance must be achieved between rendering an environment as risk free as possible and continuing to provide as nurturing an environment as feasible. Beginning in 2017, The Joint Commission convened a series of expert panels to identify suicide risks specific to inpatient units in psychiatric and acute care hospitals, as well as emergency departments and a number of behavioral health care settings.[†]

Identifying Environmental Suicide Risks

To help identify and address potential suicide risks in the environment, organizations should consider conducting walk-throughs of rooms, units, or other areas that house high-risk patients. Behavioral health care settings and psychiatric units are the primary focus; however, it is important to consider suicide risks in other areas as well. Emergency departments, ICUs, radiology departments, bathrooms, and other locations should be assessed for suicide risks.

EC professionals can walk through a unit with department directors and unit managers, consider the types of patients who occupy the space, identify issues, prioritize threats, and address those threats. During these walk-throughs, it is important to remember that what is safe for a low-risk patient

---

[†] These settings include residential treatment, partial hospitalization, intensive outpatient, and outpatient treatment programs.[2,3] These panels identified ligature risk as a major concern. One of the most common methods of suicide in a health care setting is hanging. This makes identification and removal of ligature risk tremendously important to the establishment of a safe physical environment. Joint Commission Standard EC.02.06.01, EP 1 requires that interior spaces meet the needs of the patient population and are safe and suitable to the care, treatment, and services provided.

Job Hazards Analysis Worksheet

Required by the Occupational Safety and Health Administration, job hazards analyses (JHAs) can be conducted using a worksheet such as this example. JHAs are necessary assessments to determine the safety risks associated with specific job tasks.

Note: *The complete worksheet may be adapted and is available for internal use on the flash drive (print only) or by clicking the tool link in the Risk-Assessment Toolbox (e-book only) on page 77.*

Published in *Environment of Care Risk Assessment*, Joint Commission Resources, 2018. **File Name:** 03 06 Worksheet JHA

JOB HAZARDS ANALYSIS WORKSHEET

COMPLETED BY: _______________________________________ DATE: _______________________________

JOB TITLE: ____ JOB LOCATION: ________________________

DEPARTMENT: _________________________

TASKS ASSOCIATED WITH JOB	POTENTIAL HAZARDS	HAZARD CONTROLS
1.	1.	1.

---

may not be safe for one who is at high risk for suicide. For example, a planter or piece of artwork may be appropriate in a low-risk unit; however, in a high-risk unit, it may be perceived as a potential hazard or weapon.

Some threats, such as exposed wires, glass vases, and hangers, easily can be removed. For others, such as lay-in ceiling tiles and breakable windows, removal may not be immediately possible. To address these types of threats, organizations should consider putting together a remediation plan with a schedule and budget that prioritizes repair scheduling. An organization that cannot fix something in an area right away should use risk-mitigation processes, such as direct supervision, shift or day-to-day evaluations, or other methods, for high-risk patients.

Specific Elements to Consider

To help consistently identify suicide risks in the environment, organizations may want to create a checklist for common areas of suicide risk, or include suicide risks on an environmental tour template (*see* page 78 for a suicide risk worksheet). Among the many risks that could be included on a suicide risk checklist, the following are some areas to consider:

- *Hanging risks.* Air vent grills, door hardware, fire sprinkler heads, shower heads, shower curtain rods, and cabinet door handles all can serve as hanging devices. Plumbing, piping, or ductwork that is concealed behind a dropped ceiling also can be used as hanging devices.
- *Suffocation risks.* Plastic trash can liners, plastic shower curtains, and plastic disposable gloves can serve as smothering materials.
- *Weapon risks.* Loose equipment, decorations, furniture, or fixtures may become weapons. Breakable mirrors, glass, or light bulbs also can be used as weapons.
- *Jumping or elopement risks.* Patients can jump out windows that are easily broken. This could lead to suicide or elopement.

There are specific actions within the environment of care that organizations can take to minimize the risk of patient suicide. When identifying these actions, organizations should consult local and state regulations, as well as other sources, including the 2014 edition(s)‡ of *Guidelines for Design and Construction of Health Care Facilities*[4,5] and the *Design Guide for the Built Environment of Behavioral Health Facilities*,[6] both from the Facility Guidelines Institute. Some common ideas include the following:

---

‡ For laboratory and office-based surgery settings, refer to the 2010 edition of the *Guidelines for Design and Construction of Health Care Facilities.*

- *Install hard-to-remove screens to cover any wall protrusions, such as fire sprinkler heads and air vent grills.*
- *Secure lay-in ceiling tiles so they cannot be removed.* This may involve riveting a metal lay-in framework to the tiles. Organizations also may want to replace a lay-in acoustical tiled ceiling with a strengthened, homogenous ceiling.
- *Remove exposed wires, window blinds cords, and telephone cords.* These can serve as hanging devices. Organizations may want to consider using cordless phones in high-risk areas. Even if patients are allowed to use cordless phones, they should be required to use them in supervised areas. This prevents a patient from taking the phone and using it in a harmful manner later on.
- *Install anti-suicide doors, which have large openings at the top and bottom, so nothing can be wedged into the door frame.* These doors also have continuous hinges to prevent patients from hanging anything between the door and the frame.
- *Remove plastic trash can liners.* In addition to removing liners, organizations may want to remove metal trash cans from high-risk areas and use straw trash cans because they do not serve as weapons.
- *Use cloth shower curtains that attach flush to the threshold above.* Eliminating the shower curtain rod eliminates a hanging risk. Breakaway rods are less desirable because they may be removed and may present safety risks.
- *Remove automatic door-closing hardware from patient rooms.* For doors that require this type of hardware, such as fire doors, organizations should be sure that patients are supervised when around the doors.
- *Make thoughtful furniture choices in patient rooms.* Use heavy, upholstered furniture that cannot be easily lifted and used as a weapon.
- *Install shatterproof glass on all windows and fixtures.* For mirrors, a break-free plastic can be used to provide the mirrored effect without the risks.
- *Avoid using metal hangers or rods in closets.* Shelves can be used to hold closet items without presenting a hanging risk.
- *Install hardware, such as door hardware, that slopes downward to prevent it from being used as a hanging support.*
- *Place convex mirrors in hallways to help eliminate blind spots.* In many health care organizations, nurses cannot see every portion of a hallway at one time. To eliminate locations where nurses cannot see patients, organizations may want to consider installing mirrors.

Every health care organization strives to provide a safe environment for the people they treat. However, it is unrealistic to expect organizations to be free of suicide risks. In certain settings, such as behavioral health care, identifying elements in the physical environment that could represent opportunities in an individual's intent to commit suicide may require a higher level of assessment. For patients who are assessed as low risk for suicide, the clinical environment will not be risk free. If a high-risk patient must enter areas that are not risk free, such as when a high-risk patient has a serious medical condition and must be admitted to a nursing floor, then it is important that the patient is supervised appropriately to prevent adverse situations. (*See* the real-world scenario beginning on page 85 that discusses risk assessments for a behavioral health care organization with multiple satellite locations.)

Identifying High-Risk Situations

In addition to assessing and addressing risks in the environment, EC staff should make sure that all clinical and facility staff are trained in how to recognize and resolve potentially risky situations. Should a facility staff member identify a potential hazard (for example, a grate that has dislodged from a fire sprinkler head, thus exposing the device), the staff member should be able to fix the problem or alert the department manager to the risk. Facilities managers also should be involved in educating clinicians and frontline staff on environmental risks for suicide and how those risks can be prevented. Clinicians are familiar with how to care for high-risk patients, but they may not always be cognizant of environmental implications. When a high-risk area is short staffed or requires additional coverage, the relief staff should be fully aware of the area's environmental risks.

Assessing Smoking Risks

Smoking presents several risks in the environment of care, in addition to the health hazards for individuals who smoke. For example, secondhand smoke is a threat to patient and worker safety. Smoking also can present a fire hazard because cigarettes, cigars, e-cigarettes, and other smoking devices can act as ignition sources. (*See* Chapter 6 for a discussion of fire safety risks associated with smoking, including e-cigarettes.)

All Joint Commission–accredited organizations are required to have a policy that prohibits smoking except in specified circumstances (*see* page 79 for a sample policy). This policy must apply to all of a health care organization's buildings, whether or not patient care takes place there. This includes power plants, administrative office buildings, and motor pools. The only exceptions are open-air parking structures and specifically constructed smoking shelters.

Acceptable Exceptions

Ideally, no one should smoke in a health care building; however, sometimes this is not possible. For example, the physician of a behavioral health care patient may determine that quitting smoking might be more dangerous to the patient's health than continuing it. In these cases, it is important that patients have a safe place to smoke that does not affect the safety of other people. These locations must be physically separated from areas where care, treatment, and services are provided, and they should have appropriate exhaust and fire safety features.

Organizations may allow exceptions to the no-smoking policy—under certain conditions—for patients, residents, or clients. There are no exceptions allowed, however, for staff and visitors, children and adolescents, or ambulatory health care patients. In a laboratory environment, there is no smoking permitted at all in any facilities under the laboratory's control.

Complying With Policy

The most important aspect of smoking management is to ensure that the organization's smoking policy is consistent with actual practice. If an organization's no-smoking policy states that the facility is a smoke-free campus, then no one should be smoking. If there are exceptions, these should be outlined clearly in the policy; and staff, patients, and visitors should be familiar with the policy and any exceptions.

Hospitals, ambulatory health care, behavioral health care, and nursing care centers are expected to monitor compliance with their no-smoking policies and develop strategies to eliminate policy violations. Staff members who violate no-smoking policies should be held accountable for their actions. EC management should work with human resources to determine the appropriate response to a smoking violation.

To help enforce no-smoking policies, many organizations turn to a strong education program. Organizations should cover the no-smoking policy during new staff orientation and during annual safety in-services. Some organizations have found maps that clearly identify designated smoking areas to be helpful (*see* page 81 for a sample map). Signs can be useful enforcement tools (*see* page 81 for sample signs). One example is posting a sign that says "No smoking beyond this point," and placing cigarette butt containers at these signs. Sample scripts to help articulate the smoke-free policy to patients, residents, individuals served, staff, and visitors begin on page 82.

Safety Risks Outside the Building

Safety does not stop at the health care facility's exit doors. There are many safety risks to consider outside the building. Thoughtful design and proper maintenance of outdoor spaces is an important part of minimizing safety risks to patients, visitors, and staff.

The design of a facility's grounds can vary widely depending on such factors as the geographical location, population served, and type of health care setting. For example, a nursing care center or hospital that has a higher than average percentage of elderly patients may consider outdoor features that accommodate failing eyesight and greater fall risk, such as extra lighting and frequent benches or other places to rest. Another example would be extra drainage in locations that experience a lot of rain, or awnings or roofs over pathways in hot, sunny climates.

Trash Compactors

Trash compactors are a common piece of equipment located outdoors. These machines can pose a safety risk not only to staff who use them but to others who may enter the area, either on purpose or by mistake. Although The Joint Commission does not specifically address safety issues regarding trash compactors, this equipment should be included in environmental tours and addressed using relevant risk assessments. OSHA regulates trash compactors as a machine that poses worker safety hazards due to moving parts, and therefore organizations that use trash compactors must comply with OSHA's guidelines regarding barriers and locks.

References

1. US Centers for Disease Control and Prevention. National Center for Health Statistics. Suicide and Self-Inflicted Injury. (Updated: Mar 17, 2017.) Accessed Feb 20, 2018. https://www.cdc.gov/nchs/fastats/suicide.htm.

2. The Joint Commission. Special Report: Suicide Prevention in Health Care Settings: Recommendations Regarding Environmental Hazards for Providers and Surveyors. *Joint Commission Perspectives.* 37(11):1,3–7, Nov 2017.

3. The Joint Commission. Special Report. Suicide Prevention in Health Care Settings: Recommendations from Third Expert Panel. *Joint Commission Perspectives.* 38(1):1–3, Jan 2018.

4. Facility Guidelines Institute. *Guidelines for Design and Construction of Hospitals and Outpatient Facilities.* Chicago: American Society for Healthcare Engineering, 2014.

5. Facility Guidelines Institute. *Guidelines for Design and Construction of Residential Health, Care, and Support Facilities.* Chicago: American Society for Healthcare Engineering, 2014.

6. Facility Guidelines Institute. *Design Guide for the Built Environment of Behavioral Health Facilities.* Edition 7.2. Apr 2017. Accessed Feb 20, 2018. http://www.fgiguidelines.org/wp-content/uploads/2017/03/DesignGuideBH_7.2_1703.pdf.

RISK-ASSESSMENT TOOLBOX

1. **Download** EC Committee Reporting Items Schedule
2. **Download** EC Tour Checklist
3. Corrective Action Plan Worksheet
   - **Download** Landscape
   - **Download** Portrait
4. **Download** EC Rounds Assessment Checklist
5. Worker Safety Department Assessment
   - **Download** Landscape
   - **Download** Portrait
6. **Download** Job Hazards Analysis Worksheet
7. **Download** Environmental Risks for Suicide Assessment Checklist
8. **Download** Smoke-Free Policy
9. **Download** Smoke-Free Policy Development Checklist
10. **Download** Satellite Treatment Location Risk Assessment

Environmental Risks for Suicide Assessment Checklist

When conducting environmental tours, staff can use this checklist to assess the environmental risks for suicide.

Note: *The complete checklist may be adapted and is available for internal use on the flash drive (print only) or by clicking the tool link in the Risk-Assessment Toolbox (e-book only) on page 77.*

Published in *Environment of Care Risk Assessment*, Joint Commission Resources, 2018.   **File Name:** 03 07 Checklist Suicide Risk Assess

ENVIRONMENTAL RISKS FOR SUICIDE ASSESSMENT CHECKLIST

*This checklist includes questions to ask to assess environmental risks for suicide in non–behavioral health units and emergency rooms as well as inpatient behavioral units. It can be used as a daily check or as a periodic check to see if changes need to be made. Answers to all questions should ideally be Y for **Yes** (unless they aren't applicable). If an answer is N for **No**, use the "Notes" section to document needed changes. Unless otherwise noted, this checklist is applicable to all program settings.*

ORGANIZATION: _______________________________   DEPARTMENT/UNIT: _______________________________

DATE OF REVIEW: ___________________   REVIEWER: _______________________________

QUESTIONS	YES	NO	NA	NOTES
NON–BEHAVIORAL HEALTH CARE UNITS AND EMERGENCY ROOMS AND INPATIENT BEHAVIORAL UNITS*				
General Facility Safety				
Are plastic trash can liners absent in every space accessible to patients?				
Are all doors to all service and supply rooms locked when staff members are not physically present?				
Are all chemicals, including alcohol-based hand rub, kept under direct staff observation or within a locked room or area inaccessible by patients?				
Are telephones located in corridors or common spaces for patient use securely wall-mounted and have a nonremovable shielded cord (maximum length 14 inches)?				
Are disposable medium-weight bendable plastic cutlery used—and accounted for after meals so that patients cannot take it and use it to harm themselves or others?				
Are only tamper-proof screws used in patient care areas?				
Ceilings, Walls, Windows, and Doors				
Are the ceilings and walls solid and resistant to ligature				

Smoke-Free Policy

This excerpt from a sample policy outlines the smoke-free requirements of the fictitious County Healthcare. Although The Joint Commission requires health care organizations to have a policy regarding the use of tobacco products, this format is not required. *See* page 80 for the "Smoke-Free Policy Development Checklist" to assist in the development, review, and/or implementation of tobacco-related policy.

Note: *The complete smoke-free policy may be adapted and is available for internal use on the flash drive (print only) or by clicking the tool link in the Risk-Assessment Toolbox (e-book only) on page 77.*

Published in *Environment of Care Risk Assessment*, Joint Commission Resources, 2018.   **File Name:** 03 08 Policy Smoke-Free

SMOKE-FREE POLICY

This sample policy can be used to develop a smoke-free policy for any health care organization.

POLICY TITLE:	Smoke-Free Policy	**POLICY NUMBER:**	90.013.032
ORGANIZATION:	County Healthcare	**EFFECTIVE DATE:**	11/06
APPROVED BY:	EC Committee	**REVISED DATE(S):**	11/10; 11/14; 11/16

I. PURPOSE

a. To continually provide a healthy and safe environment through the promotion and encouragement of good-quality lifestyle choices throughout the community, the use of tobacco products is prohibited in or on any of the campus facilities or properties.

b. To establish a consistent expectation, tobacco products include, but are not limited to, cigarettes, cigars, pipes, smokeless tobacco, and electronic nicotine delivery devices.

c. Use of any tobacco products are prohibited by any person (staff, patient, visitor, volunteer, vendor, and so on) in or on any of the campus facilities or properties. Signs posted throughout the campus identify the boundaries of the campus.

II. RESPONSIBILITIES

a. Everyone who is on the premises is expected to comply with and enforce this policy.

III. PROCEDURES

a. When a violation occurs, the violator will be informed of the tobacco-free policy and directed to locations where tobacco use is permitted.

- For a violation that is repeated by the same individual employed by the hospital, the repeat violator will be counseled and, when appropriate, disciplined for failure to comply.
- For a violation that is repeated by the same individual not employed by the hospital, the repeat violation will be counseled and, when appropriate, fined for failure to comply.

b. For individuals seeking assistance in smoking cessation, contact the County Healthcare Wellness Center at 888-888-8___ for info___ation a__d assistanc___

Smoke-Free Policy Development Checklist

This checklist includes elements that should be considered when developing, reviewing, revising, or implementing a smoke-free policy. Organizations may use it to evaluate their policy or use it to guide the creation of a policy (which The Joint Commission requires in most settings).

Note: *The complete checklist may be adapted and is available for internal use on the flash drive (print only) or by clicking the tool link in the Risk-Assessment Toolbox (e-book only) on page 77.*

Published in *Environment of Care Risk Assessment*, Joint Commission Resources, 2018.   **File Name:** 03 09 Checklist Smoke-Free Policy Develop

SMOKE-FREE POLICY DEVELOPMENT CHECKLIST

*This checklist can be used by organizations to ensure that the numerous steps involved in developing, implementing, enforcing, and reevaluating a smoke-free policy have been considered. Answers to all questions should ideally be **Y** for **Yes** (unless they aren't applicable). If an answer is **N** for **No**, use the "Notes" section to document needed changes. Unless otherwise noted, this checklist is applicable to all program settings.*

ORGANIZATION: ____

DATE OF REVIEW: _______________________   REVIEWER: _______________________________________

QUESTIONS	YES	NO	NA	NOTES
ANNOUNCEMENT OF INTENT				
Has senior management announced a commitment to creating a smoke-free policy?				
Have you prepared employees with an announcement on the organization intranet and by mail?				
POLICY INTEGRATION DECISION				
Do you plan to integrate the smoke-free policy into your overall health and wellness planning, including the wellness incentives your organization offers to employees?				
CREATION OF A POLICY TEAM				
Have you created an executive task force and committee to create the policy and plan implementation?				
Does your team include smokers, nonsmokers, and former smokers, as well as members of senior management, human resources, and security?				
Has the team solicited input from neighbors and the local community?				
TASK FORCE WORK				
Has the task force researched other smoke-free health care organizations to explore their legal				

Smoke-Free Resources

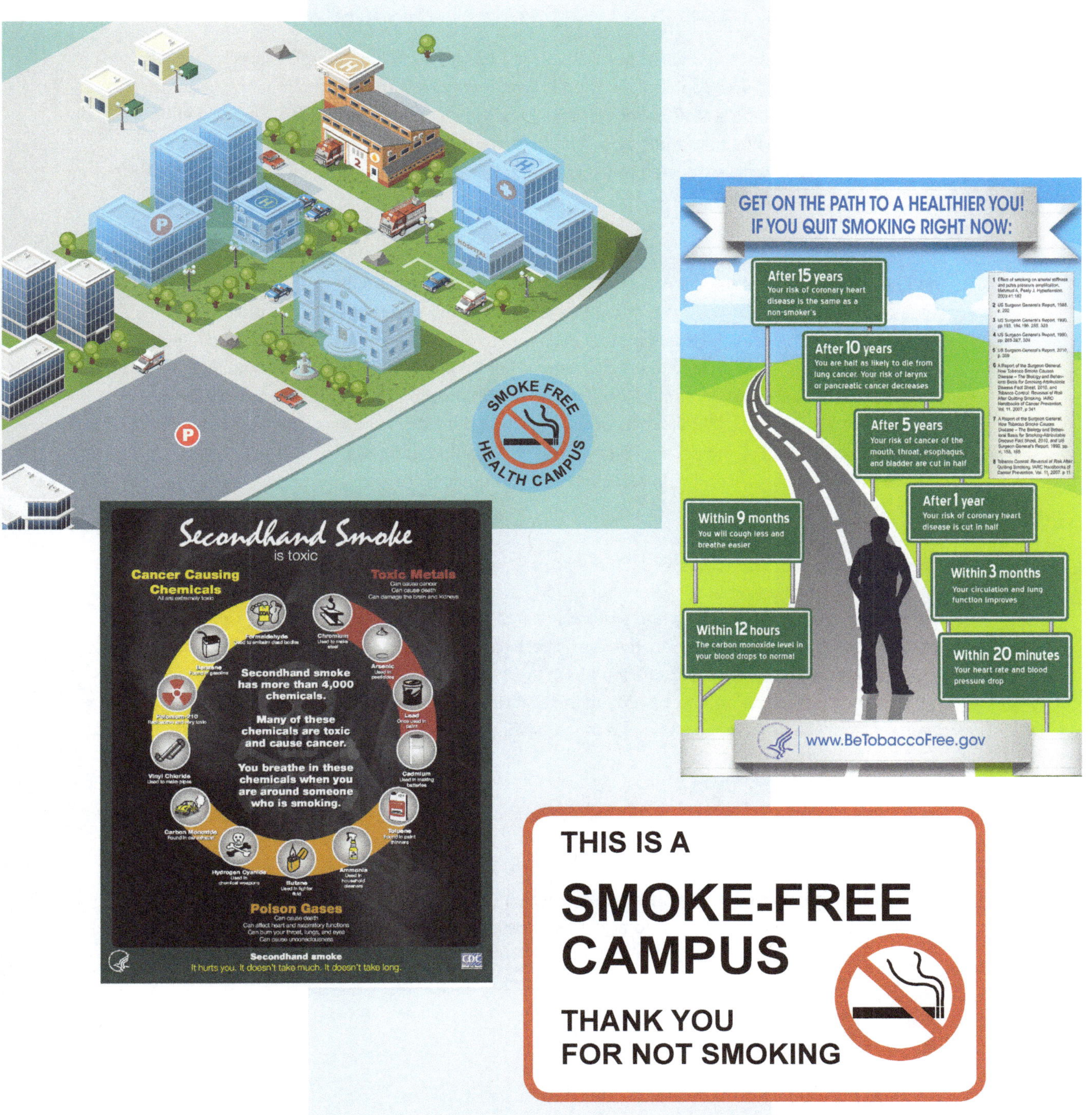

Health care organizations can use any number of resources to inform people of their smoke-free policy. Maps showing designated "smoke-free" areas and signs indicating a "smoke-free" campus are direct visual tools used to reinforce an organization's policy. Whereas posters and brochures can supplement these direct tools by providing educational information and direction to smoke-free resources.

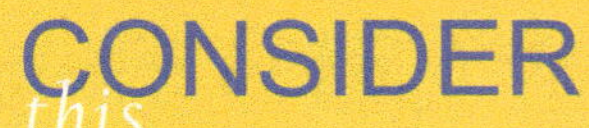

Readying Staff to Enforce a Smoke-Free Policy

When speaking with an individual about a smoke-free policy violation, organization employees should be knowledgeable about the policy and have some ready responses for whomever they encounter—whether it be a staff member, patient, individual served, or visitor. Educating staff on how best to approach individuals who violate an organization's smoke-free policy enforces the policy as well as empowers staff to help individuals maintain a healthy environment in and around the organization's facilities.

Be Prepared

Staff need to know what the smoke-free policy states so a consistent message is being spread across the organization. In addition, most health care organizations have a type of smoking-cessation program available; ensuring that staff know how to contact this program or locate its office and that staff have access to brochures or other informational materials is also useful. Staff approaching individuals about a smoke-free policy violation need to be ready with as much information as possible to explain the violation and direct the individual(s) to a desig-nated smoking area. Having access to smoking-cessation program materials is also beneficial if the individual seems receptive to receiving that information.

Literature and Signs

When speaking with individuals about the smoke-free policy, it helps to have informational materials—such as a brochure—on hand. Brochures typically include information about the organization's smoke-free policy and smoking cessation, and a map indicating the smoke-free and designated smoking areas. Poster-sized flyers also can inform individuals about the smoke-free policy, as well as information about the hazards of smoking. In addition, many organizations post signs and maps around their facilities to indicate the smoke-free policy; staff can direct individuals to these signs and maps, also. (*See* page 81 for examples.)

Engaging the Individual

Engaging an individual can be an awkward experience if a person doesn't feel comfortable. The example scripts are not meant to be memorized, but are provided as a foundation that can be used when discussing the smoke-free policy with individuals. Also, keep in mind that when approaching an individual to discuss the smoke-free policy, the goal is to deliver the policy's message nonconfrontationally, not to argue with the individual about their smoking habits.

Example Scripts

The following are scripts staff can review to give ideas on how to approach individuals about the smoke-free policy.

Note: *For the purpose of these scripts, smoking includes the use of cigarettes (including electronic cigarettes), cigars, pipes, and smokeless tobacco. When drafting its smoke-free policy, organizations should clearly indicate what types of products are restricted.*

Examples for Individuals Who Are Unaware of the Smoke-Free Policy

Example 1

Hi. I'm not sure if you are aware, but our organization has a smoke-free policy. We are a smoke- and tobacco-free campus, which includes inside our facilities and our grounds outside. May I ask you to extinguish your [cigarette, cigar, pipe] and [dispose of it in the nearest waste can/put it away]? Thank you!

Example 2

Pardon me. You may not be aware, but our organization's campus and facilities are smoke free. Here is a brochure that explains our organization's smoke-free policy and includes a map indicating designated smoking areas. If you'd like, I'd be happy to show you to the nearest designated smoking area. Otherwise, I must ask that you extinguish your [cigarette, cigar, pipe] and [dispose of it in the nearest waste can/put it away]. Thank you for your cooperation!

Example 3

Good day to you. I am an employee here at the organization. Because we are committed to providing safe, quality health care, I want to make you aware that we are a smoke-free campus, meaning we do not allow tobacco products in any of our facilities or on our grounds. Here is a brochure with information about our policy and our smoking-cessation program, as well as a map showing the areas designated for tobacco use. Please don't hesitate to ask any questions and thank you for respecting our policy.

Example for Individuals Who Are Aware of the Smoke-Free Policy

Example 1

Excuse me. I'd like to remind you that our organization has a smoke-free policy in effect for the entire campus. We consider this policy an important part of the health care, services, and treatment we provide. Please extinguish your [cigarette, cigar, pipe] and [dispose of it in the nearest waste can/put it away]. If you have questions or would like information about quitting, visit our website, which includes information about our smoking-cessation program.

Examples for an Approached Individual Who Reacts Negatively

Example 1

I can appreciate that this is difficult for you, but our policy was put in place for the health and safety of everyone who comes to our health care organization. We really appreciate your cooperation.

Note: *In cases where politeness and empathy are not effective and/or the situation escalates,* do not *continue to engage. Walk away and contact a manager or security to inform them of the situation.*

continued

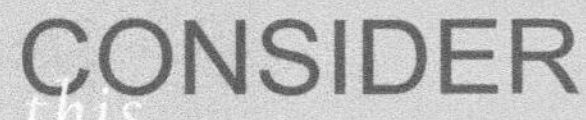

Examples for Individuals Asking to Smoke in Their Car

Example 1

Thank you for asking! Yes, according to our policy you are permitted to smoke while inside your vehicle as long as the windows are rolled up and no byproducts (cigarette butts) are left on the ground.

Example 2

No. Our smoke-free policy encompasses our entire campus. We ask that you respect our policy and not smoke in your vehicle while on campus property. If you'd like, I can provide you with a map that can direct you to designated smoking areas.

Examples for Other Situations

Example 1—Electronic Cigarettes

No, I'm afraid our policy does not allow you to smoke electronic cigarettes anywhere on our campus either, including your car. Although they don't contain tobacco or require a flame to ignite, they are still considered a fire hazard. Thanks for your cooperation.

Example 2—Vendors and Contractors

I want to let you know in advance that our organization is smoke free. The use of any tobacco products is prohibited on organization property, including parking areas. Please see the information provided for more information about our policy, including what products are prohibited and a map indicating smoke-free and designated smoking areas. Contact information is included for any questions. Thank you for respecting our smoke-free policy.

Assessing Risk in Satellite Behavioral Health Care Facilities

Organizations that provide behavioral health care services face a unique collection of risks that mix patient safety, facility security, fire safety, and emergency management. Multiply those risks across 11 different sites in varied geographical locations. Now divide them into residential and outpatient facilities, and divide them again into owned and leased spaces. This complex equation describes the situation faced by the Gateway Foundation.

The Gateway Foundation provides substance abuse treatment services to adults and adolescents at 10 locations in Illinois: 6 are in the Chicago area, including 3 in downtown Chicago; 2 are in central Illinois; 3 are in the southern part of the state; and 2 are in the St. Louis metropolitan area. The organization also offers similar services at a facility in Delaware. Gateway also provides substance abuse treatment services in a number of "satellite locations" such as nursing homes and other facilities operated by other agencies.

Mitigating Elopement Risk

According to Marty Varpa, Gateway's director of facility management, the organization's locations focus on elopement risk because of the high number of adolescents who receive this type of treatment and service.

"We have a responsibility to keep all of our clients safe, especially those who are adolescents," Varpa says.

Windows were an elopement concern at the Carbondale facility, Varpa explains. To limit the risk of a client leaving through a window, the organization wanted to restrict the opening of windows. A risk assessment raised concerns about the potential risks to fire safety and adequate ventilation.

The seriousness of these issues led the team to research requirements under the National Fire Protection Association's *Life Safety Code*®* and other local fire safety and building codes. It was determined that if a building is a fully sprinklered facility, opening windows could be restricted. In addition, the ventilation requirements could be met by mechanical means. Because the building met

---

* *Life Safety Code*® is a registered trademark of the National Fire Protection Association, Quincy, MA.

both of these exemption requirements, the risks associated with restricted window opening were mitigated. The facility was able to decrease the risk of elopement without increasing fire safety or ventilation risks.

Gateway's Lake Villa facility approached elopement risk from a different angle. At that location, the organization implemented a pilot program to document the hourly nighttime checks in adolescent bedrooms. According to Varpa, it has been the policy for staff members to check on adolescent clients every hour. Until now, though, the checks were not consistently documented. The new system requires the staff member to swipe an electronic reader located on the far side of the room. The goal is to hold staff to a higher accountability, thereby reducing the risk of elopement.

Balancing Risks

Like other behavioral health care facilities, Gateway must address a heightened risk of suicide. Many environmental risks related to suicide are found in bathrooms, such as shower curtain rods and plumbing pipes.

To minimize suicide risks, all Gateway locations have removed locks on bathroom doors, except when the bathroom is accessed from a common corridor. For example, a bathroom that serves a private room does not have a lock, but a bathroom that serves the lobby or waiting room does have a lock. Joint Commission Life Safety (LS) Standard LS.03.01.20 specifies which room can be locked in certain conditions, as well as acceptable types of locks.

The issue of shower curtain rods required the organization to balance risks. Assessment showed that breakaway shower curtain rods would reduce the risk of suicide but increase the risk of a client using the rod as a weapon.

"We needed to weigh the risks," Varpa says. "We had to determine which risk was greater, and whether the lesser risk was acceptably low." In the end, it was determined that the risk of suicide was greater, with more significant impact, and breakaway rods were installed organizationwide.

continued

Ownership of Risk

Leasing space, as many organizations do, can sometimes interfere with an organization's ability to minimize risks. There are sometimes conflicts or discrepancies between the organization's requirements and those of the building owner. Varpa emphasizes that organizations occupying leased space should be careful to ensure that the organization's risk-related requirements are being met by the party responsible for maintaining the building.

Owning or controlling a facility can make it easier for an organization to take actions to mitigate risk. When Gateway's Springfield location expanded its outpatient services, it encountered a new risk regarding security. The existing parking lot was not adequate to meet the increased need, and clients and staff were using street parking in the surrounding neighborhood. This created an increased risk to both clients and staff, as the organization could not provide security in those areas.

Gateway is responding to this situation as part of its long-term plan. It has acquired property adjacent to the facility to create a parking lot that will be managed by the organization. This will allow Gateway to have control over which measures are appropriate and effective to make sure clients, staff, and visitors are safe when parking.

One tool Gateway uses to assess risk in locations where treatment services are provided within a facility owned and managed by another agency is shown on page 87.

Managing Multiple Locations

The Gateway Foundation encompasses facilities throughout Illinois, which means greater diversity than one might think. Each site has very different needs, demographically and geographically, that affect the risks each must address. For example, facilities in the southern part of the state are near the New Madrid fault line and have emergency plans that account for seismic activity—something unnecessary for the northern facilities. Similarly, Gateway's residential facilities need to prepare for emergencies differently than its outpatient ones.

To manage the divergent needs of its multiple locations, Gateway has developed a tiered approach to managing risks. First, it utilizes a broad organizationwide plan that is applicable to all its locations. Gateway involves representatives from each location in an annual training session that focuses on The Joint Commission's Environment of Care, Life Safety, and Emergency Management standards, among other "big picture" issues. This is supplemented by plans that are generated locally. These plans deal with the unique needs of each location and are periodically reviewed by the organization.

"This system allows us to face the challenge of maintaining consistently low risk across such a diverse range of locations," Varpa says.

Satellite Treatment Location Risk Assessment

The Gateway Foundation uses tools, such as this featured tool, to assess risks for treatment services when providing them at locations owned and managed by another agency.

Note: *The complete assessment worksheet may be adapted and is available for internal use on the flash drive (print only) or by clicking the tool link in the Risk-Assessment Toolbox (e-book only) on page 77.*

Source: Gateway Foundation, Chicago, IL. Used with permission.

Published in *Environment of Care Risk Assessment*, Joint Commission Resources, 2018.   **File Name:** 03 10 Sat Treatment RA

SATELLITE TREATMENT LOCATION RISK ASSESSMENT

Satellite location	
Address	
Date conducted	
Entity that owns and/or manages the building where the services occur	
Location(s) in the building where the services occur	
Do we take a role in the building's fire and/or emergency drills?	
Building contact information in the event of an emergency	

chapter 4

Hazardous Materials and Waste

Hazardous materials and waste (also known as *hazmat*) are materials whose handling, use, and storage are guided or defined by local, state, or federal regulation, such as the US Occupational Safety and Health Administration's (OSHA's) Regulations for Bloodborne Pathogens regarding the disposal of blood and blood-soaked items and the Nuclear Regulatory Commission's regulations for the handling and disposal of radioactive waste. This also includes hazardous vapors (for example, gluteraldehyde, ethylene oxide, nitrous oxide) and hazardous energy sources (for example, ionizing or nonionizing radiation, lasers, microwave, ultrasound). Although the Joint Commission considers infectious waste as falling into this category of materials, federal regulations do not define infectious or medical waste as hazardous waste. Hazardous materials and waste are present in all sectors of business, and health care organizations are no exception; in fact, they typically store and use a wider variety of such materials than do many other industries (*see* the illustration on page 91).

Management of risks associated with hazardous materials and waste is included under The Joint Commission's Environment of Care (EC) Standard EC.02.02.01. However, because of the nature of this issue, there is some crossover into other standards chapters. For example, hazardous waste can pose an infection risk; thus Infection Prevention and Control (IC) Standard IC.02.01.01 requires organizations to minimize infection risk associated with storing and disposing of infectious waste. Similarly, some medications (such as chemotherapy agents) are considered hazardous; thus Medication Management (MM) Standard MM.01.01.03 requires organizations to safely manage the risks involving such medications.

Many agencies regulate the use of hazardous chemicals and waste, including OSHA, the US Environmental Protection Agency (EPA), and the US Department of Transportation (DOT). These agencies require health care organizations to maintain up-to-date and adequate inventories of all hazardous chemicals and waste and report annually on the types and quantities of such chemicals and the locations where they are being stored and used in the organization.

The EC standards also require organizations to create and maintain inventories of hazardous materials and waste and to consider criteria consistent with applicable laws and regulations when developing inventories.

STANDARDS *to know*

EC.02.02.01

IC.02.01.01

LD.04.01.01

MM.01.01.03

TERMS *to know*

hazardous materials

hazardous waste

Overview of Assessing Risks

The primary risk assessment associated with hazardous materials and waste is the annual inventory of hazardous chemicals. A thorough chemical inventory ensures that hazardous materials are used, stored, monitored, and disposed of according to applicable laws and regulations. This inventory process will be discussed beginning on page 92.

Participants in the Process

Organizations should have a designated individual who oversees management of hazardous materials and waste. This may be a dedicated position, such as a "hazmat officer." In other organizations, the responsibility might be included in the role of the safety officer or EC director, or possibly given to the EC committee. Whoever is designated to oversee this management, the individual will need to work with representatives from facilities management, infection control, environmental services, and any departments that handle high-risk materials and waste on a regular basis (for example, laboratory, radiology, pharmacy, oncology). With their particular perspective and specialized knowledge, these individuals are essential to identifying risks and working through the risk-assessment process.

Identifying Risks

Risks involving hazardous materials and waste can be identified through several sources. These risks should be included in an environmental tour (*see* Chapter 3 for a discussion of environmental tours). In addition, review of the required hazardous materials and waste inventory may point to potential risks.

Standardized Product Labels

Product labels, which must identify the chemical name and any hazardous ingredients, are another source to use when determining the risks associated with hazardous materials being introduced and used in a health care facility. OSHA adopted specific requirements for product labels to bring its labeling requirements into alignment with the United Nations (UN) Globally Harmonized System of Classification and Labeling of Chemicals (GHS). *See* page 93 for a sample OSHA product label. The following elements are now required on all hazardous chemical labels, known as the Hazard Communication Standard (HCS) HazCom Labels[1]:

- *Product identifier*. Typically, a code and product or chemical name, the same product identifier must match the information in Section 1 of the safety data sheet (SDS).
- *Supplier identification*. Contact information for the supplier or manufacturer, including name, address, and telephone number.
- *Hazard pictograms*. Standardized, universal symbols; selection determined by chemical hazard classification (*see* page 94).
- *Signal word*. *Danger* and *warning* are the only two words used as a "signal word"; *danger* is used to classify more severe hazards, while *warning* is used for less severe hazards.
- *Hazard statement(s)*. These warning statements include all applicable health hazards specific to the product; hazard statements may be combined, when appropriate, to reduce redundancies and are specific to hazard classifications; the same statements should be used for the same hazards regardless of what the product is or who manufactures it.
- *Precautionary statement(s)*. These statements provide recommended measures to consider to minimize or prevent adverse effects resulting from improper storage or handling practices; the four types of precautionary statements are *prevention*, *response*, *storage*, and *disposal*.

Product labels also may include supplementary information deemed helpful by the manufacturer or supplier. Information provided in this section is not required but may include the following:

- Listing the percentage of ingredient(s) with unknown acute toxicity when it is present in a concentration of 1%
- Including personal protective equipment (PPE) pictograms to inform staff handling the product what they should wear to protect themselves
- Providing directions for how to use the product
- Listing the expiration date

Safety Data Sheets

Safety data sheets (SDSs), which are provided by the company that produces the hazardous material, also should be reviewed to help identify potential risks. These informational documents are more detailed than product labels, and they include guidance on exposure limits, toxicity, fire and explosion risk, reactivity, health hazards, cleanup procedures, and PPE required while handling the material.

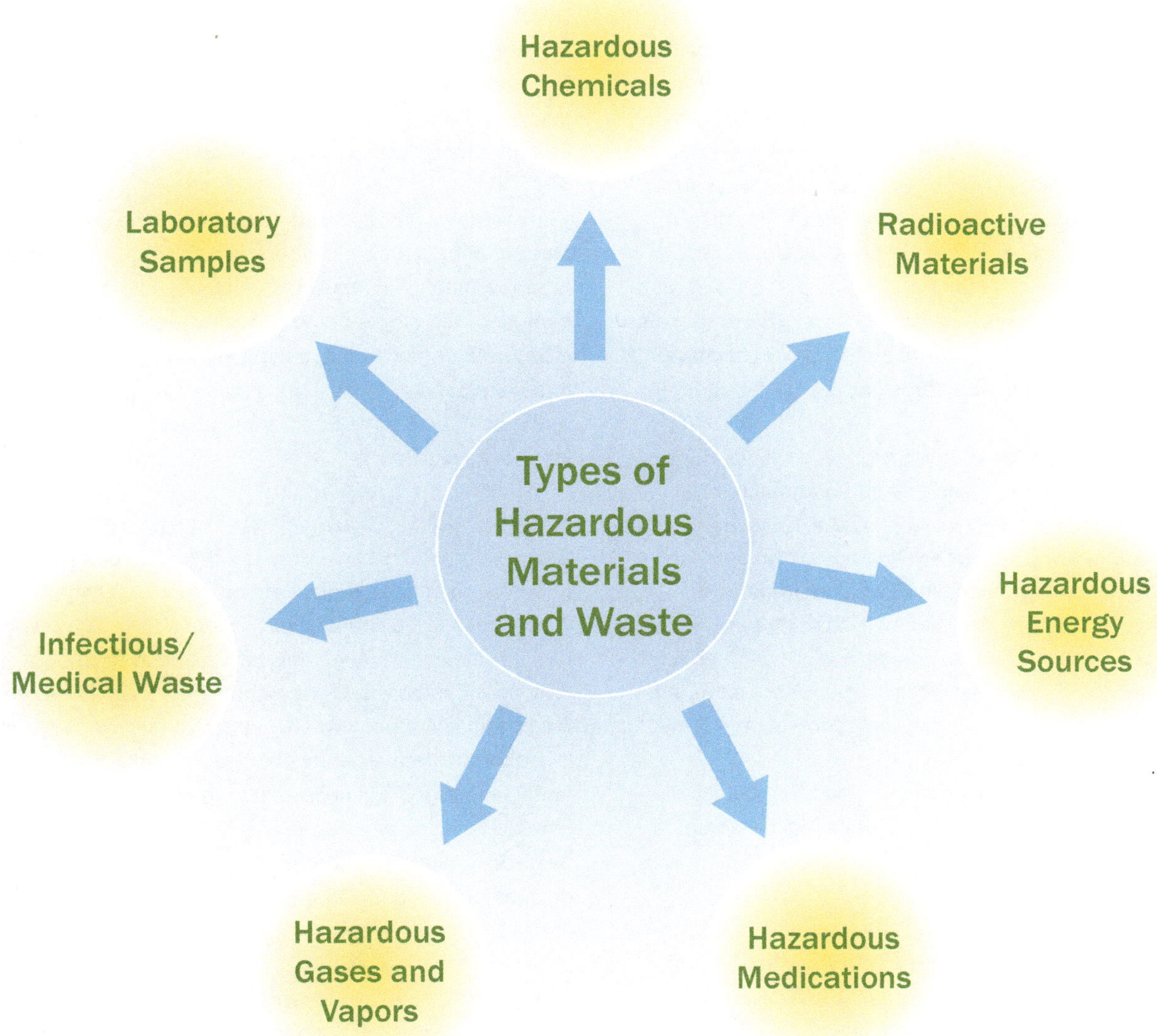

All health care settings are required in some capacity to manage risks related to hazardous materials and waste in accordance with Standard EC.02.02.01; typically, these items fall into the categories illustrated here as far as this standard is concerned. Organizations also must ensure they are in compliance with other laws and regulations, such as those set by the US Department of Transportation (DOT), the US Environmental Protection Agency (EPA), and US Occupational Safety and Health Administration (OSHA).

Manufacturers and vendors of hazardous chemicals are required by law to provide purchasers with an SDS for each product. An organization is legally required to obtain an SDS for each hazardous chemical used or stored on the premises and make these available to employees in their work areas on their work shifts (*see* page 96 for an explanation regarding the use of common household-type chemicals). Organizations should make the SDS readily available at any time to any staff member; there must not be any barriers to SDS access. This means that someone who is authorized to use the computer or fax system, for example, always must be available to obtain an SDS for employees who do not have such authorization. Access may be provided through an electronic database, or via hard copies that are kept in a central location or that are available in various departments. Any of these storage and retrieval methods is acceptable under Joint Commission standards and OSHA requirements.

In addition to standardizing product labels, OSHA's SDS requirements have been standardized and must be presented in a user-friendly format using a 16-section format. The following provides a brief explanation of the sections with a more detailed breakdown of what information is required in each section and a sample SDS on page 95.[2]

- Sections 1 through 8 contain general information about the chemical, identification, hazards, composition, safe-handling practices, and emergency control measures (for example, firefighting).
- Sections 9 through 11 contain technical and scientific information, such as physical and chemical properties, stability and reactivity, and information about toxicity and exposure control.
- Sections 12 through 15 are required to maintain consistency with the UN GHS; however, because they concern matters handled by other agencies, OSHA does not enforce the content of these sections.
- Section 16 is allotted for any additional information not already captured in the SDS.

Inventory Management

The primary risk assessment activity for hazardous materials and waste is maintaining a complete, current inventory. This inventory should be conducted annually because products are introduced and obsoleted in the health care market constantly, making the inventory potentially vary from one year to the next.

Everyone's cooperation is important to ensure an accurate record and to avoid bringing new chemicals into the facility undetected. The materials management department, through which most hazardous materials enter a facility, should be included in the chemical inventory process. Staff from this department can help identify new chemicals coming into the system and coordinate and control chemical purchases. Materials management staff should report to the EC committee any new chemicals brought into use, or chemicals that are being discontinued, as soon as possible.

The inventory process also may prevent the unnecessary storage of unused or expired chemicals that could pose a potential safety risk, particularly if these chemicals are confused with others being used in the organization. An inaccurate or incomplete chemical inventory can lead to severe consequences, such as fire, injury, illness, and death. (*See* page 97 for a hazardous waste storage inspection checklist.)

Simplify by Delegating, Standardizing

Although a physical inventory like this is an enormous undertaking in large organizations, it is necessary. To simplify the process, organizations may choose to assign responsibility for the inventory of their own areas to each department that stores and/or uses hazardous chemicals. For example, the pharmacy manager can inventory the pharmacy, while the laboratory manager inventories the hazardous materials in the laboratory. It is important to remember that designated satellite facilities around the community that house or use hazardous chemicals also must complete the inventory, and designated personnel in these facilities should be prepared to engage in this process.

To ensure a consistent inventory across an organization, define what constitutes a hazardous chemical so that all individuals completing the inventory understand what materials should be included. On page 98, the illustration provided lists some, but certainly not all, of the chemicals included on the inventory list.

Joint Commission EC standards require that organizations have a written, current inventory of hazardous materials and waste whose handling, use, and storage are addressed by law and regulation, though it does not prescribe what that inventory must look like. However, Leadership (LD) Standard LD.04.01.01 requires health care organizations to comply

OSHA Product Label

This sample label identifies the elements of the standardized product label required by the US Occupational Safety and Health Administration (OSHA) that aligns with the United Nations Globally Harmonized System of Classification and Labeling of Chemicals.

Note: *This product label is available as a template that may be adapted and is available for internal use on the flash drive (print only) or by clicking the tool link in the Risk-Assessment Toolbox (e-book only) on page 102.*

Source: US Occupational Safety and Health Administration, Washington, DC.

with laws and regulations. In the case of hazardous materials and waste, that includes local, state, and federal regulations, such as those from OSHA, EPA, and DOT.

OSHA regulations, which are referenced by EPA for chemical inventory requirements, state that the minimal chemical inventory should contain the following:

- Chemical name
- Chemical Abstracts Service (CAS) Registry Number
- Common name
- Synonyms
- Product/mixture name (if applicable)
- Percentage of ingredients in product/mixture (if applicable)

The DOT does not require a chemical inventory because the agency's focus is on the shipment of hazardous materials (that is, manifests). But because The Joint Commission requires that an organization's hazardous waste be included on its inventory, the use of the DOT UN number would be an acceptable identifier for this hazardous waste if no CAS number is available.

In addition, EPA requires some facilities to submit the chemical inventory to the State Emergency Response Commission (SERC), Local Emergency Planning Committee (LEPC), and local fire department annually by March 1, in accordance with the Emergency Planning and Community

OSHA Hazardous Materials Pictograms

Health Hazard

- Carcinogen
- Mutagenicity
- Reproductive Toxicity
- Respiratory Sensitizer
- Target Organ Toxicity
- Aspiration Toxicity

Flame

- Flammables
- Pyrophorics
- Self-Heating
- Emits Flammable Gas
- Self-Reactives
- Organic Peroxides

Exclamation Mark

- Irritant (skin and eye)
- Skin Sensitizer
- Acute Toxicity (harmful)
- Narcotic Effects
- Respiratory Tract Irritant
- Hazardous to Ozone Layer (non-mandatory)

Gas Cylinder

- Gases Under Pressure

Corrosion

- Skin Corrosion/Burns
- Eye Damage
- Corrosive to Metals

Exploding Bomb

- Explosives
- Self-Reactives
- Organic Peroxides

Environment (Non-Mandatory)

- Aquatic Toxicity

Flame Over Circle

- Oxidizers

Skull and Crossbones

- Acute Toxicity (fatal or toxic)

Source: US Occupational Safety and Health Administration, Washington, DC.

To ensure worker comprehension and reduce misunderstandings, the US Occupational Safety and Health Administration (OSHA) standardized the pictograms that accompany product labels. Each pictogram represents particular types of hazards and which pictogram is used is determined by OSHA's chemical hazard classification. Further information about labeling and pictograms is available on OSHA's website: https://www.osha.gov/dsg/hazcom/index.html.

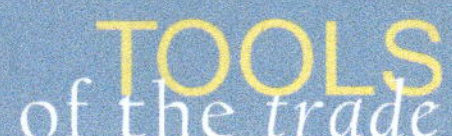

Required Information for Safety Data Sheets

The US Occupational Safety and Health Administration's (OSHA) 16-section format outlines what information is required to be included in a safety data sheet (SDS).

Note: *The complete list of requirements for SDSs and a sample SDS, as well as a template that may be adapted for internal use, is available on the flash drive (print only) or by clicking the tool link in the Risk-Assessment Toolbox (e-book only) on page 102.*

Source: US Occupational Safety and Health Administration, Washington, DC.

Published in *Environment of Care Risk Assessment*, Joint Commission Resources, 2018.   **File Name:** 04 02 SDS Requirements

REQUIRED INFORMATION FOR SAFETY DATA SHEETS

SECTION 1—IDENTIFICATION

Section 1 identifies the chemical listed on this safety data sheet (SDS), as well as its recommended uses. The required information for this section includes the following:

- Product identifier used on the label and any other common names or synonyms by which the substance is known.
- Name, address, phone number of the manufacturer, importer, or other responsible party, and emergency phone number.
- Recommended use of the chemical (for example, a brief description of what it actually does, such as flame retardant) and any restrictions on use (including recommendations given by the supplier).

SECTION 2—HAZARDS IDENTIFICATION

This section identifies the hazards of the chemical presented on the SDS and the appropriate warning information associated with those hazards. The required information consists of:

- The hazard classification of the chemical (for example, flammable liquid, category*).
- Signal word.
- Hazard statement(s).
- Pictograms (the pictograms or hazard symbols may be presented as graphical reproductions of the

Household Items

The US Occupational Safety and Health Administration (OSHA) does not require that safety data sheets be provided to purchasers of household consumer products when the products are used in the workplace in the same manner that a consumer would use them (for example, where the duration and frequency of use—and, therefore, exposure—is not greater than what the typical consumer would experience). However, this exemption in OSHA's regulation is not based on the chemical manufacturer's intended use of its product but on how it is actually used in the workplace. Employees who are required to work with hazardous chemicals in a manner that results in a duration and frequency of exposure greater than what a normal consumer would experience have a right to know about the properties of those hazardous chemicals.

Right-to-Know Act (EPCRA), Sections 311–312, Tiers I and II.[3] Facilities required to submit this inventory are those that have chemicals with quantities equal to or greater than the following thresholds (applicable to the health care environment):

- For Extremely Hazardous Substances (EHSs), either 500 pounds or the Threshold Planning Quantity (TPQ), whichever is lower
- For all other hazardous chemicals, 10,000 pounds

The inclusion of a column on the inventory that identifies a substance as a hazardous chemical (OSHA), hazardous material (DOT), or hazardous waste (EPA) is not necessary under Joint Commission standards. Organizations may choose to document this information if they find it beneficial.

A standardized form also may be helpful to ensure that complete and consistent information is collected from all departments (*see* page 101 for an inventory worksheet). The following is some important information to consider including on the worksheet:

- Name and primary responsibility of the department completing the form (for example, laboratory, clinical area, nonclinical area, off-site location, office)
- Name of the department's manager or primary contact person
- Name of the building in which the department is located
- Room number of the department
- Inventory date
- Full product/chemical name (**Note:** *Staff should write out the full chemical name of each hazardous chemical. Abbreviations and chemical nomenclature are not acceptable.*)

- Manufacturer name
- Product/catalog number
- Existence and availability of the SDS
- Maximum quantity on hand (estimated total volume or weight located in designated room number)
- Storage location (for example, building, department, and room number)
- Health, safety, or fire risks associated with or around the product
- PPE required
- Indication that staff have received training regarding the material in question

The safety manager should be available to provide assistance and training on how to conduct the inventory and complete any forms associated with the inventory.

Review for Accuracy, Completeness

After a department completes its inventory, the safety manager, EC committee, or other responsible party should review it for completeness, although this is not required. Again, using a checklist can help the reviewer identify any missing or incomplete information.

Review Existing Inventory, or Re-Create?

When conducting the chemical inventory, there are two common approaches. Some organizations may decide to just print out the current inventory form they have on file and submit it to the appropriate department for review. Other organizations may choose to have the department perform an entirely new inventory each year.

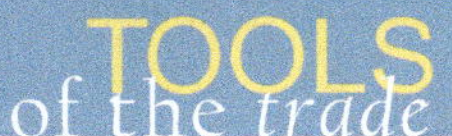

Hazardous Waste Storage Inspection Checklist

Organizations can use this checklist to ensure hazardous waste storage areas are safe.

Note: *The complete checklist may be adapted and is available for internal use on the flash drive (print only) or by clicking the tool link in the Risk-Assessment Toolbox (e-book only) on page 102.*

Published in *Environment of Care Risk Assessment*, Joint Commission Resources, 2018.   **File Name:** 04 03 Checklist Haz Waste Storage Inspect

HAZARDOUS WASTE STORAGE INSPECTION CHECKLIST

ORGANIZATION: ____

STORAGE AREA: ____

	REVIEW DATE				COMMENTS
	REVIEWER INITIALS				
CONTAINERS	YES/NO	YES/NO	YES/NO	YES/NO	COMMENTS
Is there sufficient aisle space for inspection of all containers?					
Are all waste containers closed?					
Are all containers compatible with the material stored inside?					
Are all waste containers free from damage or corrosion?					
Are containers of liquids stored in a containment system?					
Are incompatible waste containers segregated appropriately?					
CONTAINER LABELS	YES/NO	YES/NO	YES/NO	YES/NO	COMMENTS
Are all containers labeled with the appropriate waste labels?					
Are biohazardous containers red in color or labeled with a biohazardous symbol?					
Are all labels filled out completely and legibly?					

There are pros and cons to each approach. Reviewing the current inventory takes less time and may be appropriate for areas that deal with fewer hazardous materials. However, this approach may result in the department neglecting to identify anything new. Re-creating the inventory from scratch encourages a more purposeful and thorough result. On the other hand, it can be time-consuming, and there is a chance a department may forget about some items previously identified.

Organizations may consider switching the process every year. In other words, one year the department reviews the inventory on file and submits any changes, and the next year the department conducts an entirely new inventory and compares the results.

Storing Inventory Information

Storing information collected in a chemical inventory process within a computerized database can be extremely helpful in keeping the data easily accessible and user-friendly. For example, when locating information about a particular chemical with widespread use in the organization, staff members easily can access the chemical's information through a database. Likewise, when staff members are determining what chemicals are used in a particular area, a computer database can help facilitate the information-gathering process. Such a database also will make it easier to do an annual update of the inventory.

Responding to the Inventory

When the chemical inventory process is complete, the safety manager and EC committee should consider taking the following actions, as needed, to anticipate and address any risks associated with the inventory:

Identify safer alternatives to hazardous chemicals. Some products may have alternatives that are equally effective but safer or easier to use. For example, a department may list bleach on its chemical inventory. Bleach is a common disinfectant, but using it safely requires training and provision of related devices, such as eye wash stations. A safety manager may want to recommend a less corrosive disinfectant alternative.

Design safer storage practices. The inventory review may illuminate situations in which chemicals are being stored in ways that contradict the guidelines listed on the product label and/or SDS. For example, a safety manager may notice

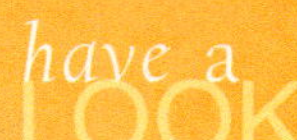

Commonly Used Hazardous Materials

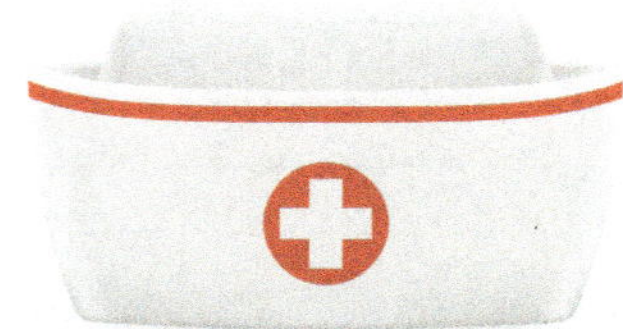

Environmental Services

- Cleansers used for surfaces
- Detergents used for laundry
- Disinfectants

Nursing Units

- Reagents – all types
  - Acids
  - Bases
  - Solvents
- Pharmaceuticals
- Alcohols
- Creams and gels

Maintenance Areas

- Paints
- Solvents
- Oils
- Fuels

Maintaining a comprehensive inventory of hazardous materials is critical for any health care organization. Knowing what hazardous materials are used in a health care facility allows personnel responsible for it to monitor its usage, storage, and disposal in accordance with state and federal regulations.

that a reactive chemical is stored in the same area with flammables and recommend that one be moved to a different location.

Enact additional security methods, when needed. Sometimes a department is using or interacting with hazardous chemicals that require additional security to preserve the safety of patients and staff. For example, if an academic medical center has a laboratory that conducts research and uses anthrax for a study, and this lab identifies anthrax on its chemical inventory, the safety manager should work with the department to implement additional security methods that may be needed to preserve patient, staff, and visitor safety.

Provide safety training for first responders. In the case of a chemical spill or leak, the first people on the scene should know what to expect and do. It is important that staff members—particularly those who work in areas that use or store the most dangerous chemicals—be trained in safe methods to respond to an incident involving hazardous materials. OSHA offers guidance on training requirements

under its Hazardous Waste Operations and Emergency Response (HAZWOPER) standard. The level and type of training will vary based on the anticipated hazards and what capabilities the staff members will need to respond to those hazards.

Eliminate unneeded or outdated chemicals. This can help reduce unnecessary hazards and provide the opportunity for more efficient use of storage space.

Review SDS inventory. Every hazardous chemical in an organization requires an SDS. Each employee should know where their department's SDSs are located and how to access them. If a particular product or chemical does not have an SDS on file, or if the SDS is outdated, the situation must be addressed immediately.

Monitor hazardous gases and vapors associated with dangerous chemicals. Frequent air monitoring is required when employees use specific products, such as formaldehyde (used in laboratories and the morgue to preserve tissue), ethylene oxide (used to sterilize surgical instruments), and waste anesthetic gas (used by surgical staff in the operating room). A chemical inventory will help an organization in identifying areas that require air monitoring.

Submit the organization's inventory to the appropriate local, state, and federal government agencies. The federal government is very concerned about where large quantities of hazardous materials are being stored and used. As previously discussed, EPA requires facilities that manage certain levels of certain materials to submit reports to state and local agencies.

Review shipping practices. DOT regulates the shipping of hazardous materials and waste on public roadways, rails, aircraft, and ships. Typically, roadways, and possibly rail, might affect an organization. Health care facilities are considered the generator of hazardous materials and waste shipped from the facility. Whoever sends out is the shipper (generator); whoever receives is the receiver.

Special Risk Considerations

The following sections explore several important issues to consider when addressing risks associated with hazardous materials and waste.

Personal Protective Equipment

PPE is one of the primary means of keeping people safe from harm caused by hazardous chemicals. PPE includes such items as gloves, gowns or aprons, masks and respirators, goggles, and face shields. Different materials require different types of PPE to ensure safety. Gloves, for example, can be made from a variety of materials that are used to perform different tasks. (*See* page 103 for the advantages and disadvantages of common glove materials.)

PPE is effective only when used properly, starting with which items are necessary for which actions with which chemicals. The SDS for each product must state what PPE is necessary during handling, use, and cleanup. Staff must know where to find this information and be trained in the right way to use PPE. Training also should include proper procedures for donning and doffing PPE, disposal, and factors that compromise the ability of PPE to effectively protect. For example, long fingernails or hand jewelry may tear gloves, and face masks that don't fit snugly may allow fluids or gases to damage skin or eyes. Staff also should know how to respond if PPE is compromised during use.

Imaging Staff

Individuals who are occupationally exposed to ionizing radiation, whether machine produced or from radioactive material, may need to have their exposure monitored. Generally, states determine the threshold for monitoring occupational radiation exposure from machine-produced radiation. The requirement for staff monitoring due to exposure from radioactive material may be regulated by either the state or the Nuclear Regulatory Commission. For those organizations that use The Joint Commission for deeming purposes, the US Centers for Medicare & Medicaid Services (CMS) Conditions of Participation (CoP) require that radiation workers be checked periodically, by the use of exposure meters or badge tests, for the amount of radiation exposure.

Protection for both staff and patients from ionizing radiation may be required in certain applications, including computed tomography (CT), positron emission tomography (PET), or nuclear medicine (NM) services. Although the risk from exposure to medical levels of ionizing radiation is low, if there is no benefit to be gained exposure should be avoided or mitigated. Proper protective apparel, such as aprons, shields, gloves, and glasses should be available for the use of both patients and staff. Such equipment should be stored, cleaned, and inspected following manufacturer recommendations and the advice of the facility's radiation safety officer.

Magnetic resonance imaging (MRI) presents unique safety risks because of its use of strong magnetic fields and radio waves. There is a risk that magnetic objects brought into the scan room could become a projectile that could injure patients or staff. In addition, there is a risk to patients of thermal injury or injury from embedded metallic objects or shrapnel. The fields also can affect devices or leads implanted in patients and there is the potential of hearing damage from noise. It is imperative that only screened individuals have access to the scan room and the area immediately outside the MRI scan room.

Eye Wash Stations and Showers

Many hazardous chemicals can severely injure or damage eyes and/or any skin they come into contact with. Therefore, eye wash stations and emergency showers are essential components of a health care organization's hazardous materials and waste risk-management effort.

Drenching Facilities

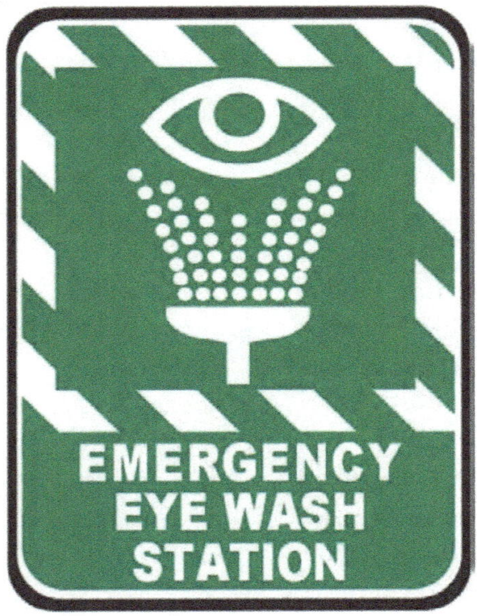

Access to drenching facilities is necessary for staff that come in contact with corrosives on the job. Drenching facilities include eye wash or eye/face wash stations and showers. What facilities an organization needs depends on the extent of possible exposure and the types of hazardous materials being handled. The US Occupational Safety and Health Administration (OSHA) requires the availability of a full-drench shower for hazardous chemicals. For requirements specific to drenching equipment, OSHA defers to the American National Standards Institute (ANSI). The standard ANSI developed for eye washes and showers requires an organization to have an emergency eye wash and shower on the same level as the hazard; in addition, the standard requires unobstructed access that is within 10 seconds of the hazard area, as well as staff training on the correct use of the equipment.

Hazardous Materials and Waste Inventory Worksheet

Hazardous materials and waste inventory can be a daunting task—especially for larger health care systems. However, the inventory is a necessary task to ensure the safety of individuals in a health care facility. Organizations can use this worksheet to collect relevant inventory information and ensure it is complete and consistent throughout its facilities.

Note: *The complete worksheet may be adapted and is available for internal use on the flash drive (print only) or by clicking the tool link in the Risk-Assessment Toolbox (e-book only) on page 102.*

Published in *Environment of Care Risk Assessment*, Joint Commission Resources, 2018.

File Name: 04 04 Worksheet Hazmat Invent

HAZARDOUS MATERIALS AND WASTE INVENTORY WORKSHEET

DATE: ______________ MANAGER: ________________________________ PHONE: ________________________

BUILDING: ________________________ DEPARTMENT: ________________ LOCATION/ROOM NUMBER: ______________

| CHEMICAL NAME | COMMON NAME/ SYNONYM | PRODUCT/MIXTURE NAME | CAS# | MANUFACTURER | SDS | % OF INGREDIENTS IN PRODUCT | QUANTITY ON SITE | | DATE | | PPE REQUIRED |
							ACTUAL	MAX	RECEIVED	EXPIRED	
					☐						☐
					☐						☐

OSHA requires eye wash stations in every facility where people may be exposed to injurious corrosive materials—including health care organizations. Eye wash stations must be located in an area that can be reached in 10 seconds or less (higher-risk hazards, such as harsh acids, may require a shorter travel distance). They must clearly be identified, well lit, and located on the same level as the hazard. OSHA references the American National Standards Institute/ International Safety Equipment Association guidelines (ANSI/ ISEA Z358.1) regarding design details—such as height, position, flow rates, and valves—that must be used in eye wash stations.[4] Personal eye wash units are considered supplementary to, and not a substitute for, traditional eye wash stations.

Emergency showers, which drench the entire body, often are found in laboratories and occasionally in plant operation areas because these areas often deal with larger volumes of chemicals, which increases the risk of large-scale spills or other incidents. If a facility determines that there is a need for an emergency shower, OSHA again references ANSI/ISEA Z358.1 for placement and design. Similar to eye wash stations, showers should be located no more than 10 seconds away from the hazard (closer for higher-risk hazards), be clearly identified and well lit, and be on the same level as the hazard.[4]

Access to drenching facilities is necessary for staff that come in contact with corrosives on the job. Drenching facilities include eye wash or eye/face wash stations and showers (*see* page 100). What facilities an organization needs depends on the extent of possible exposure and the types of hazardous materials being handled. OSHA requires the availability of a full-drench shower for hazardous chemicals. For requirements specific to drenching equipment, OSHA defers to the American National Standards Institute (ANSI). The standard ANSI developed for eye washes and showers requires an organization to have an emergency eye wash and shower on the same level as the hazard; in addition, the standard requires unobstructed access that is within 10 seconds of the hazard area, as well as staff training on the correct use of the equipment.

Transportation Requirements

Regulations regarding transportation of hazardous materials and waste fall under the DOT's Pipeline and Hazardous Materials Safety Administration (PHMSA). Overall, the regulations require hazardous materials to be "properly classed, described, packaged, marked, labeled, and in condition for shipment as required or authorized."[5]

Health care organizations need to be aware of the specific transportation requirements for all hazardous materials and waste they handle, both coming into the facility (for example, purchased products) and going out of the facility (for example, waste materials). For products coming into the facility, these transportation and disposal details will be included in the SDS. For hazardous waste, which includes chemicals, pharmaceuticals, and infectious materials, there are different requirements for organizations classified as "generators" of waste and those that will store, treat, or dispose of waste. As a hazardous waste generator, the organization is responsible for determining its generator status by types and volumes of hazardous waste—and to meet all regulatory requirements associate with that status.

Risks of Disposal

When disposing of hazardous materials and waste, it is vital that all materials be handled in a way that minimizes risks. Organizations need to implement processes that allow for the monitoring and easy reporting of identified risks. To ensure the successful disposal of hazardous materials, focus on the following steps:

- *Separation.* Keep hazardous waste storage and processing areas separate from sterile areas and clean supplies.
- *Classification.* Separate hazardous waste by type and keep it away from ordinary trash.
- *Transportation.* Establish a minimal travel distance between the site of final use and a protected disposal unit.
- *Documentation.* Track the waste collection and handling process to allow for continuous monitoring and evaluation of the organization's efforts to be in compliance with all applicable regulations.

- *Contractor.* If an organization uses a contractor, select one that is reputable and experienced; also make sure to evaluate the effectiveness on an ongoing basis.

References

1. US Occupational Safety and Health Administration. OSHA Brief: Hazard Communication Standard: Labels and Pictograms. Feb 2013. Accessed Feb 20, 2018. https://www.osha.gov/Publications/OSHA3636.pdf.
2. US Occupational Safety and Health Administration. OSHA Quick Card™: Hazard Communication Safety Data Sheets. 2016. Accessed Feb 20, 2018. https://www.osha.gov/Publications/OSHA3493QuickCard SafetyDataSheet.pdf.
3. US Environmental Protection Agency. EPCRA Sections 311–312: Emergency Planning and Community Right-to-Know Act (EPCRA) Hazardous Chemical Storage Reporting Requirements. (Updated: Nov 2, 2016.) Accessed Feb 20, 2018. http://www2.epa.gov/epcra -tier-i-and-tier-ii-reportingepcra-sections-311 -312#covered-for-more-information.
4. American National Standards Institute/International Safety Equipment Association (ANSI/ISEA). American National Standard for Emergency Eyewash and Shower Equipment. Arlington, VA: ISEA, 2014.
5. Federal Motor Carrier Safety Administration. How to Comply with Federal Hazardous Materials Regulations. (Updated: Dec 17, 2014.) Accessed Feb 20, 2018. http://www.fmcsa.dot.gov/regulations/hazardous -materials/how-comply-federal-hazardous-materials -regulations.

RISK-ASSESSMENT TOOLBOX

1. [Download] Standardized OSHA Product Label Template
2. Safety Data Sheet
   - [Download] Required Information for Safety Data Sheets
   - [Download] Safety Data Sheet Template
   - [Download] Sample Safety Data Sheet
3. [Download] Hazardous Waste Storage Inspection Checklist
4. [Download] Hazardous Materials and Waste Inventory Worksheet

Advantages and Disadvantages of Glove Materials

Gloves used in the health care environment are commonly made from the materials listed in the following table. Each has advantages and disadvantages that must be weighed when selecting the gloves that are appropriate for a given task.

Material	Pros	Cons
Latex (natural rubber)	• Good for water-based and biological materials • Tensile strength • Tactile sensitivity • Puncture/tear resistant • Elasticity	• Poor for organic solvents • Oxygen, UV light, ozone can deteriorate • Oils can degrade • Can provoke allergies
Vinyl (PVC)	• Good for bases, acids, fats, oils, amines, and peroxides • Good abrasion resistance	• Poor for most organic solvents, glutaraldehyde, and chemotherapy agents • Less durable • Vulnerable to breakdown from alcohol
Nitrile	• Good for oils, solvents, greases, and some acids and bases • Resistant to punctures, several chemicals, glutaraldehyde, and abrasion	• High modulus and stiffness • Oxygen, UV light, and ozone can deteriorate
Neoprene	• Good for alcohols, acids, bases, peroxides, fuels, hydrocarbons, phenols • Resistant to many chemicals and oil	• High modulus and stiffness • Oxygen, UV light, and ozone can deteriorate
Polyurethane	• Resistant to oil and abrasion • Tensile strength	• Vulnerable to alcohol breakdown • Slippery • Embrittles and hardens at low temperatures
Norfoil	• Suitable for most hazardous chemicals • Resists permeation by a wide range of solvents, acids, and bases	• Poor fit

UV, ultraviolet; PVC, polyvinyl chloride.

Sources

1. The Joint Commission. Glovesick. *Environment of Care® News*. 2014 Jul:17(7):5–7, 11.

2. Kimberly-Clark Health Care Education. Do the Gloves You Wear Afford Appropriate Barrier Protection for the Task at Hand? Accessed Feb 20, 2018. http://www.ibrarian.net/navon/paper/Kimberly_Clark_Health_Care_Education.pdf?paperid=21069503.

3. Office of Environment, Health and Safety, University of California, Berkeley. Glove Selection and Usage. Accessed Feb 20, 2018. https://ehs.berkeley.edu/workplace-safety/glove-selection-guide.

chapter 5

Security

When a person enters a health care organization, whether it's for treatment, for work, or to visit a friend or family member, that individual has the reasonable expectation that his or her security will be preserved. This includes protection from personal harm and loss and damage to property. An important aspect of security management within a health care organization is an assessment of the environment's security risks. Conducting a security risk assessment allows the organization to define an appropriate security program and its boundaries.

There are many different types of risks that fall under the umbrella term *security*. They often are managed in conjunction with safety risks, though they are distinct. (*See* Chapter 3 for a discussion of safety risks.) Joint Commission Standard EC.02.01.01 considers security risks to be those that put people and property at risk of harm or loss. They typically result from intentional acts by individuals from either outside or inside the health care organization.

Security is something most patients, residents, individuals served, and staff in a health care organization take for granted (*see* page 106). The security risk assessment allows environment of care (EC) staff to anticipate potential security risks and respond to any areas that need attention. Done well, the security risk assessment can improve safety, health, and satisfaction (*see* page 107).

Overview of Assessing Risks

The Joint Commission requires organizations to continually monitor their environment for, among other things, security-related incidents. These include the following:
- Injuries to individuals within the organization's facilities
- Incidents of damage to the organization's property or the property of others (patients, residents, individuals served, staff, and visitors)
- Other security incidents involving patients, residents, individuals served, staff, or others within its facilities (for example, abductions, theft)

These incidents should be reported (internally and, if applicable, externally) and investigated according to the organization's established processes.

Frequency of Assessments

To maintain a consistently high level of security in a health care facility, security risk assessments should be frequent.

Security Risks

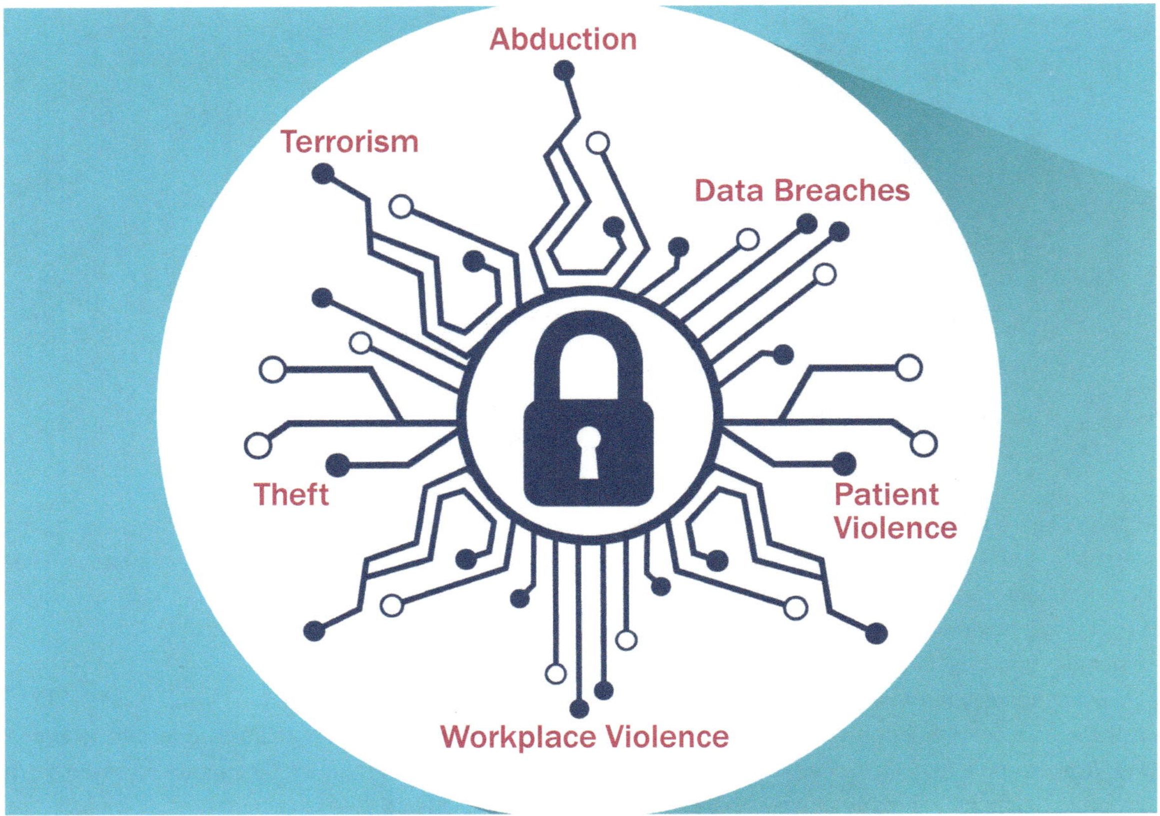

Unlike safety risks that typically are accidental, security risks are intentional acts that cause harm to people in a health care facility or disrupt an organization's functionality. This illustration lists the most commonly identified security risks in health care, but it is not an exhaustive list.

Many events can affect security risks, including the following:

- Construction of a new space
- Creation of a new department
- Implementation of new security measures
- Changes in staffing (for example, hiring, termination)
- Changes in population the health care facility serves
- Shifts in the community demographics

Security risks and plans should be evaluated as part of the required annual evaluation and review of the organization's overall EC plan (*see* pages 109 and 110 for two security risk-assessment worksheets).

Identifying Risks

Like all other types of risk assessments, the first step is identifying which risks and hazards to assess. One source is the local police department, which may have already conducted a risk assessment for the grounds and thus can help point out potential security issues that need attention. Review of *Sentinel Event Alert*s from The Joint Commission also can highlight areas that an organization may want to target for assessment.

In most cases, however, the primary sources for identifying security risks are the department managers and those who work with specific patient populations. These individuals will know best which security risks are most likely to affect their areas. For example, the nurse manager for the labor and delivery unit can help identify risks for infant abduction or domestic violence. Likewise, the facilities manager can shed light on building security risks, such as poor parking lot lighting or inappropriately placed security cameras.

Identifying Risks at the Departmental Level

When conducting security assessments in particular areas or departments, organizations should begin by determining

Elements of Security Risk Assessment

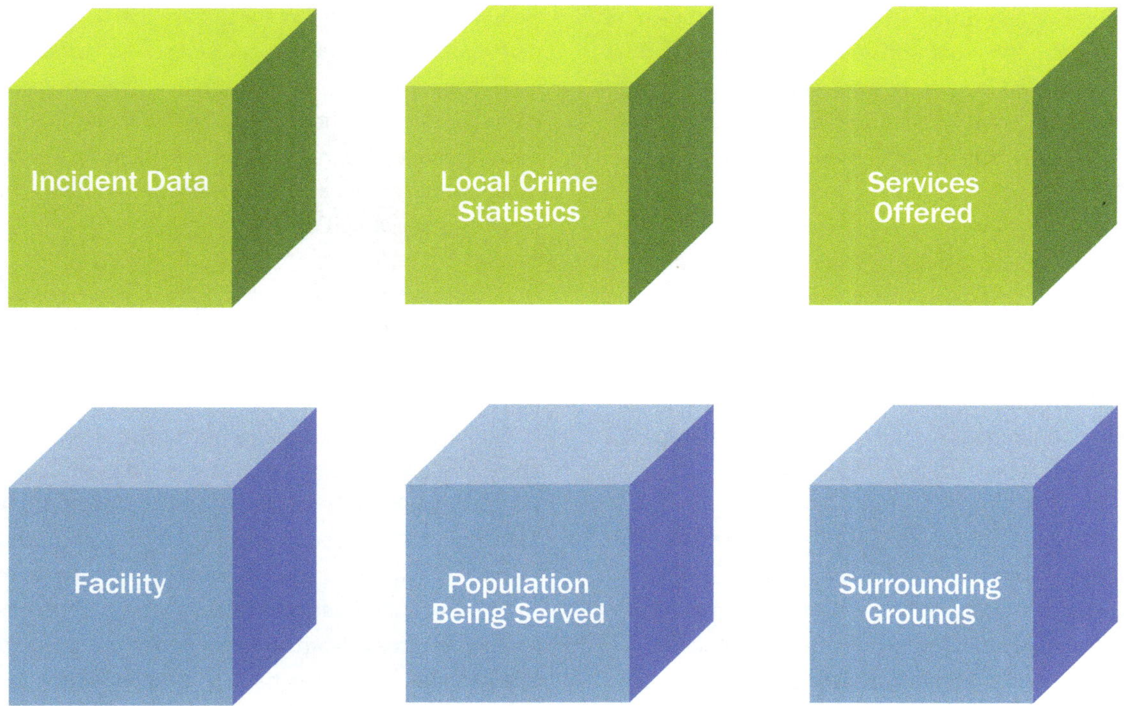

what their high-risk areas and departments are and what types of risks are possible in these areas. (*See* page 111 for a list of these types of areas and departments.)

Number and severity of security incidents within the area or department. These could include actual incidents, such as thefts, acts of violence, or abductions, as well as complaints from staff members and patients, residents, individuals served, regarding fear for their safety.

Level of access to the area or department. Some areas of a health care organization (such as admitting or reception) have open access, while others (such as the pharmacy) have secured access. Open access can create a greater potential for security incidents, such as theft, because anyone can access the area at any time. A closed access area will require consistent monitoring to ensure that no one who does not have proper access enters the area. This monitoring could be automated, such as through a key card identification system. (*See* page 113 for a medication storage and security assessment checklist.)

Security hardware present in the area. Such hardware can include monitored alarm systems, automatic door locks, closed-circuit video surveillance systems, panic buttons, call stations, and delayed egress. Security hardware can enhance security by preventing access, monitoring activity, and alerting the security department of improper activities within a space.

Degree of public traffic through the area, as well as the degree of isolation. Isolated areas may be at higher risk for some security issues, such as physical violence or sexual assault, because events can occur without other people being aware of them. Public traffic areas can present a greater risk for other security issues, such as theft, because there are more people entering and exiting the area, and any one of these people could present a threat.

Potential degree of loss associated with a security incident. For example, within the labor and delivery department, a security incident could lead to the abduction of a child. The potential loss in this area is catastrophic. This factor should influence the security plans for this area.

Risks present in the community. Different communities present different security risks. For example, a community may have known gang activity, which could present a threat to safety for home health care workers, as well as for staff within a facility—particularly the emergency department or intensive care unit (ICU). Gang members who shoot an individual who then ends up in the emergency department or ICU may show up at the facility to "finish the job."

Security needs of particular patient populations. Different patient populations have different security needs. For example, psychiatric and pediatric patients will have very specific security needs related to elopement, abduction, and violence. (*See* later sections for further discussion of these risks.)

Security risks associated with particular times of day. For example, inadequate parking lot lighting may present a security threat for second- and third-shift staff. Landscaping also can provide optimal hiding spaces during the dusk and evening hours.

Security risks associated with contraband. Within some departments, there may be a risk of patients, residents, individuals served, or families bringing articles to the facility that are against organization policies—such as weapons, drugs, or cigarettes.

Security needs when caring for criminals or prisoners. In some cases, a department will need to treat an individual who is under arrest or has been transferred from a nearby incarceration facility. Organizations should consider the security risks associated with this situation, including the risk for violence, gang activity, and elopement.

Responding to Security Risks

The security assessment should serve as the basis for the organization's security policy. When the risk-assessment process is complete, policies and procedures should be enacted to reduce any identified risks.

Security risk assessments also form the basis for performance improvement activities. After assessing risk in different departments, the safety manager or security manager may want to highlight high-risk areas to help focus security management efforts in the areas that present the most risks, such as the emergency department, pharmacy, labor and delivery, ICU, and radiology.

Security management is not the job of security staff alone. All staff in an organization should be considered part of the overall security plan and should be trained on the organization's security-related policies, procedures, and processes. In particular, staff members in security-sensitive areas should be aware that they work in such areas, and they should be able to describe the security features within their areas, such as stationed security officers, card swipe machines, alarms or security systems, and panic buttons. Also, pertinent information about any security-sensitive areas should be incorporated into new employee orientation. This ensures that employees have relevant information about their job's specific security risks and procedures from day one.

Common Security Risks in Health Care Settings

Many security risks that result from physical acts are applicable to all health care settings. These security risks create potential far-reaching issues that can compromise the quality and safety of the care, treatment, and services health care organizations endeavor to provide, as well as the safety of health care staff. The incidents can come from internal and external sources, including the following topics that are common across most settings:

- Workplace violence and bullying
- Employee response to termination
- Infant/child abduction
- Wandering and elopement concerns
- Forensic patients

Workplace Violence

Health care workers are among the populations most at risk for workplace violence. The Bureau of Labor Statistics reports that more than 11,000 health care and social assistance workers were injured by workplace violence in 2014—69% of all such injuries in private industry.[1] The National Institute of Occupational Safety and Health (NIOSH)

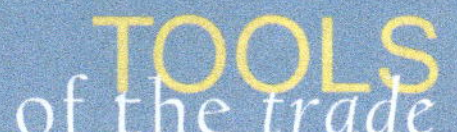

Security Event Risk-Assessment Worksheet

When assessing an organization's high-risk areas, identifying what areas pose the greatest threat help to drive performance improvement efforts. This worksheet can be used to determine what security events have the greatest risk, allowing security management to focus its efforts on the most critical areas identified.

Note: *The complete worksheet may be adapted and is available for internal use on the flash drive (print only) or by clicking the tool link in the Risk-Assessment Toolbox (e-book only) on page 122.*

Source: US Army Medical Department, Army Public Health Center, Aberdeen Proving Ground, MD. Medical Safety Template— Security Risk Assessment. (Updated: Jan 2015.) Accessed Feb 20, 2018. http://phc.amedd.army.mil/PHC%20Resource%20Library/ MedicalSafetyTemplate-SecurityRiskAssessment2015.docx.

Published in *Environment of Care Risk Assessment*, Joint Commission Resources, 2018.　　　**File Name:** 05 01 Worksheet Security Event RA

SECURITY EVENT RISK-ASSESSMENT WORKSHEET

DEPARTMENT: _______________________________________　　DATE:_______________________________

RISK ELEMENT DESCRIPTION	OCCURRENCE PROBABILITY (1–5)	OCCURRENCE IMPACT (1–5)	TOTAL IMPACT SCORE (PROBABILITY x IMPACT)
PEOPLE			
Infant/pediatric abduction			
Assault			
Elopement			
Forensic patient			

---

defines workplace violence as "the act or threat of violence, ranging from verbal abuse to physical assaults directed toward persons at work or on duty."[2] Examples of violence include threats (expressions of intent to cause harm, including verbal threats, threatening body language, and written threats), physical assaults (attacks ranging from slapping and beating to rape, homicide, and the use of weapons such as firearms, bombs, or knives), and muggings (aggravated assaults, usually conducted by surprise and with intent to rob). The US Occupational Safety and Health Administration (OSHA) defines workplace violence as "any act or threat of physical violence, harassment, intimidation, or other threatening disruptive behavior that occurs at the work site."[3]

Workplace violence can cover a variety of acts, including the following:

- Verbal threats to inflict bodily harm, including vague or covert threats
- Verbal harassment, such as abusive or offensive language, gestures, or other discourteous conduct
- Slander, including making false, malicious, or unfounded statements against other individuals, which tend to damage their reputations or undermine their authority
- Attempts to cause physical harm by striking, pushing, and other aggressive physical acts , such as sexual assault (which includes rape)
- Domestic or gang violence that follows the victims into the facility, or that occurs in a home care residence
- Disorderly conduct, including shouting, throwing or pushing objects, punching walls, and slamming doors
- Terrorism against workers

These incidents can range in scope from a skirmish in a hallway to an active-shooter situation that puts the entire facility at risk. Also, keep in mind that a small incident can escalate if not dealt with properly.

The topic of workplace violence in health care settings received a great deal of attention in 2016, due in part to a US Government Accountability Office (GAO) report titled "Workplace Safety and Health: Additional Efforts Needed to

Security Asset Risk-Assessment Worksheet

Organizations need to assess risks associated with its assets, in addition to security-related events. This worksheet provides an opportunity to assess the assets of an organization, which can lead to prioritizing revised or planned security measures for assets that potentially could have a life-threatening impact if breached.

Note: *The complete worksheet may be adapted and is available for internal use on the flash drive (print only) or by clicking the tool link in the Risk-Assessment Toolbox (e-book only) on page 122.*

Published in *Environment of Care Risk Assessment*, Joint Commission Resources, 2018.   **File Name:** 05 02 Worksheet Security Asset RA

SECURITY ASSET RISK-ASSESSMENT WORKSHEET

ORGANIZATION: ______________________________   DATE: ______________________

Risk Codes	1 = Minimal impact	2 = Significant impact	3 = Potential life-threatening impact	4 = Actual life-threatening impact
Cost Factors	2 = Easily replaceable at low cost and low risk	4 = Significant impact in financial terms or harmful to organization	6 = Very valuable in financial terms and considered a high priority	8 = Very harmful to organization if lost, damaged, or injured or extremely harmful if loss of life
To Determine Priority Score	Multiply the risk code by the cost factor; add additional risk, in accordance with security data for area			

Unit/Department	Assets*	Security Risks†	Risk Code	Cost Factors	Measures Taken	Measures Planned	Priority Score
Administration Office							
Behavioral Health Unit							
Blood Bank							
Cashier							
Cleaning and Laundry							
Computer/Mainframe Room							
Dining Facility Storage							

Help Protect Health Care Workers from Workplace Violence"[4] and a new OSHA toolkit released in December 2015 titled "Preventing Workplace Violence in Healthcare."[5]

In response to inquiries from the field, The Joint Commission created a Workplace Violence Prevention Resources portal, located on the Joint Commission website at https://www.jointcommission.org/workplace_violence.aspx. The goal of this portal is to broaden the awareness of workplace violence in health care by bringing relevant and timely information and resources applicable across health care settings to a central location. The portal provides links to materials developed by The Joint Commission as well as federal and state government resources and those from professional associations. The portal also includes information from health care organizations that have encountered events and/or effectively reduced workplace violence.

Risk Factors

There are a variety of risk factors for the incidence of workplace violence. Organizations should conduct a risk assessment specific to workplace violence that focuses on particular areas, departments, or patient populations. When conducting a workplace violence risk assessment organizations also should ensure that both the internal environment and surrounding community are included to ensure a comprehensive view of potential risk factors. (*See* page 115 for an environmental risks for workplace violence checklist.) For example, a behavioral health care unit may present risks for workplace violence because psychiatric patients can be more prone to violent activity than other types of patients.

Certain areas of a health care facility are at heightened risk for workplace violence (*see* the illustration on page 111). The emergency department, for example, is a common site

Commonly Identified High-Risk Areas

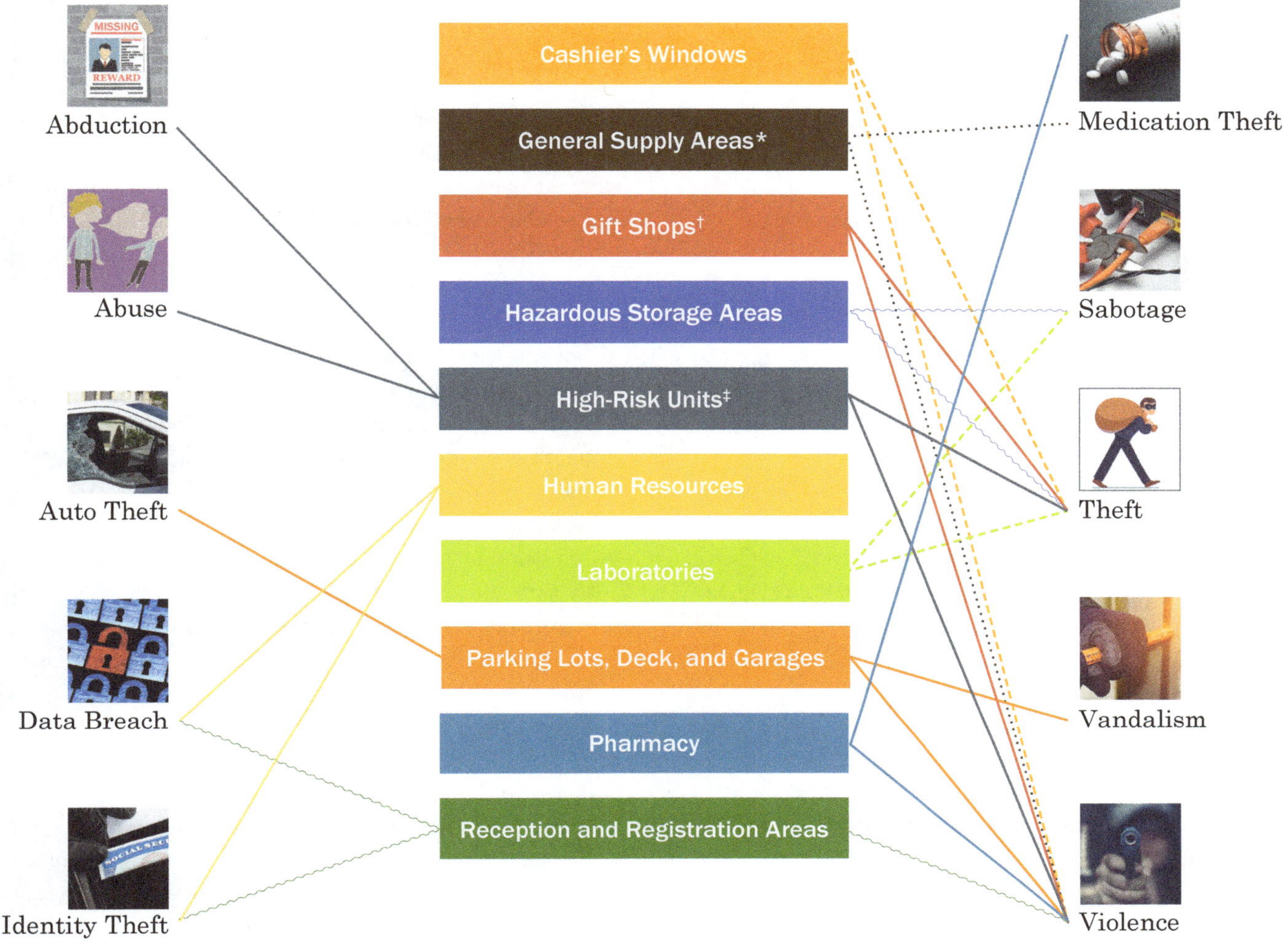

In health care organizations, the commonly identified security-sensitive areas listed in the center of this illustration have a higher potential for the issues listed on either side. Organizations need to identify which areas in their facilities are high risk and determine the types of issues that are present. While this illustration provides a sample of high-risk areas and potential issues, it is not a comprehensive list. .

---

* These types of areas could house syringes and sharp instruments.
† Gift shops typically are found only in hospital settings.
‡ Certain areas, units, or departments, such as the emergency department, intensive care unit, labor and delivery, pediatrics, and common rooms in behavioral health care organizations, are at high risk for security incidents; however, any area in a health care facility has the potential for these incidents.

for incidents of violence in a hospital. Many factors contribute to this, among them the heavy volume of patients, including those with behavioral, psychiatric, and substance use issues; 24-hour access; frequent overcrowding; the potential for external violence (for example, gang or domestic) to follow the victim into the health care facility; and patients and visitors who are under the influence of alcohol or illicit drugs.

When assessing an organization's potential for workplace violence consider the following points:
- Likelihood of patients, families, and visitors to carry a handgun
- Presence of gangs or gang activity in the community
- Temptations—such as drugs and money—found in a health care environment

- Lower staffing levels during times of increased activity, such as meal and visiting times
- Change of shifts that occur in the darkness
- Lighting of parking areas
- Vegetation around the building that could be a place for someone to hide during evening hours
- Staff training to recognize and manage hostile and aggressive behavior
- Accessibility of security hardware, such as panic buttons and call stations

All these factors can affect security and workplace violence, either alone or in combination.

Because home care requires staff to enter an individual's residence, there is a greater risk for domestic and/or gang violence from the individual, family, friends, and the community. Home care organizations should train staff on assessing the environment and, if necessary, modify schedules to avoid placing staff in harm's way.

Many organizations have a variety of policies, procedures, and features in place that directly or indirectly relate to workplace violence prevention. These may include a program for nonviolent crisis intervention, call buttons for summoning help in the parking lot, and a code to call for assistance in an emergency situation. All of these can be drawn together under the umbrella of workplace violence prevention. The resulting program must be clearly communicated to staff members, and it must have the support of organization leadership. Suggestions for preventing violence in health care facilities are found on page 116; for proactive ideas using safety-enhancing design and equipment to prevent workplace violence, *see* page 117.

Active-Shooter Situations

One of the most terrifying and widely publicized security incidents is when a person with a gun opens fire or someone with a knife starts attacking. These individuals are known as "active shooters." US government agencies—including the White House, US Department of Justice/Federal Bureau of Investigation, US Department of Education, and US Department of Homeland Security/Federal Emergency Management Agency—define an active shooter as "an individual actively engaged in killing or attempting to kill people in a confined and populated area."[6(p. 5)] These events are often seen as unpredictable and sudden. Although this is in some

ways true, it does not mean that there are not ways to mitigate the risk and prepare for such an incident.

Developing a plan to respond to active shooters, as well as training and educating staff about that plan, is critical. This might be handled through the existing security team or by a dedicated threat assessment team. The plan should address the following:

- Training staff to identify individuals who may commit a violent act
- Procedure for reporting an active-shooter incident
- When to utilize the run, hide, and fight responses
- Evacuation policy and procedure, including escape route assignments and alternative routes if primary routes are unusable
- Lockdown procedures
- Communications, both internally and with community law enforcement, during an active-shooter incident
- How to interact with first responders and emergency personnel
- Procedures to follow in the immediate aftermath of an incident

Staff should be trained on all aspects of the plan, know how to use security features such as alarms and door locks, and should be empowered to report on any behavior or situation they feel might be unsafe. (To help your organization prepare for an active-shooter event, *see* page 118 for resource tools and page 128 for a real-world scenario.)

Workplace Bullying

Workplace bullying (also referred to as lateral or horizontal violence)[7] is "repeated, health-harming mistreatment of one or more persons (the targets) by one or more perpetrators."[8] Bullying is abusive conduct that takes one or more of the following forms: verbal abuse; threatening, intimidating, or humiliating behaviors (including nonverbal); and/or work interference—sabotage—that prevents work from getting done.[8]

To correct bullying behaviors that can undermine a culture of safety, all health care facilities should consider taking the following specific safety actions:

- Educate all team members on appropriate professional behaviors that are consistent with the organization's code of conduct.
- Hold all team members accountable for modeling desirable behaviors.

Medication Storage and Security Assessment Checklist

This checklist can be used to assess an organization's storage and security of medications and to determine if there are any risks. In addition, this checklist can be used on a daily basis to ensure the consistent storage and security of medication in various health care settings.

Note: *The complete worksheet may be adapted and is available for internal use on the flash drive (print only) or by clicking the tool link in the Risk-Assessment Toolbox (e-book only) on page 122.*

Published in *Environment of Care Risk Assessment*, Joint Commission Resources, 2018. **File Name:** 05 03 Checklist Med Store Assess

MEDICATION STORAGE AND SECURITY ASSESSMENT CHECKLIST

*This checklist includes questions to assess an organizations' storage and security of medication and can be used to determine risks that require attention. Answers to all questions should ideally be **Y** for **Yes** (unless they aren't applicable). If an answer is **N** for **No**, use the "Notes" section to document needed changes. Unless otherwise noted, this checklist is applicable to all program settings.*

ORGANIZATION: _________________________________ DEPARTMENT/UNIT: _________________________________

DATE OF REVIEW: _________________________ REVIEWER: _________________________________

QUESTIONS	YES	NO	NA	NOTES
ALL MEDICATIONS*				
Are all medications stored per manufacturer's recommendations?				
Are all stored medications labeled with the contents, expiration date/time, and any applicable warning?				
Are multidose vials stored properly and labeled with an end-of-use date/time and initials in accordance with policy?				
Are all storage areas (including cabinets and carts) locked/secured when not in use?				
Are medications for external use stored separately from medications for internal use?				
Have all expired, damaged, and/or contaminated medications been removed?				
Is the medication storage area clean and uncluttered, with no excess debris?				
Are keys or lock combinations for storage areas under the control of authorized staff?				
Are syringes and needles kept secured or in an area away from patient/family access?				
CONTROLLED SUBSTANCES*				

Develop and implement policies and procedures/processes that address bullying, reducing fear of retaliation; responding to patients, residents, or individuals served, and families who witness bullying; and beginning disciplinary actions (how and when).

Employees and Staff

Like any business, health care organizations are made up of individuals who work together toward common goals. Occasionally those individuals can turn against each other or their employer out of anger, frustration, greed, or other motivating factors. These individuals can pose a variety of security risks, including the following:

- Violence
- Theft of materials or sensitive data
- Sabotage of the physical structure or technology
- Vandalism

Employees may engage in these activities for several reasons. Most incidents of internal security risks are cases in which an individual sees an opportunity and feels he or she is unlikely to get caught. Sometimes an individual is emotionally upset and wants to make a statement— commonly revenge against the employer. Occasionally a person is motivated by personal gain or is employed by a third party. Family and friends may take advantage of their personal familiarity with an employee to gain access or get information. Terrorism, while rare, can be difficult to deter because the individual is usually trying to make a very public statement, is highly skilled, and is willing to accept high risk.[9]

Organizations should consider these various types of internal attackers when assessing risks and designing security plans.

Terminations

Letting an employee go can be an emotionally charged experience for both employer and employee. The individual being terminated may feel angry or hurt over the decision, and in some cases he or she chooses to seek to retaliate against the employer. These incidents may take place at the moment of termination, or the individual may return at a future time to act. Therefore, it is important that plans address both immediate and long-term risks.

One of the best ways to mitigate these risks is to identify potentially high-risk terminations. For example, employees who have engaged in violence in the past may resort to it

again when faced with job loss. Other examples include individuals with access to sensitive, restricted, or dangerous materials or information (for example, patient billing files or clinical records; medications, including those available through automated dispensers; hazardous materials or chemicals).

How an organization manages terminations in general, and high-risk terminations in particular, can have a significant impact on minimizing security risks. Actions to consider taking when terminating an employee include the following[10]:

- Conduct the termination meeting in a neutral place, with a third party present. If physical violence is identified as a risk, notify security personnel ahead of time and have them nearby.
- Have all paperwork ready, including final paycheck and information on the organization's procedure for reporting grievances.
- Be prepared to remove the individual from the property as quickly as possible. If theft is a concern, a supervisor may clean out the workspace and ship personal items to the employee.
- Collect any property owned by the organization, particularly electronics such as laptops or tablets, as these may contain sensitive or confidential information.
- Revoke access to the organization's network and databases, including automated medication dispensing devices, and change system passwords, if applicable.
- Collect keys, keycards, or other physical access items; or re-key or reprogram locks.
- Alert security staff to any incidents that occur at the time of termination so they can be prepared if the individual returns to the facility. Other staff may be asked to report to security if a potentially dangerous individual is seen on the property.

Of course, it is likely that even an individual identified as a high security risk will not require any of these measures. However, it's good to be prepared.

Specific Patient Populations

As previously mentioned, particular patient populations can have specific security needs. The following sections discuss some population-specific security issues. Organizations should consider these issues carefully in their security assessments.

Environmental Risks for Workplace Violence Assessment Checklist

This US Occupational Safety and Health Administration (OSHA)–adapted checklist can help an organization assess valuable information to determine the environmental risks for workplace violence. Organizations also can consult the resources developed by OSHA and other organizations—accessible through The Joint Commission's Workplace Violence Prevention Resources portal—to identify additional examples of effective strategies for preventing and mitigating the impact of workplace violence.

Note: *The complete worksheet may be adapted and is available for internal use on the flash drive (print only) or by clicking the tool link in the Risk-Assessment Toolbox (e-book only) on page 122.*

Source: Adapted from OSHA. Guidelines for Preventing Workplace Violence for Healthcare and Social Service Workers. Washington, DC: OSHA, 2016. Accessed Feb 20, 2018. http://www.osha.gov/Publications/osha3148.pdf.

Published in *Environment of Care Risk Assessment*, Joint Commission Resources, 2018. **File Name:** 05 04 Checklist Environment Risk for Violence

ENVIRONMENTAL RISKS FOR WORKPLACE VIOLENCE ASSESSMENT CHECKLIST

*This checklist can be used to assess environmental risks for workplace violence in a health care organization. Answers to all questions should ideally be Y for **Yes** (unless they aren't applicable). If an answer is N for **No**, use the "Notes" section to document needed changes. Unless otherwise noted, this checklist is applicable to all program settings.*

ORGANIZATION: _______________________________   DEPARTMENT/UNIT: _______________________________

DATE OF REVIEW: _______________   REVIEWER: _______________________________

QUESTIONS	YES	NO	NA	NOTES
GENERAL APPROACH				
Are safety and security issues specifically considered in the early stages of facility design, construction, and renovation?				
Does the current violence prevention program provide a way to select and implement controls based on the specific risks identified in the workplace security analysis? How does this process occur?				
NEIGHBORHOOD				
Do crime patterns in the neighborhood influence safety in the facility?				
Do workers feel safe walking to and from the workplace?				
PUBLIC ACCESS				
Are entrances visible to security personnel and are they well lit and free of hiding places?				
Is there adequate security in parking or public transit waiting areas?				
Is public access to the building controlled, and is this system effective?				
Can exit doors be opened only from the inside to prevent unauthorized entry?				

Tips for Preventing Patient Violence

Here are some suggestions for preventing patient violence:

- Provide comfortable waiting rooms.
- Adopt measures to decrease waiting times.
- Provide sensitive, timely information to people who are waiting.
- Minimize the furniture and accessories (for example, pictures, vases, ashtrays) in interview rooms or crisis treatment areas.
- Establish a system for identifying patients with a history of violence (be conscious of privacy and confidentiality issues).
- Discourage staff from wearing necklaces to prevent strangulation.
- Discourage staff from carrying items that may be used as weapons (for example, keys and pens).
- Ensure that nurses and physicians are not alone when providing care that involves close contact with the patient.
- Treat and/or interview agitated patients in areas that are relatively open but still maintain privacy (rooms with removable partitions, for example).
- Survey the facility regularly to remove items that could be used as weapons, such as maintenance tools or abandoned visitor possessions.

Source: US Occupational Safety and Health Administration (OSHA). *Guidelines for Preventing Workplace Violence for Healthcare and Social Service Workers*. Washington, DC: OSHA, 2016. Accessed Feb 20, 2018. https://www.osha.gov/Publications/osha3148.pdf.

Infant/Child Abduction

The issue of infant/child security, and particularly that of infant/child abduction, has perhaps the highest profile of all health care security concerns. Fortunately, thanks mainly to the work done by the National Center for Missing & Exploited Children (NCMEC), the health care industry knows more about the crime of infant/child abduction and how to prevent it than perhaps any other health care security issue. NCMEC also offers specific guidance for health care professionals (*see* page 121 for additional information about NCMEC).

Infant/child abductions fall into two broad categories: those perpetrated by a stranger and those perpetrated by a family member, often referred to as a domestic abductor. Domestic abduction, by far the more common type of abduction, is often the result of a custody issue between parents or between a parent and a government child welfare agency. In contrast with abductions by strangers, health care organizations often have advance information about the possibility of domestic abduction.

Although infant/child abduction happens rarely in health care organizations, and such incidents almost always end happily, infant and pediatric abductions are security risks that all organizations that treat infants or children must address. The EC security standards require organizations to identify potential security risks and implement security procedures that address the handling of an infant or pediatric abduction, as applicable. Security managers may want to meet with the staff of relevant departments, including labor and delivery, neonatal intensive care, pediatrics, and even obstetrics. These staff members may be in the best position to identify potential abduction risks. In addition, the security manager should walk around the department and other areas of the organization, specifically looking for potential infant/child abduction risks.

Addressing risks

When any risks are identified, the organization should address them as quickly as possible. The consequences of an inadequate security system to prevent infant/child abduction can be severe. Methods to address abduction risks include the following:

- Infant and mother identification systems, such as band matching, DNA identification, and antibody profiles
- Restricted access devices

Proactive Engineering Approach to Preventing Workplace Violence

Following are safety-enhancing design and equipment ideas to help prevent workplace violence.

Architectural adaptations that can be made to existing floor plans include the following:
- Closed-circuit television monitoring and video recording of high-risk units
- Electronic access controls for emergency treatment areas
- Metal detectors—installed or handheld, where appropriate—to detect guns, knives, or other weapons
- Enclosed nurses' stations, deep service counters, or bullet-resistant, shatterproof glass in reception, triage, and admitting areas or client service rooms
- Employee "safe rooms" for use during emergencies
- "Time-out" or seclusion areas with high ceilings without grids for patients who "act out"
- Separate rooms for forensic patients
- Comfortable client or patient waiting rooms designed to minimize stress
- Locks on counseling rooms, treatment rooms, and staff bathrooms
- Efficient closers on doors (shouldn't be too slow)
- Bright, effective lighting, both indoors and outdoors
- Minimal furniture, arranged to prevent entrapment, without sharp corners or edges and affixed to the floor, if possible
- Limited number of pictures, vases, or other items that can be used as weapons
- Curved mirrors for hallway intersections or concealed areas

Alarm systems and other monitoring/response devices include the following:
- Panic buttons (at nurses' stations, triage stations, registration areas, hallways, nurse lounge areas)
- Handheld alarms or noise devices
- Cellular phones, particularly for home health care workers
- Private-channel radios

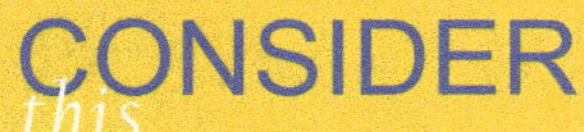

Preparing for an Active Shooter Event—Online Resource Tools

For additional information or tools to prepare your organization for an active-shooter event, visit the following links:

- "Preventing Workplace Violence in Healthcare" (US Occupational Safety and Health Administration)
  https://www.osha.gov/dsg/hospitals/workplace_violence.html

- "Workplace Violence Prevention Resources" portal (The Joint Commission)
  https://www.jointcommission.org/workplace_violence.aspx

- "Preparing for Active Shooter Situations" (*Quick Safety*, Issue 4, The Joint Commission)
  http://www.jointcommission.org/assets/1/23/Quick_Safety_Issue_Four_July_2014_Final.pdf

- "Preventing Violence in the Health Care Setting" (*Sentinel Event Alert*, Issue 45, The Joint Commission)
  http://www.jointcommission.org/assets/1/18/sea_45.pdf

- "Active Shooter Planning and Response in a Healthcare Setting," 3rd edition (Healthcare and Public Health Sector Critical Infrastructure Protection Partnership)
  https://www.fbi.gov/file-repository/active_shooter_planning_and_response_in_a_healthcare_setting.pdf

- "Hospital Code Silver Activation: Active Shooter Planning Checklist" (California Hospital Association)
  http://www.calhospitalprepare.org/sites/main/files/file-attachments/cha_active_shooter_checklist_12-19-12.doc

- "Active Shooter: How to Respond" (US Department of Homeland Security)
  http://www.urmc.rochester.edu/MediaLibraries/URMCMedia/flrtc/documents/active_shooter_booklet.pdf

- "Active Shooter Drill Materials" (Hospital Association of Southern California)
  http://www.hasc.org/active-shooter-drill-resources

Note: *All websites were accessed Feb 20, 2018.*

- Video cameras and surveillance
- Tagging mechanisms—these systems usually relate to infant/child abduction and involve a band attached to the infant or child by the ankle, wrist, or umbilical cord. Movement of the infant/child past any of the strategically located sensors triggers an alarm to initiate staff response.
- Delayed-egress door hardware, including alarms
- Staff education about security measures—a knowledgeable and aware staff is instrumental in helping prevent infant/child abductions.
- Requiring staff to wear easily recognizable, clearly displayed photo identification badges—these must be surrendered upon termination of employment, and all missing badges must be immediately reported and an appropriate security response initiated.

Staff should be trained on all security procedures and on the use of any high-tech devices.

Education of new parents also is paramount to preventing infant abductions. The parents should be introduced to general security precautions at prenatal classes and given more specific information at the time of admission. Parental education may include some general security tips, such as refraining from publishing birth announcements in newspapers and not giving out personal information on social media. Organizations also should consider posting information about preventing infant abduction within the mother's room. In any event, caregivers will want to reinforce the security safeguards during their initial and follow-up care of the mother.

Staff on pediatric units also may want to screen the parent or guardian who accompanies an infant or child to the organization in order to identify potentially disruptive family situations, such as estrangement or a custody battle that might affect unit security. The better informed the entire unit staff, the safer the unit.

Patient Wandering and Elopement

Patient wandering and/or elopement can happen in any health care setting, but the risk is greatest in situations in which patients are fully mobile but cognitively limited or impaired. For example, it is not uncommon for individuals being served in locked behavioral health care units to try to escape. Likewise, geriatric patients who are physically capable but mentally impaired (for example, patients

with Alzheimer's or dementia) also are at risk for wandering or elopement.

The mismanagement of a patient's whereabouts ranges from a minor situation in which a patient, briefly, cannot be located readily, to a major situation in which a patient has actually left the facility. Most often, the patient who is missing has gone for tests as scheduled, is with family on a walk or in the cafeteria, or is visiting with another patient in that patient's room.

The gravity of an elopement situation depends to a certain extent on who is missing: The disappearance of a behavioral health care patient or a nursing care center resident can be very serious, whereas the decision to leave the facility by a rational, voluntary adult medical/surgical patient is not as much of a problem. Some wanderers suffer from Alzheimer's disease or another form of dementia; others experience disorientation as a result of a drug.

The goal in managing the wandering individual is to prevent elopement—leaving the premises without permission and/or without understanding the consequences of doing so. Elopement may be intentional or unintentional. To prevent elopement, security managers should assess their organizations for potential wandering and elopement threats. Talking with department managers of units that are at high risk for elopement, such as behavioral health care areas, geriatric units, and so forth, can help pinpoint organization risks.

When risks have been identified, organizations can work to address them. Possible interventions include the following:

- Thorough patient assessment for possible wandering and/or elopement potential
- Use of technology to monitor patients, or track or limit their movements through the facility (for example, closed-circuit television, alarmed exits, window protection, locked exits, personal electronic tracking systems)
- Assigning high-risk individuals to rooms near the nursing station
- Maintaining vigilance among caregivers

Forensic Patients

Health care organizations sometimes treat patients who are under legal or correctional restrictions. These are known as forensic patients or prisoner patients. They typically require supervision by law enforcement officers and may enter the facility through the emergency department or be admitted directly for surgery or other procedures. Some facilities may see a greater number of forensic patients due to location, but all health care organizations should be prepared for the security risks that come with these cases.

Caring for these types of patients involves the heightened potential for security issues, such as violence, elopement, and presence of contraband. Forensic patients may be wearing personal monitoring devices or be physically restrained with devices such as handcuffs or shackles brought into the facility by law enforcement. Most security incidents occur when these restraints are partially or completely removed, either to perform a medical procedure or when the patient asks to use the bathroom or must change into a gown. During these times, the patient may attempt to escape, potentially using physical violence or weapons. One study conducted by the International Association for Healthcare Security and Safety found that most escape incidents that resulted in injuries occurred when the patient was able to gain control of the law enforcement officer's own weapon (firearm, Taser, pepper spray, or baton). The study also found that the restraints themselves may be used as a weapon to disable an officer or clinical personnel.[11]

Responding to risks

Forensic patients can be unpredictable, and security incidents can occur suddenly and without warning. Therefore it is important to manage risks through preparation. Health care organizations should work with the correctional facilities that transfer and monitor these patients to develop policies and procedures that address the varied concerns of both institutions. With the policies and procedures in place, health care organizations should educate and teach staff— particularly those in emergency departments and any medical/surgical unit that would be caring for such patients—to manage high-risk situations with this specific patient population.

It is important that staff be able to recognize situations that present the highest risk. For example, as previously mentioned, risk increases whenever restraints are removed. Other high-risk situations include when the patient is moved and when a health care worker must be in close physical proximity to the patient to provide care. Extra caution should be exercised whenever sharps or other potentially dangerous items are used. If an organization determines that it treats

a high volume of forensic patients, it may wish to evaluate its own security staff to ensure that it is adequate to meet needs.

Familiarity with procedures is another important factor in maintaining security. Organizations may want to run "prisoner escape" drills with staff who are likely to encounter forensic patients. These drills can be very helpful in translating knowledge into action. Also, staff should know what to expect from law enforcement officers and how to interact with them appropriately and effectively. In addition, law enforcement or corrections officers that accompany forensic patients should receive orientation and training on what to expect in the health care setting.

Finally, the physical environment itself can be used to mitigate risks from forensic patients. Organizations should ensure that they have facilities that are appropriate to house and treat forensic patients. For example, hospitals— particularly small or rural ones—do not have well-secured areas designated specifically for inmates. In these cases, a standard room must be prepared before the patient is admitted. Preparations may include removing or securing any items or equipment that could be used as a weapon. Also, the room must be large enough to accommodate any officers who accompany the patient.

Technology and Data Security

As information technology continues to expand, health care organizations are relying more and more on electronic data storage and transfer. Everything from prescriptions to financial documents, clinical records to employee files, has moved from paper to electronic documents. This transition has resulted in a similar expansion in the number, seriousness, and scope of threats to those data. Add to this the necessity of confidentiality surrounding an individual's health information, and data security emerges as a primary concern for modern health care organizations.

Technology-related risks are varied and can originate from individuals within the organization (that is, employees) or outside the organization. Risks include the following:

- Identity theft
- Sabotage of networks or data systems, such as intentional infection with viruses or malware
- Exposure of sensitive patient medical data, such as diseases, medical conditions, and treatments

The National Center for Missing & Exploited Children

The National Center for Missing & Exploited Children (NCMEC)—the leading nonprofit organization in the United States dedicated to issues related to missing and sexually exploited children—publishes *For Health Care Professionals: Guidelines on Prevention of and Response to Infant Abductions*. This free online resource, now in its 10th edition, provides the following to health care organizations:

- Summary guidelines—not legal advice—to assist the prevention of infant abductions
- "Typical" abductor profile, with a warning that an abductor may not fit such a profile
- Physical security measures and development of a response plan in the event of an abduction
- Potential abduction for additional health care settings, including the home, after an infant is discharged from a maternal/child care unit
- Self-assessment tool for hospitals to determine risks associated with infant abduction

For Health Care Professionals: Guidelines on Prevention of and Response to Infant Abductions is accessible through the NCMEC website at https://www.missingkids.org/ourwork/publications/missing/nc05 (Accessed Feb 20, 2018).

- Unauthorized access to restricted medications
- Potential for unauthorized control of portable and implantable medical devices, such as insulin pumps and pacemakers
- Adverse patient safety events that result from incorrect or miscommunicated information entered into an electronic health record

Assessing and addressing these risks require the combined efforts of information technology and security staff members. However, like all security issues, maintaining technology security should be part of every staff member's job responsibilities. Individuals should be encouraged and empowered to report, through established organizational procedures, anything they feel may put technological security in jeopardy (*see* page 123 for a cybersecurity checklist). The discussion beginning on page 124 outlines the top 10 myths of security risk analysis.

Although software has been known to fail, most data security risks are a function of access. Health care organizations should focus their risk-management efforts accordingly. Many risks can be minimized through simple, practical measures, such as installing a lock on a door to prevent unauthorized access to certain equipment, updating the virus protection software, or locating printers close to computers to minimize the risk of unattended documents. (For health information technology (IT) and new technology checklist tools, *see* pages 126 and 127, respectively.)

Other actions that can help maintain data security include the following:

- Requiring strong passwords and/or frequent updates to user passwords
- Updating software patches only as authorized by the manufacturer
- Encrypting data both in storage and in transit
- Limiting access to critical systems as much as possible, without compromising safety
- Educating and training staff members on use of technology at hiring, when new devices or systems are introduced, and/or periodically to refresh skills
- Reporting security incidents to the device manufacturer or software publisher to give insight into existing weaknesses and point to solutions

References

1. Bureau of Labor Statistics. Table R4: Number of Nonfatal Occupational Injuries and Illnesses Involving Days Away from Work by Industry and Selected Events or Exposures Leading to Injury or Illness, Private Industry, 2014. Accessed Feb 20, 2018. http://www.bls.gov/iif/oshwc/osh/case/ostb4370.pdf.

2. US Centers for Disease Control and Prevention, National Institute for Occupational Safety and Health. Occupational Violence. (Updated: Dec 13, 2016.) Accessed Feb 20, 2018. https://www.cdc.gov/niosh/topics/violence/default.html.

3. US Occupational Safety and Health Administration. Workplace Violence. Accessed Feb 20, 2018. https://www.osha.gov/SLTC/workplaceviolence/.

4. US Government Accountability Office. Report to Congressional Requesters. Workplace Safety and Health—Additional Efforts Needed to Help Protect Health Care Workers from Workplace Violence. Mar 2016. Accessed Feb 20, 2018. http://www.gao.gov/assets/680/675858.pdf.

5. US Occupational Safety and Health Administration. Preventing Workplace Violence in Healthcare. Dec 2015. Accessed Feb 20, 2018. https://www.osha.gov/dsg/hospitals/workplace_violence.html.

6. US Federal Bureau of Investigation. A Study of Active Shooter Incidents in the United States Between 2000 and 2013. Sep 16, 2013. Accessed Feb 20, 2018. https://www.fbi.gov/file-repository/active-shooter-study-2000-2013-1.pdf/.

7. The Joint Commission. Bullying has no place in health care. *Quick Safety*. No. 24. Jun 2016. Accessed Feb 20, 2018. https://www.jointcommission.org/assets/1/23/Quick_Safety_Issue_24_June_2016.pdf.

8. Workplace Bullying Institute. Healthy Workplace Bill. The Problem: What Is Workplace Bullying? Accessed Feb 20, 2018. http://healthyworkplacebill.org/problem/.

9. Tripwire. Identifying and Preventing Insider Threats. Zinatullin L. Oct 19, 2014. Accessed Feb 20, 2018. http://www.tripwire.com/state-of-security/incident-detection/identifying-and-preventing-insider-threats/.

10. i-Sight. 6 Tips to Lower Risk in High-Risk Employee Terminations. Dimoff T. Accessed Feb 20, 2018. http://i-sight.com/resources/6-tips-to-lower-risk-in-high-risk-employee-terminations/.

11. Security Magazine. Managing Security for Emergency Departments with High-Risk Patients. Warren B. May 1, 2014. Accessed Feb 20, 2018. http://www.securitymagazine.com/articles/85454-managing-security-for-emergency-departments-with-high-risk-patients.

RISK-ASSESSMENT TOOLBOX

1. [Download] Security Event Risk-Assessment Worksheet
2. [Download] Security Asset Risk-Assessment Worksheet
3. [Download] Medication Storage and Security Assessment Checklist
4. [Download] Environmental Risks for Workplace Violence Assessment Checklist
5. [Download] Cybersecurity Checklist
6. [Download] Health IT Security Decision Checklist
7. [Download] New Technology Decision Checklist

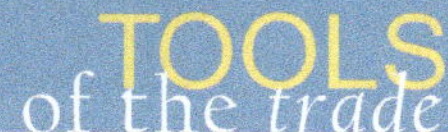

Cybersecurity Checklist

With various forms of technology housing protected health information (PHI), electronic health records (EHRs), and so on, assessing the risks of a health care facility's cybersecurity is paramount. This checklist provides organizations with a tool to determine how effective its cybersecurity is and identify its risks.

Note: *The complete checklist may be adapted and is available for internal use on the flash drive (print only) or by clicking the tool link in the Risk-Assessment Toolbox (e-book only) on page 122.*

Source: Adapted from US Department of Health & Human Services (HHS). *Top 10 Tips for Cybersecurity in Health Care.* Washington, DC. Accessed Feb 20, 2018. https://www.healthit.gov/sites/default/files/Top_10_Tips_for_Cybersecurity.pdf.

Published in *Environment of Care Risk Assessment,* Joint Commission Resources, 2018.   **File Name:** 05 05 Checklist Cybersecurity

CYBERSECURITY CHECKLIST

*This checklist can be used to assess cybersecurity risks in a health care organization. Answers to all questions should ideally be Y for **Yes** (unless they aren't applicable). If an answer is **N** for **No,** use the "Notes" section to document needed changes. Unless otherwise noted, this checklist is applicable to all program settings.*

ORGANIZATION: _________________________________   DEPARTMENT/UNIT: _________________________________

DATE OF REVIEW: _________________   REVIEWER: _________________________________

QUESTIONS	YES	NO	NA	NOTES
MOBILE DEVICES				
Policies are in place prescribing use of mobile devices.				
All staff members understand and agree to abide by mobile device policy and procedures.				
Mobile devices are configured to prevent unauthorized use.				
Protected health information (PHI) on mobile devices is encrypted.				
Connections between authorized mobile devices and electronic health records (EHRs) are encrypted.				
MAINTENANCE				
Policies are in place prescribing electronic health record (EHR) system maintenance procedures.				
Staff with responsibilities for maintenance understand and agree to system maintenance policies and procedures.				
Computers are free of unnecessary software and data files.				
Remote file sharing and printing (including remote printing) are disabled.				
Vendor remote maintenance connections are documented and fully secured.				

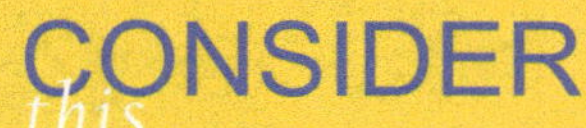

Security Risk Analysis—Top 10 Myths

The Health Insurance Portability and Accountability Act (HIPAA) Security Rule requires covered health care entities to conduct a security risk analysis (also known as risk assessment) of its organization. This risk analysis allows organizations to ensure their compliance with HIPAA security regulations, as well as identify potential threats to protected health information (PHI).

HIPAA's risk-analysis requirement comes with misunderstandings and misinformation. The following are the top 10 myths of security risk analysis according to the US Department of Health and Human Services' (HHS) Office of the National Coordinator for Health Information Technology.

1. *Security risk analysis is optional for small health care providers.*
   False. All providers considered "covered entities" under HIPAA are required to conduct a risk analysis.
2. *Installing a certified electronic health record (EHR) program fulfills the security risk analysis meaningful use (MU) requirement.*
   False. Providers must perform a full security risk analysis regardless if they use a certified EHR. Security requirements address all electronic protected health information (e-PHI) an organization maintains—not just what is included in an EHR.
3. *All privacy and security concerns can be addressed and handled by the EHR vendor.*
   False. EHR vendors may provide information, assistance, and training on the privacy and security aspects of the product, however they are not responsible for ensuring compliance with HIPAA Privacy and Security Rules.
4. *Security risk analysis must be outsourced.*
   False. Smaller providers may be able to conduct a security risk analysis using self-help tools. To ensure that a thorough and professional risk analysis that will stand up to compliance review is performed, expert knowledge is needed that may be obtained through an experienced outside professional.
5. *Providing a checklist will demonstrate compliance with the risk analysis requirement.*
   False. Checklists are useful tools, but fall short of performing a systematic security risk analysis or providing the required documentation that the risk analysis has been performed.
6. *There is one security risk analysis method that must be followed.*
   False. There are countless methods available to perform a security risk analysis. HHS provides resources to assist organizations identify and implement the most effective and appropriate safeguards to secure e-PHI.
7. *A security risk analysis only needs to review EHRs*
   False. All electronic devices that store, capture, or modify e-PHI should be included in a security risk analysis. EHR hardware and software, as well as devices that have access to EHR data (for example, tablet or mobile phone) also should be included in the analysis.
8. *Only one risk analysis is required.*
   False. To ensure compliance with HIPAA, organizations must continuously review, correct, modify, and update security protections.

9. *All risks must be fully mitigated before attesting an EHR incentive program.*

   False. The EHR incentive program requires correcting any deficiencies identified during the risk analysis when reporting as part of the risk-management process.

10. *Security risk analysis must be completely redone each year.*

    False. The full security risk analysis should be performed when an organization adopts an EHR. Each year following or when changes to the practice or electronic system occur, review and update the prior analysis to determine any new risks. Under the MU programs, reviews are required for each EHR reporting period; for eligible professionals, the EHR reporting period is 90 days or a full calendar year (depending on the eligible professional's year of participation in the program).

Source: US Department of Health and Human Services. Top 10 Myths of Security Risk Analysis. (Updated: Mar 28, 2014.) https://www.healthit.gov/providers-professionals/top-10-myths-security-risk-analysis (**Accessed:** Feb 20, 2018.)

Health IT Security Decision Checklist

Providing a secure environment is more than the physical facility. Organizations must protect their patients' privacy also. Organizations can use this checklist as part of the Health Insurance Portability and Accountability Act (HIPAA)–required security risk analysis to ensure HIPAA compliance and identify potential risks to protected health information.

Note: *The complete checklist may be adapted and is available for internal use on the flash drive (print only) or by clicking the tool link in the Risk-Assessment Toolbox (e-book only) on page 122.*

Published in *Environment of Care Risk Assessment*, Joint Commission Resources, 2018.   **File Name:** 05 06 Checklist Health IT Security

HEALTH IT SECURITY DECISION CHECKLIST

*This checklist can be used when contracting with data security firms, manufacturers, or vendors. It also can be used during mergers and acquisitions. This checklist helps to ensure HIPAA compliance and data security when two organizations work together or merge together and have potential access to protected health information. Answers to all questions should ideally be **Y** for **Yes** (unless they aren't applicable). If an answer is **N** for **No**, use the "Notes" section to document needed changes. Unless otherwise noted, this checklist is applicable to all program settings.*

ORGANIZATION: _________________________________   DEPARTMENT/UNIT: _________________________________

DATE OF REVIEW: ______________________   REVIEWER: _________________________________

TYPE OF REVIEW (FOR EXAMPLE, CONTRACTING, MERGER/ACQUISITION): _________________________________

QUESTIONS	YES	NO	NA	NOTES
Is there proof that the organization is compliant with HIPAA regulations, including HIPAA X12 5010?				
Does it provide HIPAA training?				
Has the organization had any security data breaches?				
If so, can the organization provide a summary of what happened and how it was resolved?				
Is there a process to safeguard confidential information and to protect your organization's PHI?				
Can the process provide strong encryption for data transfers or conversions?				
Can it provide encryption for confidential information or PHI sent through e-mail?				
Does it have encryption key management systems with access control?				
Will it deny third parties access to your data?				
Is it able to prevent data leaks (has it been tested and is it monitored and maintained for this purpose)?				

New Technology Decision Checklist

Organizations can use this checklist when making decisions about purchasing or adopting new technology, ensuring risks are discussed before acquiring new technology.

Note: *The complete checklist may be adapted and is available for internal use on the flash drive (print only) or by clicking the tool link in the Risk-Assessment Toolbox (e-book only) on page 122.*

Published in *Environment of Care Risk Assessment*, Joint Commission Resources, 2018.   **File Name:** 05 07 Checklist New Technology

NEW TECHNOLOGY DECISION CHECKLIST

This checklist includes questions to consider when an organizations is making a decision about purchasing or adopting new technology. It can ensure that all the necessary questions have been discussed regarding the new technology. Answers to all questions should ideally be **Y** *for* **Yes** *(unless they aren't applicable). Unless otherwise noted, this checklist is applicable to all program settings.*

ORGANIZATION: _________________________   DEPARTMENT/UNIT: _________________________

DATE OF REVIEW: _________________   REVIEWER: _________________________

TYPE OF TECHNOLOGY: _________________________

QUESTIONS	YES	NO	NA	NOTES
Does the new technology meet the needs of a specific environment in your organization?				
Will it improve patient care, streamline work, and/or automate mundane tasks?				
Have you asked end users for input as you have been exploring options related to the new technology?				
Have you examined product safety reviews or alerts for the new technology?				
Have you consulted a third party using the technology to confirm the manufacturer's or vendor's claims?				
Have you conducted a failure mode and effects analysis or human factors analysis on the technology?				
Is it interoperable with current technologies in your organization?				
Can changes be made to the technology to address organizational policies/protocols?				
Will it fit into your current work-flow processes or can you adjust work-flow processes to fit?				
Have you analyzed its impact on your security and confidentiality protocols as well as HIPAA compliance?				

Assessing Risk of Shooting

It is an unfortunate fact that people do bring weapons into health care organizations with the intent of causing injury or harm. The threat of a shooting incident is one that all hospitals must prepare to manage, whether the shooter is a staff member, patient, family member, or someone from the community.

According to Paul Ford, director of Safety, Security and Transportation at Tampa General Hospital in Florida, 146 shootings have taken place in hospitals over the past 10 years. None of those shootings have been active-shooter situations. By definition, an active shooter is an individual who actively engages in killing or attempting to kill people in a confined and populated area. Although an active shooter in a hospital is a possibility, the statistics say that hospital shooters have a particular purpose and a target.

Types of Shootings in Hospitals

Hospital shootings fall into four categories:
1. Prisoners who try to take a gun away from a police officer, primarily in the emergency department
2. Domestic violence situations involving a patient or staff member as the victim
3. Suicide shootings, in which a patient with a long-term or painful disease shoots himself or herself, or is shot by a family member, in an effort to relieve suffering
4. Grudge shootings, or incidents in which an individual seeks revenge

"Grudge shootings and domestic violence incidents are where I do most of my work with hospitals," Ford says. "That is usually where hospitals need to improve the way they assess shooter risks."

Areas of Special Risk

When assessing shooter risks, the following are considered critical focus areas:
- *Physical space.* This includes the building itself and all of its security features. How easy is it to enter the facility? What types of access controls are used? Are there security cameras and other surveillance systems, and how are they set up?

- *Neighborhood.* What is it like around the hospital? Is there significant gang activity? Does the state allow people to carry weapons?
- *Types of services offered.* Does the hospital offer historically high-risk services, such as pharmacies and transplant units? Does the hospital have any arrangements with law enforcement to care for forensic patients, or children who are removed from a dangerous home environment?

Type of organization. Trauma is another area of care that carries a high risk of violence—is the hospital a Level 1 trauma center, and how many trauma patients does the hospital see? Teaching hospitals, with their mix of physicians and residents with varying levels of experience, are at elevated risk.

Type of security personnel. Is the security staff employed by the hospital, or is it a contracted service? How much turnover is there in the security staff? What kind of training do they receive? Are they trained on how to assist police during a shooter situation?

History of violence. What kinds of incidents have happened at the facility in the past? Keeping records of all violent incidents enables the organization to track trends and better identify risks.

Organizational atmosphere regarding staff. Have there been layoffs at the hospital? Are there individuals in the organization who are difficult to work with? What is the termination procedure? Is employee health being managed appropriately?

Patient satisfaction. If an organization consistently receives negative comments about patient experiences, it may indicate a risk for retaliatory violence.

Creating Plans

All these items should be used to identify which areas are most likely to present risk of a shooting incident, and they should form the basis of a global (organizationwide) risk-management plan. According to Ford, this plan should address the following issues:

- Communication, such as what types of announcements will alert staff, patients, and visitors and keep them informed during an incident
- How to interact with police, including which staff members meet them at arrival and assist with navigation and access
- Training for all employees, with special focus for those working in high-risk areas, and incorporating realistic exercises or drills

Global (organizationwide) assessment must be combined with assessment that addresses risks in specific areas. These historically include the emergency department, pharmacy, transplant units, and human resources. The specific risks associated with these areas should be assessed separately. Staff working in these areas should be trained to recognize and respond to these particular risks and to be familiar with the communication process.

Responding to Risks

Each organization will have a unique mix of risks that will require a unique response. However, there are some systems that can strengthen an organization's preparedness.

Ford advocates for the following elements to mitigate the risk of injury or death during a shooter situation:

- First, Ford says hospitals should have a standardized system for reporting all incidents of violence to help track trends and be proactive in preventing violence from occurring.
- Second, he recommends a standardized, plain-language announcement system for shooting situations. Coded alerts protect staff, he explains, but leave patients and visitors unaware of the dangers.
- Third, he encourages organizations to create training exercises that use real-world strategies, including running or hiding in patient rooms or bathrooms.
- Finally, Ford recommends that all nursing stations have panic buttons and that staff know how and when to use them.

Ideally, risk assessments will not only help the organization effectively and safely respond to shooter situations but also prevent them from happening in the first place.

chapter 6

Fire Safety and Life Safety

A fire in a health care facility can be devastating. All health care facilities must be designed, constructed, maintained, and operated to minimize the possibility of a fire emergency. And yet, fire and life safety standards are among the most challenging for organizations to meet.

Fire Safety and Life Safety

Managing fire and smoke risks are addressed by The Joint Commission in two chapters of the *Comprehensive Accreditation Manual* (*CAM*) or E-dition: Fire safety is included in the Environment of Care (EC) standards, while the Life Safety (LS) standards are included in a separate, dedicated chapter (*see* page 132 for a checklist to assist with compliance with Standard EC.02.03.05). Fire safety and life safety are related concepts, but there are differences as they relate to Joint Commission purposes. (**Note:** *Because LS risks vary across health care settings, different accreditation programs have different LS requirements. When assessing LS risks,* see *the LS requirements in the applicable* CAM *or E-dition or program-specific requirements.*)

Fire safety standards address the minimum requirements for protecting against injury to life and/or property damage due to fire. They deal with general fire prevention and building construction issues, including fire drills, maintenance of firefighting and prevention equipment, and which measures to use during construction and other lapses in regular fire safety measures.

Joint Commission LS standards, by contrast, are written specifically to conform to the requirements of the National Fire Protection Association's (NFPA) *Life Safety Code*®* (NFPA 101–2012). The *Life Safety Code* is applicable only to threats of injury to life (not property) and encompasses incidents of panic as well as fire. LS standards are more detailed than the fire safety standards. They include requirements for systems, construction, and hardware issues, as well as building layout, design elements, and exits.

---

* *Life Safety Code*® is a registered trademark of the National Fire Protection Association, Quincy, MA.

STANDARDS to *know*

EC.01.01.01	LS.01.01.01
EC.02.01.01	LS.01.02.01
EC.02.01.03	LS.02.01.70
EC.02.03.03	LS.03.01.20
EC.02.05.01	LS.03.01.70
EC.02.06.05	

TERMS to *know*

barrier

fire watch

interim life safety measures (ILSM)

Life Safety Code®

occupancy

Checklist for Compliance with Standard EC.02.03.05

This checklist can help organizations ensure continuous compliance with Joint Commission Environment of Care (EC) Standard EC.02.03.05 and its requirements to inspect, test, and maintain fire equipment and fire safety building features, in addition to the frequency these tasks should be completed. *See* the *Comprehensive Accreditation Manual* or E-dition for additional information about this standard and its requirements.

Note: *The complete checklist may be adapted and is available for internal use on the flash drive (print only) or by clicking the tool link in the Risk-Assessment Toolbox (e-book only) on page 142.*

Published in *Environment of Care Risk Assessment*, Joint Commission Resources, 2018.   **File Name:** 06 01 Checklist Standard EC020305

CHECKLIST FOR COMPLIANCE WITH STANDARD EC.02.03.05

*This checklist can be used to determine compliance with The Joint Commission Environment of Care (EC) Standard EC.02.03.05, which requires organizations to maintain fire safety equipment and building features. Answers to all questions should ideally be Y for **Yes** (unless they aren't applicable). If an answer is N for **No**, use the "Notes" section to document needed changes. Check the Comprehensive Accreditation Manual or E-dition to determine specific program/setting applicability.*

ORGANIZATION: _________________________________ DEPARTMENT/UNIT: _________________________________

DATE OF REVIEW: _________________ REVIEWER: _________________________________

QUESTIONS	YES	NO	NA	NOTES
Do you have a complete inventory of all devices to be tested?				
Do you have a mechanism to confirm that all the appropriate devices have been tested and that none have been overlooked?				
Do you have a mechanism to ensure that the testing occurs in the required time frame and that the testing and results are documented in accordance with requirements?				
Do you have a method to make sure that service personnel are qualified and experienced in inspection, testing, and maintenance activities?				
Do you generate a deficiency report from any testing?				
Do you document any corrective actions to be taken, based on the report?				
Do you have a time line for these corrective actions?				
If repairs are made, do you have a mechanism to "close the loop," documenting the "who," "what," "where," and "when" of the repairs?				
Do you commission the system after the repairs?				

Overview of Assessing Risks

LS standards require an individual (or individuals) to be assigned to manage *Life Safety Code* compliance. This responsibility involves three areas:

1. Assessing the building for *Life Safety Code* compliance
2. Creating and maintaining the Statement of Conditions™ (SOC), as appropriate in accordance with Standard LS.01.01.01 (*see* "The Statement of Conditions™" section beginning on page 42 in Chapter 2)
3. Managing the resolution of any *Life Safety Code* deficiencies.

These three tasks may all be assigned to one person, or they may be assigned to different people. For example, an organization may put a building engineer in charge of assessing the building, an administrative professional in charge of the SOC, and the maintenance manager in charge of resolving any deficiencies.

No matter how the responsibilities are divided, representatives from various departments should be involved, as they will have insight into the fire risks that are most common in their areas. For example, surgical teams will be familiar with the fire risks associated with the use of supplemental oxygen and lasers, kitchen staff will know about risks from grease fires, and information technology staff will have experience with overheated electronics or static discharge.

Assessment Opportunities and Frequencies

There are several methods for assessing fire risks. These approach fire safety from both environmental and process-related perspectives. The primary methods (environmental tours, construction assessment, and fire drills) are described in this section, including their respective frequencies.

Environmental Tours

Fire safety can be assessed as part of an environmental tour, which could occur at frequencies defined by the organization relative to patient care areas and non–patient care areas. Any deficiencies noted can be entered into the work order system, the Building Maintenance Program (BMP), the Plan for Improvement (PFI) (*see* Chapter 2 for more information on PFIs), or other equivalent process, as appropriate (*see* page 134 for additional information about the BMP).

During Construction and General Maintenance

EC and LS standards require organizations to assess, manage, and take action to minimize fire safety risks during any demolition, construction, renovation projects, or general maintenance activity. Typically, areas under construction are inspected daily. Work that involves wiring or cabling is particularly prone to risk because it often requires the penetration of fire and smoke barriers. Any documentation or checklists used in the risk assessments should include anticipated code deficiencies based on the work at hand, as well as verification that any appropriate interim life safety measures (ILSM) or other mitigating actions have been put into place and are being enforced. More information on ILSM can be found later in this chapter.

Fire Drills

Fire drills must be used to identify fire safety risks according to Standard EC.02.03.03. Organizations are required to critique fire drills to evaluate the effectiveness of relevant equipment, building features, and staff response. Some examples of issues to watch for during fire drills are the release of the automatic hold-open devices on smoke barrier doors and audibility of the alarm system and associated overhead pages. Fire drill evaluations must be documented.

Fire drill–related standards also provide required frequencies for fire drills, which vary depending on the type of occupancy (*see* page 55 in Chapter 2 for a more detailed discussion for determining occupancy). Effective in 2018 all fire drills must be unannounced, in accordance with The Joint Commission and 2012 *Life Safety Code* requirements, and drills must be held at unexpected times and under varying conditions. Also, organizations must comply with new and revised requirements for managing fire and life safety hazards.[†] For health care and ambulatory health care occupancies, The Joint Commission does not require the evacuation of patients, residents, or individuals served during a drill. Also, drills must be held at unexpected times and under varying conditions (*see* the sample fire drill matrix beginning on page 135). When drills are conducted between 9:00 P.M. and 6:00 A.M., the organization does not have to use audible alarms to notify staff; alternative methods may be used to avoid disrupting sleeping patients.

[†] *See* the "Environment of Care" (EC) and "Life Safety" (LS) requirements of the *Comprehensive Accreditation Manual* or E-dition for setting-specific requirements.

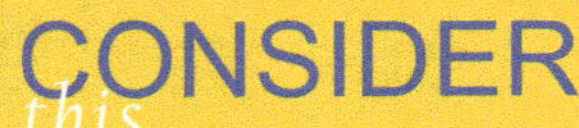

The Building Maintenance Program

As a proactive approach to Life Safety (LS) chapter compliance, an organization can choose to create a Building Maintenance Program (BMP)—an optional, planned way to appropriately and effectively manage certain features of fire protection in a health care facility. An effective BMP includes the following:

- Written strategies to manage the items covered in the program
- A documented schedule for the frequency of maintenance
- Processes for evaluating the effectiveness of the program

Although a BMP is not a requirement of the standards, The Joint Commission recommends creating one as a best practice to help proactively address potential repair and maintenance issues and prevent compliance problems. It is important to note that although organizations are encouraged to use this type of program, doing so will no longer provide a scoring advantage during an on-site survey.

BMPs do not apply to items that are lacking at a required location, but rather to those that are out of repair and, indeed, by virtue of their nature, may fail at any time. These may include issues with the following elements:

- Fire doors: automatic/self-closing, gaps, and undercuts
- Corridor separation: slab-to-slab/penetrations
- Corridor doors: positive latching, gaps, and undercuts
- Smoke barriers: slab-to-slab/penetrations
- Smoke barrier doors: self-closing devices, gaps, and undercuts
- Linen and waste chute doors
- Means of egress: illumination, snow, and ice
- Exit signs: illumination
- Grease-producing devices: inspection and cleaning

If any items on this list are found to be out of compliance, they should be repaired promptly, typically through a work order system.

The BMP is designed to allow health care organizations to manage risks appropriately and yet maintain the features of fire protection. Surveyors require evidence of ongoing maintenance or they will not accept it as a means of ensuring fire safety. Documentation of routine inspections and associated corrective maintenance should be used to demonstrate the effectiveness of a BMP.

Example Fire Drill Matrix

A fire drill matrix can pull together information from several sources to allow an organization to see any patterns that may be present. By collecting all the days, dates, and times from various shifts, a clear picture is formed of where the lack of variation occurs. In this sample matrix, there is a clear lack of variation. Three of the organization's four first-shift fire drills were conducted on Thursday mornings between 8:00 A.M. and 9:00 A.M. Similarly, the second-shift fire drills were conducted about the same time on Thursdays predominantly. This lack of variation demonstrates noncompliance with the required standards.

Note: *This matrix may be adapted and is available for internal use on the flash drive (print only) or by clicking the tool link in the Risk-Assessment Toolbox (e-book only) on page 142.*

Published in *Environment of Care Risk Assessment*, Joint Commission Resources, 2018.

File Name: 06 02 Fire Drill Matrix

Fire Drill Matrix

Organization: County Health Care

Score at: EC.02.03.03, EP 3

			Quarterly Fire Drills											
			Q1			Q2			Q3			Q4		
Day = M, Tu, W, Th, F, Sa, Su Time: 24-hour format			Jan	Feb	Mar	Apr	May	Jun	Jul	Aug	Sep	Oct	Nov	Dec
1st Shift	Normal	Location/Building	fl/main											
		Day	M											
		Date	1-2-16											
		Time	0700											
	ILSM	Location/Building												
		Day												
		Date												
		Time												
2nd Shift	Normal	Location/Building												
		Day												
		Date												
		Time												
	ILSM	Location/Building												
		Day												
		Date												
		Time												
3rd Shift	Normal	Location/Building												
		Day												
		Date												
		Time												
	ILSM	Location/Building												
		Day												
		Date												
		Time												

continued

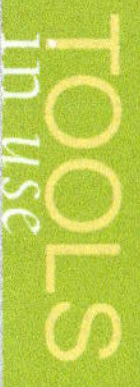

Published in *Environment of Care Risk Assessment*, Joint Commission Resources, 2018.

File Name: 06 02 Fire Drill Matrix

Previous and Current High-Risk Fire Drills (recommended, not required)
(e.g., kitchen, surgery, cath/EP lab, MRI, plant)

Location	Kitchen		Location			Location			Location			Location		
	Previous	Current		Previous	Current		Previous	Current		Previous	Current		Previous	Current
Day	W	Th	Day			Day			Day			Day		
Date	10-15-15	10-9-16	Date			Date			Date			Date		
Time	0900	1200	Time			Time			Time			Time		

Quarterly Ambulatory Fire Drills

1st Shift		Q1	Q2	Q3	Q4		Q1	Q2	Q3	Q4
	Location/ Building	AST				Location/ Building				
	Day	Tu				Day				
	Date	2-15-16				Date				
	Time	1200				Time				

Annual Business Occupancy Fire Drills (2 Years of Drills)

Building	Medical Office Bl		Building			Building			Building			Building		
	Previous	Current		Previous	Current		Previous	Current		Previous	Current		Previous	Current
Day	W	Th	Day			Day			Day			Day		
Date	5-14-15	6-10-16	Date			Date			Date			Date		
Time	0900	1300	Time			Time			Time			Time		

Definitions of Shifts

Using the following table, provide timeframes for shift hours
(e.g., 1st shift: 0700–1600; 2nd shift: 1600–2400; 3rd shift: 2400–0700

1st shift	
2nd shift	
3rd shift	

NA   Not applicable for no shift, building, location, or ILSM.

NC   Not completed or missed.

EC, environment of care; cath/EP lab, cardiac catheterization/electrophysiology laboratory; MRI, magnetic resonance imaging; ILSM, interm life safety measures.

If an organization operates in rented or leased space, these drills need to be conducted only in the areas occupied by the organization.

Identifying Risks

Fire safety risks can be identified in several ways. As previously described, they can come from environmental tours or required fire drills. Preconstruction risk assessments are another source, as fire safety is frequently affected by common construction activities and maintenance activities, such as opening walls or ceilings, or interrupting utilities such as electricity and water. These risks must be identified and managed before and during any demolition, construction, renovation, or general maintenance.

Engineering and maintenance staff who make periodic rounds of the building or who perform building assessments should be aware of *Life Safety Code* issues. Any deficiencies discovered should be addressed promptly. These rounds should address issues such as damaged smoke or fire barrier doors, burned-out exit lights, inappropriate door wedges, broken latches, and so on. (These are the types of deficiencies that often are included in a BMP, addressed earlier in this chapter.) Inspections by state and local fire control agencies, as well as third-party entities such as insurance companies, also can reveal risks. (*See* page 138 for a life safety mock tracer worksheet that can be used as a tool to identify risks.)

The SOC tool was designed with the sole purpose of helping organizations identify EC and LS risks and deficiencies to maintain a constant state of safety and compliance. Although the SOC is no longer mandatory to maintain a record of deficiencies and improvements made outside the on-site survey, The Joint Commission highly encourages health care organizations to use this tool to more efficiently maintain *Life Safety Code* compliance. (*See* Chapter 2 for a detailed discussion about the SOC.)

Interim Life Safety Measures

Sometimes a building code deficiency identified within the SOC cannot be corrected immediately. Construction or renovation projects or maintenance activity create temporary deficiencies that must be addressed. During such times, the safety of patients, staff, and others (for example, vendors, construction workers) coming to an organization's facilities is diminished.

To address these potential safety risks, health care organizations need to proactively identify administrative actions to be taken to preserve patient, staff, and visitor safety. The Joint Commission has created several such administrative actions—called ILSM—that can help organizations temporarily compensate for significant hazards posed by deficiencies, construction, or maintenance activities. Certain ILSM are designed for construction and renovation; however, most can be applied to any situation that compromises life safety. Examples of ILSM include additional fire drills, fire watches, signage to indicate alternate exits, and ensuring unobstructed exits.

For accreditation programs that are required to have an ILSM policy, failure to implement this policy can cause an adverse decision for the organization that will result in a follow-up survey to assess the organization's resolution of this failure.

Creating an ILSM Policy

Although not all ILSM must be implemented for every *Life Safety Code* deficiency and/or every construction project, all assessments and implementations must be documented. Hospital and critical access hospital programs are required to develop a policy as to which of the ILSM are appropriate for deficiencies and projects of various scope and duration, while ambulatory health care (ambulatory occupancy) and behavioral health care programs are recommended to develop a policy. The policy must include written criteria for evaluating various deficiencies and construction hazards to determine when and to what extent the different ILSM apply. It is recommended that the policy be approved by the organization's EC committee. (*See* page 140 for a sample of such a policy.)

ILSM Risk Management

The need for ILSM can be determined by conducting an ILSM risk assessment. Similar to other risk assessments, this process is used to mitigate risks identified during an LS–deficient situation. Some organizations use a form to assess the need for ILSM (*see* page 141 for an ILSM matrix).

Identifying Participants

When determining the appropriate ILSM, working with staff in the area where ILSM are needed is beneficial because they are more familiar with the location and the needs of those within that location. They also may identify some obstacles in

Life Safety Mock Tracer Worksheet

Organization's can use or create a mock tracer worksheet focused on fire and life safety issues to determine risks. Mock tracers are another tool organizations can add to their risk-assessment arsenal to identify fire and life safety risks.

Note: *The complete worksheet may be adapted and is available for internal use on the flash drive (print only) or by clicking the tool link in the Risk-Assessment Toolbox (e-book only) on page 142.*

Published in *Environment of Care Risk Assessment*, Joint Commission Resources, 2018.　　　**File Name:** 06 03 Worksheet Life Safety Tracer

LIFE SAFETY MOCK TRACER WORKSHEET

This tracer worksheet is filled in with questions pertinent to life safety, but can be revised to fit a particular program setting or health care facility. Review the relevant standards listed in the next section to determine what requirements are applicable to specific programs and settings.

Relevant Standards for these questions include the following: LS.01.01.01, LS.02.01.10, LS.02.01.30, LS.02.01.35, LS.02.01.40, LS.02.01.50, LS.03.01.10, LS.03.01.30, LS.03.01.35, and LS.03.01.40. Relevant standards cited are not necessarily applicable to every question; determine applicability within a specific program/setting. Check the comprehensive

implementing ILSM that need to be addressed. When assessing for ILSM, organizations should consider consulting the construction manager, engineers, architects, infection control, and other individuals closely associated with the project or corrective action, as they may have an in-depth understanding of the implications associated with the potential LS deficiencies.

Identifying Areas That Require ILSM

Organizations need to implement ILSM only in areas of the building that are affected by a construction project or deficiency. For example, additional fire drills might be required only in areas where one of the egress paths is temporarily unavailable.

To determine if ILSM are necessary, organizations should continuously monitor for potential EC and LS deficiencies. This can be done in a variety of ways, including by regularly reviewing the SOC, conducting optional environmental tours and building maintenance rounds, listening to staff reports, and continually examining construction and renovation plans.

When a potential deficiency is discovered, individual(s) within the organization, such as the facilities manager or the safety officer, must determine what ILSM can address the deficiency appropriately and thoroughly.

By their very nature, ILSM are intended to be temporary and should be in place only while the deficiencies exist. When an organization is in compliance with the EC or LS requirements, the ILSM can be eliminated.

Ensuring Compliance with ILSM

While ILSM are in place, organizations may post information about those measures implemented (via website, posters, or communication boards) so that staff and others affected are aware. In addition, staff should be trained on the ILSM, how to identify potential safety risks, and how to report activities that occur without the proper risk-prevention measures.

Organizations also should establish ways to ensure ongoing compliance with the designated ILSM and the need for further training or additional measures. This may involve periodic tours of the site, feedback from staff working in the area, or the use of a checklist.

Equivalencies

Sometimes, an assessment may identify a *Life Safety Code* deficiency that is impossible or impractical to correct due to time, logistics, or structural or financial restrictions. In these cases, an organization may request an equivalency, rather than pursuing repair or renovation to correct the deficiency.

An equivalency is a documented recognition that the intent of a *Life Safety Code* provision has been met, but the manner in which it is met is different from the design prescribed by the *Life Safety Code*. Waivers from state or local fire marshals are not recognized by The Joint Commission as approved equivalencies.

Equivalency Types

There are two types of equivalencies: traditional equivalencies and Fire Safety Evaluation System (FSES) equivalencies:

1. *Traditional equivalencies* propose alternative solutions to a single deficiency or a small group of similar deficiencies. For example, an organization's laundry chute does not have sprinklers at the top, bottom, and every other level of the building. A proposed equivalency might be to install hardwired smoke detectors within 10 feet of the chute inlet door in the appropriate rooms on every floor.

2. *FSES equivalencies* are based on an evaluation system developed by the Building and Fire Research Laboratory at the National Institute of Standards and Technology. These equivalencies address situations in which multiple deficiencies within a single building cannot be corrected in a practical manner, or when a single deficiency affects the entire building—for example, noncompliance in a construction area of a building that is fully protected by an approved automatic sprinkler system.

Both traditional and FSES equivalencies must be requested through The Joint Commission. Requests are reviewed only for survey-related deficiencies. If approved, it will remain valid until activities—such as construction, renovation, or reorganization—correct the deficiency.

The Human Factor

While fire protective elements can provide the basis for fire safety in the environment of care, risk assessments must take into account human action in that environment. Activities such as smoking, overloading an electrical outlet, cluttering corridors, and decorating an area with combustible decorations can compromise fire and life safety. The following sections will discuss these common human factors in fire safety.

Smoking

As discussed in Chapter 3, smoking in a health care facility can increase safety risks. Cigarettes, cigars, and other smoking devices that burn tobacco also create fire safety risks from lighting, use, and disposal of the item.

The Joint Commission fire safety standards in the EC chapter require organizations to have written policies that prohibit smoking in all buildings, except in specific circumstances. If the health care organization allows these exceptions, smoking must be contained in designated smoking areas that are physically separate from patient care areas and contain all appropriate fire safety features.

E-Cigarettes

E-cigarettes are gaining in popularity, and health care organizations need to make sure their policies reflect this new technology. Though e-cigarettes do not use a traditional ignition source, such as a match or lighter, or burn tobacco, they still pose a potential fire hazard.

E-cigarettes use a battery to send a small electrical current to the atomizer, which vaporizes the nicotine solution for inhalation. The hazard is associated with the conversion of the current into heat to vaporize the liquid. Some models include a rechargeable battery that can malfunction and cause explosions and fires. Although fires and explosions are rare, the US Fire Administration notes that there were 25 incidents between 2009 and 2014 that resulted in nine injuries, two with serious burns; most of the incidents occurred while the batteries were charging.[1]

The Joint Commission's standard that prohibits smoking except in specific circumstances applies to e-cigarettes, as well as other forms of smoking. Health care organizations should be prepared to deal with patients, staff, and visitors who may want to use an e-cigarette in the facility.

Organizations are encouraged to update their existing policies to include e-cigarettes and to be sure those policies are enforced. Tips on how to do this effectively can be found in the free Joint Commission publication *Keeping Your Hospital Property Smoke-Free: Successful Strategies for Effective Policy Enforcement and Maintenance*, which is available at http://www.jointcommission.org/assets/1/18/Smoke_Free_Brochure2.pdf.

Electrical Overload

Electrical devices are everywhere in a health care facility. Medical equipment, light fixtures, computer components, and charging devices for portable electronics all require electrical outlets. In many health care facilities, the need for electrical power has outpaced the number of available outlets. This can lead to shortcuts and workarounds, such as overloading outlets or misusing power strips, which create fire hazards. Organizations must ensure that every staff member is

Interim Life Safety Measures Policy

To ensure safety when building code deficiencies cannot be corrected immediately, organizations must have an interim life safety measures (ILSM) policy (such as this sample) to outline the administrative actions to ensure safety.

Note: *The complete policy may be adapted and is available for internal use on the flash drive (print only) or by clicking the tool link in the Risk-Assessment Toolbox (e-book only) on page 142.*

Source: Adapted from US Army Medical Department, US Army Public Health Center, Aberdeen Proving Ground, MD. Medical Safety Template—Interim Life Safety Measures Policy (Updated: Feb 2015.) Accessed Feb 20, 2018. http://phc.amedd.army.mil/PHC%20 Resource%20Library/MedicalSafetyTemplate-InterimLifeSafetyMeasuresPolicy.docx.

Published in *Environment of Care Risk Assessment*, Joint Commission Resources, 2018.   **File Name:** 06 04 Policy ILSM

INTERIM LIFE SAFETY MEASURES POLICY

This sample policy can be used to develop an interim life safety measures (ILSM) policy for any health care organization.

SOP No: ____

DISK FILE NAME: ____

EFFECTIVE DATE: ____

DATE REMOVED FROM SERVICE: ____________________________

---

vigilant about safe electrical usage practices to avoid those that might lead to electrical fires.

Plan Ahead for Usage

Ideally, an organization will add electrical outlets as need increases. This is not always feasible, though, as electrical work involves major construction activities, such as opening walls and ceilings and interrupting power. Such activities are lengthy and costly. However, if an organization is planning a construction or renovation project, it can use the project as an opportunity to not only meet current electrical needs but also anticipate future needs.

Safe Use of Power Strips and Extension Cords

Misuse of power strips (also known as relocatable power taps, or RPTs) and extension cords is a common cause of electrical fires. Two common misuses are "daisy chains" (one power strip or extension cord plugged into another to provide more outlets or reach greater distances), and the "mixed daisy chain" (power strips and extension cords interconnected). Both of these practices can create an electrical current overload, which can result in a fire. (*See* page 143 for additional information on RPTs.)

The US Occupational Safety and Health Administration (OSHA) requires that electrical equipment be used in accordance with the conditions under which it was approved by a recognized testing organization. In addition, NFPA provides regulations for electrical usage in health care facilities, including use of ground fault circuit interrupters (GFCIs) in locations near water, minimum number of outlets, and when and how power strips may be used.

Areas at Heightened Risk

Some areas of a health care facility are at greater risk for electrical fires due to the nature of the work done in those areas or to the type of patients inhabiting those areas. These locations include utility systems and maintenance areas, laboratories, pediatric units, surgical units, hyperbaric facilities, and any place medical gases are used.

Non-Hospital Grade Equipment

Of the many pieces of electrical equipment used in health care organizations, some are available in various grades that reflect the needs of a particular environment. For example, a power strip that is commercial grade may not be suitable for use in a health care environment. The Joint Commission has no standards that specifically address whether equipment must be hospital grade. All equipment must comply with NFPA codes. In particular, NFPA 99, *Health Care Facilities Code*, requires that all receptacles in patient care areas be tested after initial installation, replacement, and servicing of the device. Those that are hospital grade must be tested at regular intervals that are determined by performance data. By contrast, receptacles not listed as hospital grade must be tested not less than every 12 months.

Interim Life Safety Measures Matrix

Use this matrix to identify what interim life safety measures (ILSM) are applicable to mitigate existing *Life Safety Code®** deficiencies, demolition, construction, renovation, and maintenance activities, as well as noting which areas of the facility are impacted.

Note: *The complete matrix may be adapted and is available for internal use on the flash drive (print only) or by clicking the tool link in the Risk-Assessment Toolbox (e-book only) on page 142.*

** Life Safety Code®* is a registered trademark of the National Fire Protection Association, Quincy, MA.

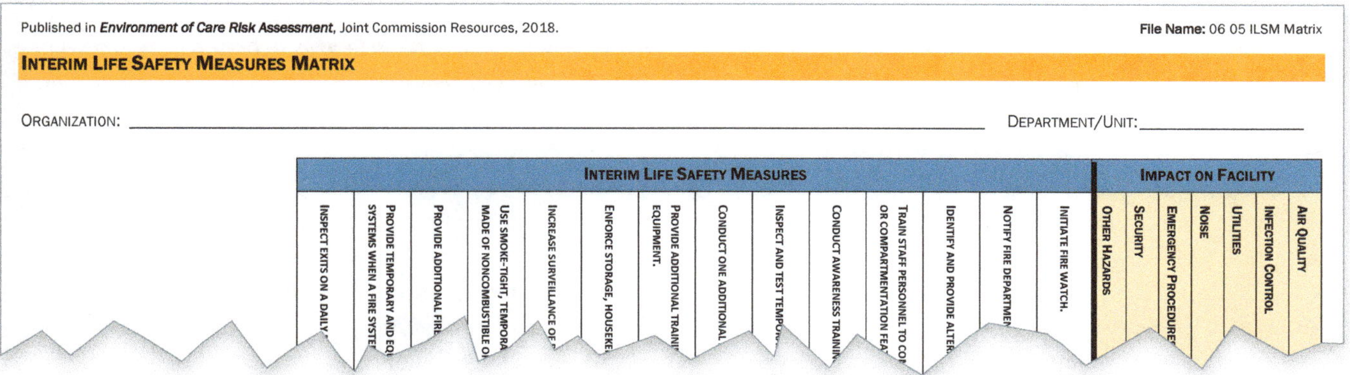

Published in *Environment of Care Risk Assessment,* Joint Commission Resources, 2018.

File Name: 06 05 ILSM Matrix

INTERIM LIFE SAFETY MEASURES MATRIX

ORGANIZATION: ____   DEPARTMENT/UNIT: _______________

INTERIM LIFE SAFETY MEASURES															IMPACT ON FACILITY						
INSPECT EXITS ON A DAILY…	SYSTEMS WHEN A FIRE SYSTE…	PROVIDE TEMPORARY AND EQ…	PROVIDE ADDITIONAL FIRE…	MADE OF NONCOMBUSTIBLE O…	USE SMOKE-TIGHT, TEMPORA…	INCREASE SURVEILLANCE OF…	ENFORCE STORAGE, HOUSEKE…	PROVIDE ADDITIONAL TRAINI… EQUIPMENT.	CONDUCT ONE ADDITIONAL…	INSPECT AND TEST TEMPOR…	CONDUCT AWARENESS TRAINI…	TRAIN STAFF PERSONNEL TO CO… OR COMPARTMENTATION FEA…	IDENTIFY AND PROVIDE ALTER…	NOTIFY FIRE DEPARTMEN…	INITIATE FIRE WATCH.	OTHER HAZARDS	SECURITY	EMERGENCY PROCEDURE…	NOISE	UTILITIES	INFECTION CONTROL	AIR QUALITY

Corridor Clutter

When a fire or other emergency occurs, staff and patients must have the ability to move unencumbered. The standards require that the means of egress is not inhibited in any way. Health care organizations are required to maintain free and unobstructed access to exits in addition to limiting wall projections into corridors.

It is not always easy to know what constitutes "clutter" in a corridor. In general, if a corridor looks cluttered, it most likely *is* cluttered. One of the practices that causes clutter is storing items in a corridor. An item is considered stored if it has not been used for patient care in the past 30 minutes. This also applies to patients, who are sometimes staged on gurneys or in wheelchairs in corridors due to overcrowding in areas, such as an emergency department or an imaging depart-ment. The *Life Safety Code* explicitly prohibits patient sleeping or treatment in corridors.

A common item stored in corridors is mobile workstations, such as computers on wheels. At certain times, such as during morning charting, these items may be in constant use, moving frequently. At other times, however, such as over-night hours, they may not be in use at all. Organizations that use mobile workstations must manage them properly to avoid storing them in corridors when not in use. Also, it is important to make sure the mobile workstation does not attract other items, such as chairs or wastebaskets.

The *Life Safety Code* makes exceptions for very specific items, such as emergency, "in use," and transport equipment (for example, crash carts). The Joint Commission also allows other kinds of carts, such as isolation carts or chemo carts, to be stored outside the associated patient's room until that patient is discharged.

Managing Corridors

There are several simple ways organizations can effectively manage corridor clutter:

- ◉ *Educate staff.* Be sure everyone understands the how and why of keeping corridors clear.
- ◉ *Reduce unused equipment.* For example, return items from other departments that are kept in corridors as a convenience, and ensure that patient care items are kept in patient rooms.
- ◉ *Maximize dead-end corridors.* If a section of corridor does not support egress, such as the space between the end wall of a hallway and the first set of doors, it is considered a "dead end." If a dead-end space is used for storage of equipment, organizations are limited to 50 square feet of storage before it must be protected as a hazardous space. Storage in dead-end corridors requires use of other features as well, either quick-response sprinklers or standard sprinklers and smoke detection.

See page 145 for a real-world project to manage corridor clutter.

Projections into the Corridor

Items are frequently mounted to corridor walls, including hand rub dispensers, computer work desks, and display monitors. If these project into the corridor, they may interfere with people or equipment moving through the hallway during a fire or other emergency situation. If a corridor is 6 feet wide or greater, the *Life Safety Code* allows certain items to project into the corridor space, though they must not be greater than 36 inches wide and project no more than 6 inches into the corridor. Headroom also must be considered, as items that are mounted near the ceiling, such as monitors, may obstruct not only movement but also visibility of exit signs. Alcohol-based hand rub (ABHR) dispensers must be mounted no less than 48 inches from another ABHR dispenser.

Decorations

Many organizations decorate their facilities for holidays: lights at Christmas, pumpkins at Halloween, streamers for the Fourth of July. These can be a welcome change from the sometimes unwelcoming health care environment. However, they must be selected and placed thoughtfully to maintain fire safety.

Only noncombustible decorations are allowed under the provisions of the *Life Safety Code*. Christmas trees, for example, must be artificial and fire-retardant; live trees are prohibited. Similarly, use of straw, branches, gauze, or similar materials is not allowed. Open flames, such as candles, are not acceptable, though battery-operated candles are permitted.

In addition, the placement of decorations can affect fire safety. Attaching items to walls, doors, floors, ceiling, or any fire protective devices (for example, sprinkler heads, exit signs, fire extinguishers, fire-rated doors)—although seemingly convenient and festive—creates fire hazards or obstructs fire protective devices. Freestanding items should be secured so they do not topple over, and they must not obstruct doors or corridors. Combustible decorations should not be placed on fire-rated door assemblies and should not prevent any type of door from closing or latching.

Most of these guidelines are common sense. If there is doubt about what decorations may be used or where, organizations are encouraged to either consult the local fire regulatory agency or simply err on the side of caution and forgo the item in question. (*See* page 144 for a decorations assessment checklist.)

Reference

1.   US Fire Administration, Federal Emergency Management Agency. Electronic Cigarette Fires and Explosions, July 2017. Accessed Feb 20, 2018. https://www.usfa.fema.gov/downloads/pdf/publications/electronic_cigarettes.pdf.

RISK-ASSESSMENT TOOLBOX

1. **Download** Checklist for Compliance with Standard EC.02.03.05
2. **Download** Fire Drill Matrix
3. **Download** Life Safety Mock Tracer Worksheet
4. **Download** Interim Life Safety Measures Policy
5. **Download** Interim Life Safety Measures Risk-Assessment Matrix
6. **Download** Decorations Assessment Checklist

Relocatable Power Taps

NFPA 99-2012, 10.2.3.6 allows for multiple outlet connections, also known as relocatable power taps (RPTs) or power strips, to be used with electrical equipment in health care facilities. Requirements for use differ when these devices are used in the patient care vicinity versus outside of the patient care vicinity, as well as for use with patient care–related electrical equipment versus non-patient care–related electrical equipment.

Power strips may be used outside of the patient care vicinity for both patient care–related electrical equipment and non-patient care–related electrical equipment.

General requirements include, but are not limited to, the following:
- Ensuring they are never "daisy-chained"
- Preventing cords from becoming tripping hazards
- Installing internal ground fault and over-current protection devices
- Using power strips that are adequate for the number and types of devices used

Patient Care Vicinity

Power strips may be used in a patient care vicinity to power rack-, table-, pedestal-, or cart-mounted patient care–related electrical equipment assemblies, provided all of the following conditions are met:
- The receptacles are permanently attached to the equipment assembly.
- The sum of the ampacity of all appliances connected to the receptacles does not exceed 75% of the ampacity of the flexible cord supplying the receptacles.
- The ampacity of the flexible cord is suitable in accordance with the current edition of NFPA 70, *National Electrical Code®*.
- The electrical and mechanical integrity of the assembly is regularly verified and documented through an ongoing maintenance program.
- Power strips may not be used in a patient care vicinity to power non-patient care–related electrical equipment (such as personal electronics).
- Power strips providing power to patient care–related electrical equipment must be Special-Purpose Relocatable Power Taps (SPRPTs) listed as UL 1363A or UL 60601-1.

Outside of the Patient Care Vicinity

Power strips may be used for non–patient care equipment, such as computers, monitors, or printers, and in areas such as waiting rooms, offices, nurses' stations, support areas, corridors, and so forth.

Power strips providing power to non-patient care–related electrical equipment must be Relocatable Power Taps (RPTs) listed as UL 1363.

Decorations Assessment Checklist

Organizations can use this checklist to assess the safety of holiday or celebratory decorations by determining whether the decorations pose an increased risk in the physical environment.

Note: *The complete checklist may be adapted and is available for internal use on the flash drive (print only) or by clicking the tool link in the Risk-Assessment Toolbox (e-book only) on page 142.*

Published in *Environment of Care Risk Assessment*, Joint Commission Resources, 2018.　　**File Name:** 06 06 Checklist Decorations Assess

DECORATIONS ASSESSMENT CHECKLIST

*This checklist includes questions that will assess the safety of holiday or celebratory decorations. Use this checklist to determine whether decorations increase environmental risks. Answers to all questions should ideally be **Y** for **Yes** (unless they aren't applicable). If an answer is **N** for **No**, use the "Notes" section to document needed changes. Unless otherwise noted, this checklist is applicable to all program settings.*

ORGANIZATION: ______________________________　　DEPARTMENT/UNIT: ______________________________

DATE OF REVIEW: __________________　　REVIEWER: ______________________________

HOLIDAY OR CELEBRATION: ______________________________

QUESTIONS	YES	NO	NA	NOTES
GENERAL				
Did the safety officer oversee the installation of the decorations?				
MATERIALS*				
Are all trees, wreaths, and other similar decorations artificial?				
Are all trees, wreaths, and other similar decorations fire/flame retardant?				
Are all combustible decorations (paper cutouts, banners, posters) flame retardant?				
Are all flame-retardant combustible decorations retreated with appropriate retardant every five years, with documented proof?				
Are you completely avoiding the use of open flame devices, such as candles?				
Are all electric candles battery operated?				
Are all decorations free of hazards related to choking or harm/injury (for example, from broken glass)?				

Assessing Risk of Corridor Clutter

Corridor clutter is a challenge for many health care organizations. Clutter accumulates easily but is a major hazard when there is an emergency. In a fire, for example, staff may need to move or evacuate patients and their beds, monitors, and pumps, sometimes in reduced visibility. Cluttered corridors can make that task much more difficult.

Northwestern Memorial Hospital in Chicago, an academic medical center, was like many other health care organizations in its struggle to maintain clear corridors. In 2014 the organization launched a compliance improvement initiative to eliminate clutter in areas staff identified as particularly prone to accumulation.

Forming the Team, Creating a Plan

The project began at the Environment of Care Committee meetings. From that group, a multidisciplinary team was formed comprising representatives of the facilities management, transport, environmental services, and security departments. These individuals brought their firsthand, day-to-day experiences to the task.

First, the team needed to identify which areas would benefit the most from corridor decluttering. After some discussion, 10 areas emerged as focus areas—some on patient floors, others in "behind the scenes" areas. All corridors chosen were 8-foot-wide exit/access corridors.

For four months, these 10 corridors would be monitored regularly, while the organization actively encouraged those departments to declutter. Members of the security team would incorporate corridor clutter checks, unannounced, into their normal rounds.

Training the Inspectors

The security staff who would be responsible for these inspections were trained to recognize which items are acceptable to store in which areas, and which are not. This training included identifying dead-end corridors that may be used for storage, as well as which items are acceptable to store.

As Rene Catalano, accreditation coordinator for the team, says, "It's not just the amount of material in a space, but what that material is." For example, cardboard boxes or wooden pallets are never acceptable to store in corridors because they present a combustion hazard.

Inspectors also needed to be able to recognize whether items were attended or unattended, which is a large part of determining whether an item is considered clutter. "If someone is actively working with the material, that's fine. It's considered 'attended.' It's not storage or clutter," explains Jeff Meyer, facilities compliance manager and driving force behind the project. "However, if it's just stowed in the corridor and no one is working with it, that would raise a red flag."

The security staff designated as clutter inspectors toured each of the 10 target areas with Meyer. This activity allowed them to see the actual space and items for which they would be responsible and to think about those from the standpoint of clutter.

Inspections were only one aspect of the project. The other, to encourage departments to declutter their areas, was initiated before the first inspection took place. Meyer used e-mail to announce the project to the management responsible for each of the 10 target areas (*see* page 147). That message explained project goals, how progress would be tracked, and generally what those areas should expect during the project's four-month span.

Corridor Compliance Checkpoints

A "Corridor Compliance Checkpoint" sign was placed at each of the 10 targeted locations. These signs served a double purpose. First, they heightened awareness of clutter on an organizationwide scale, which was intended to encourage cooperation among staff members and to eliminate clutter before it happens. Second, each checkpoint sign was labeled with a unique bar code that the inspector could scan with a handheld device. At each checkpoint, the inspector would assign a pass/fail grade. If the area failed, the specific reason was noted; for example, "accumulation of boxes."

This information, managed by a third-party database provider, made collecting, compiling, and analyzing the data easy and efficient.

continued

Sustained Support

Throughout the four-month project, the team used e-mail to keep in contact with management of the target areas. These messages offered encouragement when an area did not receive a passing grade, and congratulations when it did.

Meyer sees this as a key factor. As he says, "People get tired of hearing that their corridors are out of compliance. They need encouragement as well." Recognizing effort and improvement keeps the momentum of the project going and helps staff stay engaged in the project without feeling discouraged.

Assessing the Impact

Though corridor clutter is an issue that requires continual vigilance, the team at Northwestern Memorial Hospital believes it has developed an effective method for raising consciousness and generating improvements (*see* page 147 for before and after images). The team plans to expand the program to other areas of the facility.

"This kind of change is very visible," Catalano says. "It made us all feel so good to see the improvement." This good feeling can flow into other improvement efforts, leading to greater buy-in and teamwork among staff members.

Northwestern Memorial has done just that. The organization has introduced an "Environmental Excellence" program for patient care areas. In this program, staff assess their surroundings for potential problems and report their observations on a monthly basis.

"When a team representing the whole organization tackles the problem," says Meyer, "it's easier to get each department to want to be part of permanent solutions."

Launching the Initiative

E-mail Project Announcement

Good Afternoon,

In support of our continued efforts to maintain code-compliant, obstruction-free egress corridors, the Environment of Care Committee is beginning a new initiative focused on regular inspections in select areas of the hospital. The intent of this program is to visually inspect these selected corridors **on a weekly basis** and report the findings of these inspections to the EOC committee, and ultimately to **The Joint Commission**, as part of our improvement plan for LS.03.01.20, **to provide a clear means of egress**.

Attached to this e-mail is an image of an Inspection Point that you will see posted at each of these locations. When the corridor inspection is performed, the unique bar code you see on the poster will be scanned, and the corridor will be given a Pass/Fail rating for that visit. You will be notified of the inspection results to determine if a follow-up action is required. These weekly inspections will begin prior to the end of this month and will continue for a minimum of 4 months. **Our goal for this program is a 90% compliance rate or greater**.

Upon latest visits to these areas, items that were typically seen were wooden pallets, cardboard boxes, IV poles, biomed equipment, beds, and similar items. Some areas have already seen drastic improvement in the past couple weeks (thank you, CSS!), but we will continue to monitor these areas to maintain our compliance.

Please make every effort to visit these areas frequently to help keep our corridors and elevator lobbies safe and clutter free!

If you have any questions or concerns, please do not hesitate to contact me.

Thank you for your cooperation.

To announce this initiative to maintain code compliance and reduce corridor clutter, facilities compliance manager Jeff Meyer outlined the project and its goal.

Before and After

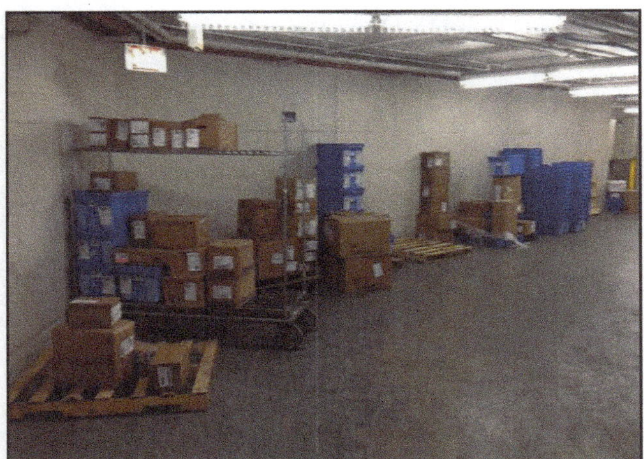

Before

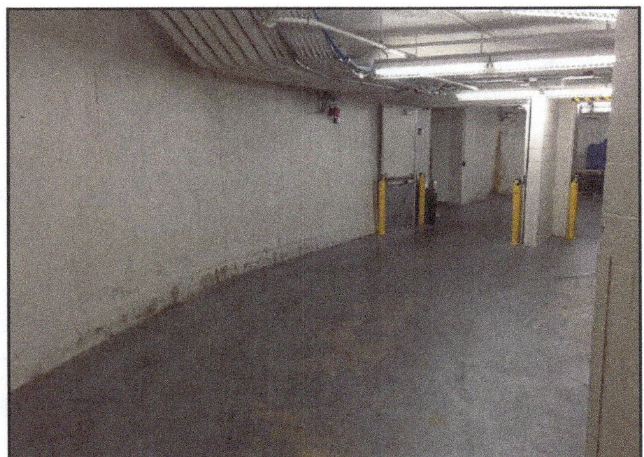

After

These before-and-after images demonstrate not only the end result of a strong risk-assessment program but also the safety improvements that were a result.

chapter 7

Medical Equipment

Medical equipment is an essential component of providing health care (*see* page 150). Properly used, medical equipment can assess, diagnose, and treat patients safely and effectively. However, equipment also has the potential for significant safety risks, the negative consequences of which can be very serious. This chapter looks at the area of medical equipment and the risk assessments associated with its use.

The term *medical equipment* applies to all equipment used in treatment, diagnostic activities, patient monitoring, or direct patient care. Medical equipment may include, but is not limited to, the following:

- *Life support.* For sustaining life or maintaining bodily function
- *Monitoring.* For recording and tracking patient conditions
- *Treatment.* For direct patient care
- *Diagnostic.* For analysis and diagnosis
- *Patient support.* For supporting patient health during diagnosis and treatment
- *Laboratory.* For use in diagnosing disease or other conditions

Overview of Assessing Risks

The primary method of assessing medical equipment risks is creating and maintaining an inventory. This is required by The Joint Commission's Environment of Care (EC) standards—the inventory must be current and in writing.

Inventory

Requirements for the inventory vary, depending on whether the organization uses Joint Commission accreditation for deemed status purposes. The following sections describe the inventory requirements. Be aware that different settings may have different requirements. For example, the option of using an alternative equipment maintenance (AEM) program is not available to ambulatory health care centers. It is important to refer to the appropriate accreditation manual to determine setting-specific requirements.

For Hospitals and Critical Access Hospitals

These organizations must identify on their equipment inventory which devices are classified as high risk, including all life-support devices. A high-risk device poses a risk of serious injury or death to the patient or staff if it were to fail. Organizations should use risk criteria to evaluate which pieces of equipment are identified as high risk. These criteria involve the following issues:

- Equipment function, such as for diagnosis, care, treatment, life support, and monitoring
- Physical risks associated with equipment use
- Maintenance requirements for the equipment
- Equipment incident history

Examples of Medical Equipment

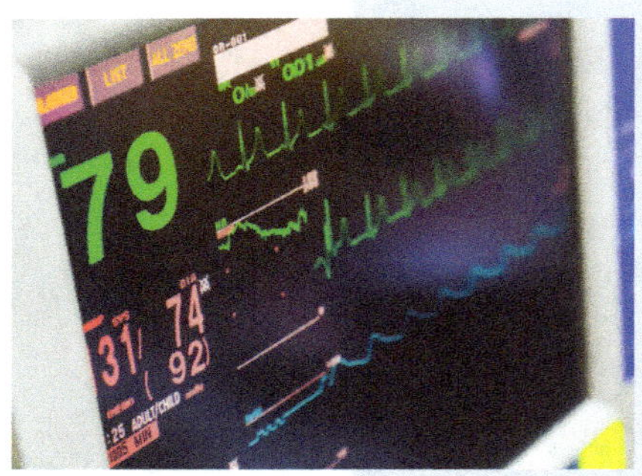

Medical Monitors

- ECG
- EEG
- Blood pressure
- Fetal monitor

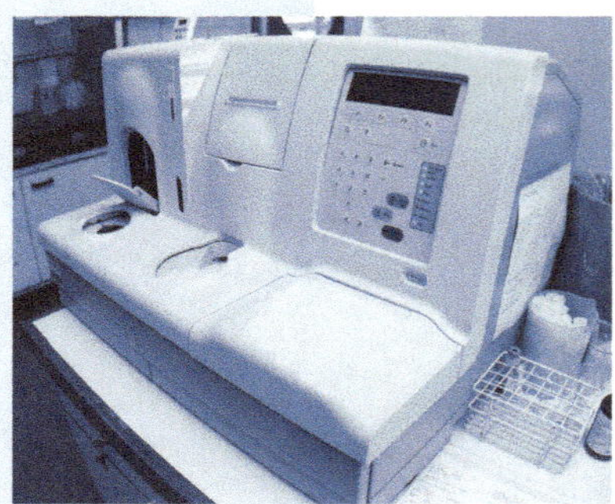

Medical Laboratory Equipment

- Blood gas analyzer

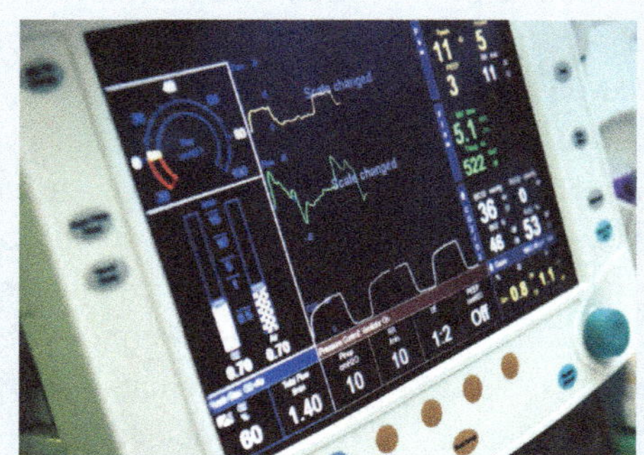

Life-Support Equipment

- Medical ventilators
- Incubators
- Anesthetic machines
- Heart-lung machines
- ECMO
- Dialysis machines

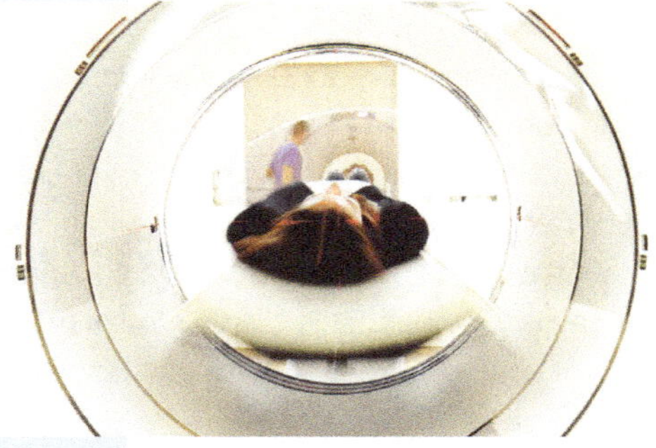

Diagnostic Equipment

- Ultrasound
- MRI machines
- PET scanners
- CT scanners
- X-ray machine

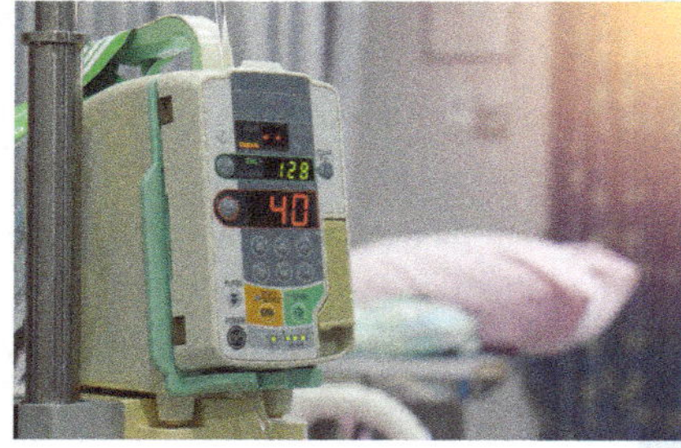

Treatment Equipment

- Infusion pumps
- Medical lasers
- LASIK surgical machines

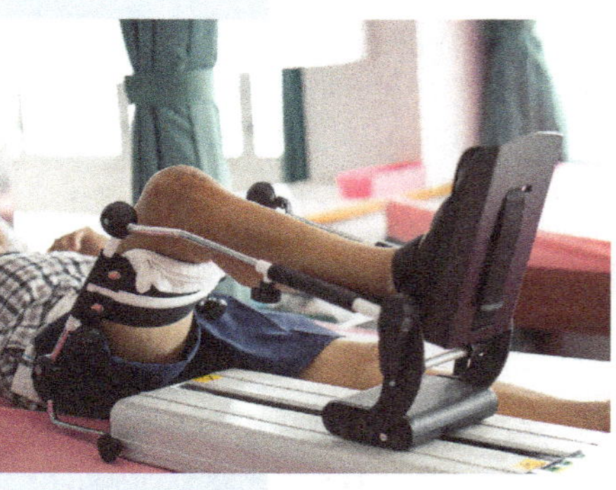

Patient Support

- CPM machines

ECG, electrocardiogram; EEG, electroencephalogram; ECMO, extracorporeal membrane oxygenation; LASIK, laser vision correction; MRI, magnetic resonance imaging; PET, positron emission tomography; CT, computerized tomography; CPM, continuous passive range of motion.

There is a vast amount of medical equipment available to health care organizations. This small sampling illustrates the great range of equipment organizations may have to manage in their facility.

Inspection, testing, and maintenance (ITM) activity must correlate to the equipment listed on the inventory. Organizations are encouraged to include the ITM frequency for the inventoried equipment as well.

If a qualified individual determines that a piece of equipment can be safely maintained under an AEM program (*see* page 152 for more information about AEM programs), it must be identified as such in the inventory. The decision to use an AEM program must be supported by written details on the following:

- How the equipment is used and the seriousness and prevalence of harm related to normal use
- Likely consequences if the equipment fails or malfunctions, including seriousness and prevalence of harm
- Availability of alternative or backup equipment in case of failure or malfunction
- Incident history of identical or similar equipment
- Maintenance requirements of the equipment

Hospitals and critical access hospitals that do not use Joint Commission accreditation for deemed status purposes
The inventory may include all medical equipment; or it may include selected equipment categorized by physical risk associated with its use (including all life-support equipment). Also, before a new type of equipment is put into use, the organization should evaluate it to determine whether or not it will be included in the inventory.

Hospitals and critical access hospitals that use Joint Commission accreditation for deemed status purposes
For these organizations, all medical equipment must be included in the inventory. Certain types of equipment must be maintained, inspected, and tested in accordance with the manufacturer's recommendations for specific activities and frequencies. These types include the following:

- Medical laser devices
- Imaging and radiologic equipment that is used for diagnostic or therapeutic purposes
- New medical equipment that does not have enough maintenance history (for example, records from the hospital's contractors or the hospital's own experience, or information from nationally recognized sources) to support use of alternative maintenance strategies
- Any equipment that is subject to federal or state law, or the US Centers for Medicare & Medicaid Services (CMS)

Conditions of Participation (CoPs), in which inspecting, testing, and maintaining must be in accordance with manufacturer's recommendations, or if these agencies have more stringent requirements

Participants in the Process

As medical equipment becomes more sophisticated, effectively assessing risks associated with that equipment requires health care engineers and clinical staff to work together. Risk assessments should involve a joint effort between clinical care services, clinical engineering, and risk management. Such interaction requires both clinical staff and engineering staff to be able to understand the operation, maintenance, and application of equipment in the care environment. Engineers and clinical staff must exchange information to educate each other and other departments on any risks associated with medical equipment.

In most health care organizations, some medical equipment is departmentalized. Typically, the laboratory and radiology departments maintain their own pieces of diagnostic equipment, and other departments may do so as well. This decentralization is appropriate, but there must be some feedback mechanism, even if by exception, into the medical equipment management program to allow all related data to be considered. This is simply another aspect of the "regardless of ownership" axiom.

In cases in which an outside vendor is in charge of maintenance and testing, the person responsible for the medical equipment still should be aware of what decentralized equipment is being tested and maintained and how it is being tested and maintained. Proper documentation on all testing and maintenance activities must be maintained by the organization. Some organizations have a quarterly meeting of all medical equipment providers conducting maintenance to reconcile their documentation and make sure everything is up to date.

All activity associated with the medical equipment should be shared through the organization's multidisciplinary improvement team for the environment of care to ensure that it is being managed to the organization's expectations.

Identifying Risks

Updating the inventory provides an opportunity to identify medical equipment risks. Any equipment labeled high risk is

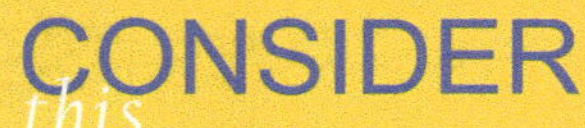

Alternative Equipment Maintenance Program

Joint Commission standards require health care organizations to manage risks associated with medical equipment. This includes proper maintenance, which generally means following manufacturers' recommendations. However, in some cases, following manufacturers' recommendations can put an unnecessary burden on a facility. The US Centers for Medicare & Medicaid Services (CMS) policy and associated Joint Commission standards now allow organizations some flexibility in their equipment maintenance program. The option of using this process, known as an alternative equipment maintenance (AEM) program, is available to hospitals and critical access hospitals that use Joint Commission accreditation for deemed status purposes.

An AEM program enables hospitals to adopt a maintenance approach that deviates from manufacturers' requirements. The Joint Commission offers the American National Standards Institute/Association for the Advancement of Medical Instrumentation document ANSI/AAMI EQ56–13, *Recommended Practice for a Medical Equipment Management Program*, as an example of standards for an AEM program. An AEM program must not compromise safety or put patients at increased risk. The decision to use an AEM program must be based on a risk assessment performed by a qualified individual. The organization must keep documentation supporting its AEM approach, and must announce its use of an AEM program at the beginning of the accreditation survey.

For hospitals and critical access hospitals that use Joint Commission accreditation for deemed status purposes, AEM programs are not permissible when any of the following conditions are present:
- Federal or state laws, or a hospital's Conditions of Participation (CoPs), require adherence to manufacturers' recommendations.
- Equipment is new and does not have a sufficient amount of maintenance history to use as a basis for a risk assessment.
- Equipment is imaging or radiologic, or a medical laser device.

In addition, AEMs may not be permissible in all settings (for example, ambulatory health care centers).

Information on AEM programs as they apply to utility systems can be found in Chapter 8.

See page 153 for an AEM program checklist.

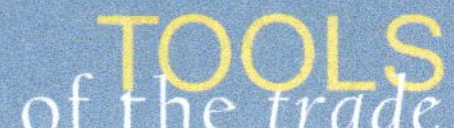

Alternative Equipment Maintenance Checklist—For Use by Hospitals for a CMS–Approved AEM Program

This checklist requires organizations to assess key questions related to the effectiveness of its alternative equipment maintenance program (AEM).

Note: *The complete checklist may be adapted and is available for internal use on the flash drive (print only) or by clicking the tool link in the Risk-Assessment Toolbox (e-book only) on page 164.*

Published in *Environment of Care Risk Assessment*, Joint Commission Resources, 2018.　　　　　**File Name:** 07 01 Checklist AEM Program

ALTERNATIVE EQUIPMENT MAINTENANCE CHECKLIST—FOR USE BY HOSPITALS FOR A CMS–APPROVED AEM PROGRAM*

This checklist can be used to identify risks in a hospital's alternative equipment maintenance program. Note that this checklist is applicable to facilities that elect to use the Joint Commission deemed status option. Answers to all questions should ideally be **Y** *for* **Yes** *(unless they aren't applicable). If an answer is* **N** *for* **No**, *use the "Notes" section to document needed changes.*

DATE OF EVALUATION: _______________________　　EVALUATOR(S): _____________________________________

EQUIPMENT INVENTORY:　　☐ MEDICAL　　☐ FACILITY

QUESTION	YES	NO	NA	NOTES
EQUIPMENT INVENTORY EVALUATION†				
Every Item of Equipment in the Inventory				
Is it identified as part of an AEM program?				
Equipment in an AEM Program				
Is it identified as critical (poses a direct threat to health and safety if it malfunctions)?				
Is it identified as required to meet everyday patient needs?				
Is it identified as likely to be needed in an emergency situation?				
Does it include a unique identification number?				
Does it identify the equipment manufacturer?				
Does it indicate if the manufacturer's recommendations are available?				
Does it include the equipment model number?				
Does it include the equipment serial number?				

a natural target for a risk assessment. Also, any equipment that is new or does not have much maintenance history may be a good candidate for assessment. The same is true for any piece of equipment that has experienced a failure or malfunction in the past.

Equipment also should be assessed for risks particular to its use. For example, disinfection and sterilization devices should be assessed for infection control risks (*see* page 155 for an endoscope reprocessing assessment checklist). Similarly, any device that uses a clinical alarm might be assessed for its effectiveness in the face of alarm fatigue and excessive noise levels.

The following risk criteria should be considered when making a decision:
- *Function.* What is the equipment supposed to do?
- *Physical risk.* What level of risks—to patients, residents, individuals served, or staff—are associated with its use? What might happen if it fails?
- *Incident history.* How many adverse events have involved this equipment? What level of severity is each event?
- *Maintenance requirements.* What is involved in making sure the equipment is always functioning properly? If it requires preventive maintenance, what might happen if it does not have it?
- *Cleaning requirements.* Who cleans the equipment (clinical staff or environmental services) and who ensures that instructions for use are followed?
- *Regulations and requirements.* Are there state or other accreditation requirements that influence whether this item needs to be in the inventory?

Equipment Selection

Managing equipment risks begins with the careful selection of that equipment (*see* page 156 for an equipment security assessment and selection decision checklist.). Each health care organization should have an established process to follow for the selection and acquisition of medical equipment. Usually the request will originate in the department that will use the equipment, and it clearly must follow the budgeting guidelines of the organization. After a request has been made, there should be a formal review process prior to the acquisition to assess any risks associated with the equipment. The complex technology of today's medical equipment calls for a thorough and detailed evaluation prior to issuing a purchase order.

Is It Appropriate?

Clinical engineering should be involved in a formal review process to ensure that the equipment requested is appropriate, that it will meet the user need, and that it is compatible with existing equipment. For some equipment, organizations can search existing databases to determine if there is a reported history of problems or failures. Should such a review reveal problems, clinical engineering should review the use and limitations of the equipment with the requesting department and explore possible alternatives.

Can It Be Properly Maintained?

Maintenance requirements also should be evaluated, in addition to the availability of parts, documentation, and repair services. In addition, organizations should consider the need for and cost of disposables. Perhaps most importantly, organizations should evaluate the human factor regarding the use of the equipment by the organization's staff in its intended environment.

Does It Require Special Support Structures?

For some pieces of medical equipment, space and special utilities are issues. It is not unusual to construct a specialized room for pieces of imaging equipment, whether just to provide the physical space or to provide appropriate shielding (such as for magnetic resonance imaging [MRI] equipment or a linear accelerator). Consequently, major pieces of diagnostic laboratory equipment must be assessed for the availability of space and utilities within the department.

How Will Staff Be Trained to Use It?

An important aspect to consider when acquiring medical equipment is training. The organization should determine whether specialized training is required for the equipment and, if so, how to provide that training. Often the vendor will provide on-site classes, or perhaps a few individuals will attend a class at the manufacturer's location. In this case, it may be helpful to send people who are users, as well as maintainers, of the equipment. This establishes a train-the-trainer situation to bring the information back to the health care organization.

Endoscope Reprocessing Assessment Checklist

Organizations can use this checklist to assess the endoscope reprocessing method and determine its effectiveness. Examining this process can help organizations identify infection control risks—on a daily or periodic basis.

Note: *The complete checklist may be adapted and is available for internal use on the flash drive (print only) or by clicking the tool link in the Risk-Assessment Toolbox (e-book only) on page 164.*

Published in *Environment of Care Risk Assessment*, Joint Commission Resources, 2018.   **File Name:** 07 02 Checklist Endoscope Reprocessing

ENDOSCOPE REPROCESSING ASSESSMENT CHECKLIST

*This checklist includes questions for assessing infection control in an organizations' endoscope reprocessing methods. Use this checklist to identify infection control risks on either a daily or periodic basis. Answers to all questions should ideally be Y for **Yes** (unless they aren't applicable). If an answer is **N** for **No**, use the "Notes" section to document needed changes. Unless otherwise noted, this checklist is applicable to all program settings.*

ORGANIZATION: _______________________   DEPARTMENT/UNIT: _______________________

DATE OF REVIEW: _______________   REVIEWER: _______________________

TYPE OF ENDOSCOPES REPROCESSED IN THE FACILITY: _______________________

QUESTIONS	YES	NO	NA	NOTES

The Medical Equipment Management Program

An effective medical equipment management program will incorporate thorough risk assessments. It also depends on good judgment and experience with various types of medical equipment.* Often health care organizations only reflect biomed responsibilities in their medical equipment management program. However, it is important to make sure sterilizers, hemodialysis and water testing equipment, laboratory equipment, and the like are also included in the plan (as described at the beginning of this chapter).

The objectives of a medical equipment management program include the following:

- Develop an equipment maintenance strategy, commensurate with risk, for each type of equipment.
- Make equipment available to clinical staff.
- Readily identify and report suspected problems.
- Readily obtain replacements.
- Schedule and deliver required maintenance activities.

Complexities of today's equipment and increased technological advancements also may lead organizations to consider risks associated with cyber threats and the accessibility and use of medical equipment through wireless technology. Organizations should also be aware of the Wireless Medical Telemetry Service (WMTS) spectrum that is used for remote monitoring of a patient's health. Organizations that use this technology are required to register these devices with the Federal Communications Commission (FCC) (*see* page 158 for additional information on WMTS).

Inclusion in the medical equipment management program does not necessarily mean that the equipment must have a scheduled maintenance activity. If the organization develops appropriate maintenance strategies that minimize risk to patients, then it is not always necessary for each item on the inventory to have an obligatory preventive maintenance or inspection event scheduled.

Important considerations when developing the medical equipment management program include how the equipment will be used and the negative consequences to the delivery of care if the equipment fails or is unavailable. An organization may use a variety of methods to complete this risk-assessment process, including a simple proactive risk assessment or a more formalized tool, such as failure mode and effects analysis (FMEA) (*See* page 21 in Chapter 1 for additional information about FMEA). It is common practice for most organizations to develop a risk ranking score for

---

* For laboratory settings, this is in regard to laboratory equipment.

Medical Equipment Assessment and Selection Decision Checklist

Organizations may use this checklist to assess the security risks associated with current medical equipment, as well as determine what potential security-related issues could arise from new medical equipment or vendors.

Note: *The complete checklist may be adapted and is available for internal use on the flash drive (print only) or by clicking the tool link in the Risk-Assessment Toolbox (e-book only) on page 164.*

Published in *Environment of Care Risk Assessment*, Joint Commission Resources, 2018.   **File Name:** 07 03 Checklist Med Equipment Asses

MEDICAL EQUIPMENT ASSESSMENT AND SELECTION DECISION CHECKLIST

This checklist includes questions for assessing the security risks associated with current medical equipment and security-related questions about potential new medical equipment or vendors. Answers to all questions should ideally be Y for **Yes** *(unless they aren't applicable). If an answer is* **N** *for* **No**, *use the "Notes" section to document needed changes. Unless otherwise noted, this checklist is applicable to all program settings.*

ORGANIZATION: _________________________________   DEPARTMENT/UNIT: _________________________________

DATE OF REVIEW: _________________________   REVIEWER: ____

TYPE OF EQUIPMENT: ____

QUESTIONS	YES	NO	NA	NOTES
FOR EXISTING EQUIPMENT*				
Does the equipment/vendor meet FDA guidelines?				
Is the equipment registered with the FCC WMTS)?†				
Do staff know how to recognize anomalies that may signal a security risk?				
Does equipment without off-the-shelf functionality operate behind your organization's firewall?				
Does wireless equipment incorporate encryption technology?				
Does the transmissions of wireless equipment stand up against electromagnetic interference?				
Does your organization have a clearly defined process for assessing new medical equipment before purchase?				
Do you have a testing process that demonstrates what "normal" and "abnormal" operations look like?				
Does your process include a system of documenting problems and reporting them to the manufacturer?				
FOR NEW EQUIPMENT*				

each type of equipment and establish a lower cutoff to help guide the decision of which devices might be identified specifically in the inventory.

Regardless of the method used to identify risk, it is important to apply prudent professional judgment to determine what equipment should be included in the medical equipment management program. Also note that when a given type of equipment is included in the program, it is included regardless of ownership. In other words, if a similar piece of equipment is on loan from a vendor, is owned by a patient, or comes into the facility in any other manner, it must fall under the medical equipment management program (*see* page 160 for additional information about equipment from outside the organization).

Maintenance Strategies

As technological advances proliferate, the characteristics defining modern medical equipment have changed as well, making the medical equipment management process more complex. For example, consider the following:

- More and more complex devices have safeguards that prevent them from failing in a manner that could harm a patient.
- Many pieces of equipment are made up of modular subassemblies that make them cost-prohibitive to repair at a component level.
- Equipment often becomes clinically obsolete before frequent, significant patterns of breakdown can occur.

The vast majority of today's digital and microprocessor-based equipment is not as susceptible to drift or worn-out components as it was years ago when the devices were analog. Therefore, when today's microprocessor equipment crashes, the failure is usually fairly obvious to the user. In addition, many devices incorporate self-diagnostics, error detection, and internal calibration, thus facilitating fault detection and correction of imminent failure. Fixing equipment typically involves resetting software or, in rare cases, swapping out defective modules or subassemblies. Very little can be done by maintenance to predict or prevent failures in this new-generation, microprocessor-based equipment.

As a result of advances in technology, an organization's medical equipment management program no longer consists of maintenance schedules requiring preventive maintenance

inspections of all equipment. Instead, it relies heavily on proactive risk assessment, sound professional judgment, and organizational experience with various types of equipment.

Determining Strategies

The EC standards require organizations to look critically at their equipment inventories and determine what maintenance strategies will be the most effective to ensure that clinical staff members have the functional and appropriate equipment they need to deliver care.

Determining appropriate maintenance strategies requires an understanding of how the equipment operates, how it might fail, how a failure mode is identified, and how different failure scenarios affect clinical operations. The concepts rely not only on trying to prevent failure (which may or may not always be possible) but also on rapidly detecting and minimizing the impact of equipment failure.

When determining maintenance strategies for different types of equipment, organizations should consider multiple types of strategies, such as interval-based maintenance, predictive maintenance, metered maintenance, run-to-fail maintenance, and corrective maintenance. (*See* page 162 for additional information on these different types of maintenance strategies.)

Not every strategy is appropriate for every piece of equipment. It is important that the decisions made about medical equipment maintenance be carefully considered, reviewed, and approved by pertinent individuals within the organization, such as the following:

- Facilities engineering leadership
- Multidisciplinary improvement team
- Risk management
- Clinical staff members

With all the data considered, a decision that reflects the consensus should be reached and implemented. (*See* page 163 for a simple equipment maintenance checklist.)

Factors to Consider

One way to refine maintenance strategies is to assess the effectiveness of the current maintenance program. For each type of equipment, organizations should take a look at the maintenance history. How often was periodic maintenance performed with no problems found and no parts replaced?

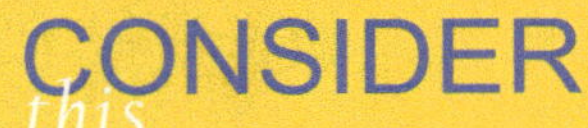

Operating and Registering a Wireless Medical Telemetry Device

According to the US Federal Communications Commission (FCC), only authorized health care providers are eligible to operate Wireless Medical Telemetry Service (WMTS) devices, and WMTS devices may be used only within a health care facility. WMTS devices must be registered with the FCC's designated frequency coordinator, the American Society for Healthcare Engineering of the American Hospital Association.[1]

An *authorized health care provider* is one of the following:
- A physician or other individual authorized under state or federal law to provide health care services
- A health care facility operated by or employing individuals authorized under state or federal law to provide health care services
- Any trained technician operating under the supervision and control of an individual or health care facility authorized under state or federal law to provide health care services

A *health care facility* is defined as a hospital or other establishment that offers services, facilities, and beds for use beyond a 24-hour period in rendering medical treatment, or an organization regularly engaged in providing medical services through clinics, public health facilities, and similar establishments, including government entities and agencies such as US Department of Veterans Affairs hospitals and health care facilities on tribal lands.

Reference
1. US Federal Communications Commission. Wireless Medical Telemetry Service (WMTS). (Updated: Mar 8, 2017.) Accessed Feb 20, 2018. https://www.fcc.gov/general/wireless-medical-telemetry-service-wmts.

Each of these experiences could be considered to be an ineffective preventive maintenance activity and, therefore, possibly a poor use of time and resources. If the majority of encounters with a piece of equipment are ineffective, it is appropriate to consider an alternative strategy. Conversely, if analysis of corrective maintenance suggests a recurring pattern of failures for a certain type of device, then a return to, or modification of, scheduled maintenance activities (in other words, preventive maintenance) is indicated.

Organizations also may want to consider manufacturers' maintenance recommendations when designing maintenance strategies. If an organization has no experience with a type of medical equipment, the manufacturer's recommendations are a good source of guidance in the establishment of a maintenance strategy, and these recommendations should be followed until some history is developed. It is also recommended that manufacturers' schedules be followed through the warranty period on any new piece of equipment.

Manufacturers' recommendations are often conservative. An individual organization's experience might show that many of these recommended schedules can be lengthened with no adverse impact on the equipment. Hence, the guidance provided by the recommendations may be helpful to establish maintenance strategies appropriate for the equipment and the situation. As always, sound professional judgment based on organizational experience is critical.

Special Considerations

The following sections explore several important issues to consider when addressing medical equipment risks.

When Equipment Fails

In addition to assessing risk for medical equipment use and maintenance, organizations should consider contingency plans should medical equipment fail. Procedures for these types of emergencies should address the following:

- What to do in the event of equipment disruption or failure
- When and how to perform emergency clinical interventions when medical equipment fails
- Availability of backup equipment
- How to obtain repair services

An emergency clinical intervention is the ultimate backup procedure for medical equipment failure—the incidents that require more than a simple call for a replacement piece of equipment. Although not required for each piece of equipment, a planned emergency clinical intervention should be established for those critical devices that affect the safety of the patient. For example, organizations should have plans in place to address hand-ventilating patients if a ventilator fails. Organizations also must ensure that any supplemental equipment needed for clinical interventions is available and functional.

Diagnostic Imaging

Diagnostic imaging is an integral part of modern health care, and it takes many forms: x-rays, MRI scans, ultrasound, nuclear medicine (NM) scans, computed tomography (CT) scans, positron emission tomography (PET) scans, and others. Many include radiation of one form or another, and all carry risks to patient and staff safety if not used properly. These risks include burns, fires, cancer, and other injuries due to radiation overexposure through inappropriate dosing or unnecessary repeated exposure. However, using too small a dose can result in misdiagnosis, delayed treatment, or even the necessity of repeating the scan and therefore exposing the patient to more radiation.

Supporting safe use of diagnostic imaging equipment entails knowledge of the equipment and how to use it, frequent inspection and testing, and cooperation between departments that use radiation-producing equipment (for example, radiology, operating room, cardiac catheterization suite), EC professionals, and patient safety staff. (*See* page 165 for a diagnostic imaging compliance checklist.)

Using the Inventory

The medical equipment inventory is a useful tool in managing diagnostic imaging risks. These devices can be located in many places throughout the facility, and the inventory should identify radiation-producing devices (particularly those that involve ionizing radiation), where they are located, and which departments are responsible for them. Keeping the inventory current also can help identify recalled items quickly so they can be removed from service before they can cause harm.

Careful Maintenance

Diagnostic imaging equipment is sophisticated and sensitive and can therefore require expert maintenance. Some organizations may assign preventive maintenance to EC staff or the radiology department, but many choose to use outside vendors to perform these tasks. No matter who performs the preventive maintenance, the EC staff should understand the overall how and when of the activities and ensure that whoever is responsible is competent and is following the established frequencies indicated in the equipment management program. Tracking maintenance and service can help the organization see larger patterns in function that might need to be addressed, such as ventilation problems, user errors, and poor equipment design or location.

Catching Malfunctions

Anyone who uses the diagnostic imaging equipment must be able to catch malfunctions before they can affect patients. This may include how to use and read radiation monitors. EC staff and equipment service professionals should provide education and training on recognizing malfunctions and reporting them in accordance with established procedures. In addition, staff should understand how to use personal protective equipment (PPE), such as lead aprons, which can reduce harm from exposure to radiation.

Diagnostic Imaging Service

In its constant effort to improve safety, The Joint Commission has introduced new and revised standards regarding diagnostic imaging services. Found in the EC, HR, MM, PC, and PI chapters[†] of the *Comprehensive Accreditation*

[†] "Environment of Care" (EC); "Human Resources" (HR); "Medication Management" (MM); "Provision of Care, Treatment, and Services" (PC); and "Performance Improvement" (PI) chapters.

Equipment from Outside the Organization

Ideally, when a patient enters a health care organization, staff should transfer the patient off any medical equipment brought from home and use the organization's equipment instead. This ensures that staff interacting with the equipment are properly trained to operate it, that the equipment is maintained appropriately, and that the equipment is clean and free from contamination. However, the decision to transfer a patient off his or her own equipment might not be so simple.

An Example

A 52-year-old cancer patient enters a hospital for a five-day stay. She is using a chemotherapy pump with a research protocol. The hospital does not use that particular type of pump when treating cancer patients and does not own a similar pump. The organization faces a decision. Do staff transfer the woman off her pump for the five days and put her on a hospital-owned pump? Or does the hospital leave the woman on her own pump for the duration of her stay? If the organization chooses to transfer the patient off her pump, her research protocol—and her treatment—will be disrupted. This transfer might affect the quality of care provided to the patient. On the other hand, leaving the patient on her pump can raise a patient safety concern if staff are not trained on the proper use of the patient's equipment. What if the woman's condition deteriorates to the point that she can no longer operate her own pump? What if the nurses treating the patient are not familiar with the pump? What if the equipment breaks? What if the pump needs to be replaced?

This scenario raises complex questions that organizations should consider when managing medical equipment from any source outside the organization itself, whether it be brought from the patient's home or provided by a vendor. There are no right or wrong answers; however, avoiding these questions is not wise. The time to think about and address them is before a patient walks into the facility with an unfamiliar piece of equipment.

Joint Commission Requirements

The Joint Commission does not dictate that staff must transfer a patient from his or her own equipment to the organization's equipment when entering a health care facility. However, organizations should have a policy in place regarding whether they will allow equipment owned by patients or vendors. If the organization decides to use this equipment, the maintenance, education, and cleanliness requirements of Joint Commission standards apply.

For equipment brought in from outside the organization, the requirements of the standards can present challenges and possible risks. In some cases, meeting these challenges is worthwhile, given the potential benefits to patient care. In other cases, transferring the patient to the organization's equipment might be more practical. Be sure to include the patient's physician when determining the use of the patient's own equipment or the organization's equipment. The physician's input also can be valuable when determining how to handle equipment associated with research protocols.

Staff Competency

An organization must ensure that staff members understand how to use any equipment brought in by patients for use in the organization. This includes all staff who will interact with the equipment, such as nurses, physicians, respiratory care therapists, and, in some cases, ancillary staff such as physical, occupational, or speech therapists. You can anticipate the education needs of staff by offering training sessions on different versions of standard equipment, such as multiple brands of ventilators. However, if a piece of equipment on which staff have not received training is brought to the facility for use, arrangements must be made to train staff on that piece of equipment before the equipment is used.

Proper Maintenance

To determine proper maintenance of equipment brought from outside the organization, the maintenance history should be reviewed with the patient as well as with the provider of the equipment, if possible. If the patient owns the equipment, he or she may be the best source of information on the equipment's maintenance history. The organization also must plan how it will obtain supplies for the equipment, address potential repairs, and obtain backup equipment, if necessary.

To ensure that a piece of equipment is clean and free of contamination, an organization should decontaminate the equipment as soon as it enters the facility. There should already be a procedure in place that requires all equipment coming on-site to undergo disinfection procedures. Equipment brought in from patients would be subject to this policy.

Deciding to Transfer

If an organization decides to transfer a patient to organization equipment, it is important that staff educate the patient about the reasons behind the decision—that transferring to organization equipment helps the organization better ensure patient safety. By educating patients on the risks involved with staying on their own equipment, the organization can help encourage transfer, when appropriate.

*Manual*s or E-dition, these new and revised standards are applicable to hospitals, critical access hospitals, and ambulatory health care organizations.

At least annually, a diagnostic medical physicist measures the radiation computed tomography dose index (CTDI) for four CT protocols: adult brain, adult abdomen, pediatric brain, and pediatric abdomen (if one or more of these is not used by the organization, other common CT protocols may be substituted). The medical physicist must verify that the CTDI is within 20% of the CTDI, as indicated on the CT console.

Further, diagnostic CT imaging equipment must undergo a performance evaluation at least annually. The evaluation includes the use of phantoms to assess a series of imaging metrics.

Similar annual performance evaluations of MRI, NM, and PET imaging equipment are required. These evaluations are intended to ensure the quality of the images being produced by the machine.

All of these processes must be documented thoroughly. The medical physicist (or possibly, in the case of MRIs, the MRI scientist) is responsible for performing these measurements and evaluations, but he or she may be assisted by individuals with appropriate training and skills.

Sterilizers

Knowing where your sterilizers are located throughout your organization is crucially important. This requires keeping an accurate inventory and conducting an inventory risk assessment.

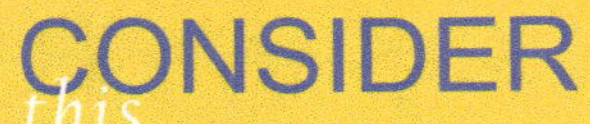

Types of Maintenance Strategies

Following is a discussion of several types of maintenance strategies. Health care organizations should consider using a combination of these to develop effective medical equipment maintenance programs that will meet the needs of the organizations.

Interval-Based Maintenance

This is the predominant strategy used by most health care organizations. It calls for given pieces of equipment to be maintained on a regular, calendar-based schedule, such as weekly, monthly, or semiannually. It is most effective for equipment with components that routinely wear out (belts, tubing, brushes). This strategy is supported easily by most information management systems.

Predictive Maintenance

This strategy is based on an if-then algorithm. Some simple measurements are made to determine if additional maintenance (typically parts replacement) is required. A predictor is selected that is sensitive to the impending failure of the equipment. This strategy allows the adjustment of maintenance cycles based on the presence or absence of the predictor. In most cases, predictive maintenance is used for equipment containing parts that experience mechanical wear, such as brushes on a centrifuge, power fluctuation in an x-ray tube, or vibration in a motor. This strategy does not apply well to electronic systems, which are the predominant devices in medical equipment inventories; hence, there are few examples in medical equipment maintenance. However, this strategy commonly is employed in utility management.

Metered Maintenance

This is based on a cycle count or hours of service instead of calendar days. Some pieces of medical equipment have methods—such as counters that indicate the number of uses—to track the cumulative length of time they have been in operation. In these cases, the maintenance schedule can be set up for specific intervals, such as every 500 cycles or every 1,000 hours of service. Common uses of metered maintenance include the number of hours of operation of ventilators or balloon pumps, or the number of slices taken by a computed tomography (CT) scanner. Although most effective, it may be very difficult to manage with computerized scheduling systems.

Run-to-Fail Maintenance

This is basically running the equipment until it malfunctions, at which time it simply is replaced or exchanged with a functional device. Run-to-fail maintenance is appropriate for medical equipment that is obviously in failure mode (for example, a blood glucose check meter with an error code displayed) and will do no harm to the patient when it fails because another meter is made available. This strategy is most effective for low-risk, low-cost commodity items, such as sphygmomanometers or thermometers, that may be uneconomical to repair. If a blood pressure cuff leaks, it is replaced by another. Ample spares are the key to this strategy.

Corrective Maintenance

Within this strategy, when equipment fails, it will be assessed, repaired, and returned to service as quickly as possible. The objective of most service organizations is to minimize unexpected corrective maintenance events. One way to do this is to assess corrective maintenance events continuously and determine if other maintenance strategies can be employed to reduce their frequency.

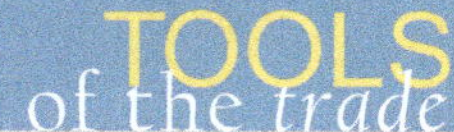

Equipment Maintenance Checklist

Organizations can use this simple equipment maintenance checklist to determine what maintenance strategies should be considered to ensure equipment safety.

Note: *The complete checklist may be adapted and is available for internal use on the flash drive (print only) or by clicking the tool link in the Risk-Assessment Toolbox (e-book only) on page 164.*

Published in *Environment of Care Risk Assessment*, Joint Commission Resources, 2018.   **File Name:** 07 04 Checklist Equipment Maintenance

EQUIPMENT MAINTENANCE CHECKLIST

*This checklist can be used to evaluate and asses an organization's equipment maintenance program and identify any areas of risk. Answers to all questions should ideally be **Y** for **Yes** (unless they aren't applicable). If an answer is **N** for **No**, use the "Notes" section to document needed changes. Unless otherwise noted, this checklist is applicable to all program settings.*

ORGANIZATION: _______________________________   DEPARTMENT/UNIT: _______________________________

DATE OF REVIEW: ______________   REVIEWER: _______________________________

QUESTIONS	YES	NO	NA	NOTES
Is there a complete inventory of equipment, regardless of ownership?				
Is all high-risk equipment (risk of serious injury or death to a patient or staff member should the equipment fail) identified on the inventory?				
Has the organization identified any equipment on the inventory that must be maintained in accordance with the manufacturer's recommendations? Such equipment might include any new equipment, diagnostic imaging or therapeutic radiologic equipment, or equipment specifically covered under state or federal law or CoP.				
Has the organization identified equipment that is maintained, inspected, and tested in accordance with manufacturers' recommendations or an AEM program?				
When using manufacturers' recommendations, does the organization have access to documentation (manufacturers' operation and maintenance manuals, standards, studies, guidance, recall information, service records) of the defined activities and frequencies for maintaining, inspecting, and testing the equipment?				

It also requires keeping the sterilizer manufacturer's instructions for use in an accessible location, adhering to those instructions when it comes to cleaning and preventive maintenance, and properly documenting that you have followed those instructions. Lapses or omissions in or failure to conduct these practices may contribute to a potential health care–associated infection and harm a patient.

Clinical Alarms

The number and volume of clinical alarms has been steadily increasing, and health care organizations find themselves at risk of missing critical patient alarms due to alarm fatigue.

To minimize these risks, The Joint Commission implemented National Patient Safety Goal (NPSG) NPSG.06.01.01 for hospitals and critical access hospitals. The goal and its related elements of performance (EPs) include the following requirements:

◉ Establish alarm safety as a priority.
◉ Identify which alarms are the most important to manage based on the organization's own particular situation and based on the following:
  • Input from clinical staff and clinical departments
  • Risk to patients if the alarm signal is not attended to or if it malfunctions
  • Whether specific alarm signals are needed or unnecessarily contribute to alarm noise and alarm fatigue
  • Potential for patient harm based on internal incident history
  • Published best practices and guidelines‡

◉ Establish policies and procedures related to clinical alarm management whose components include the following:
  • Clinically appropriate settings for alarm signals
  • When alarm signals can be disabled
  • When alarm parameters can be changed, and who in the organization has the authority to change them
  • Who in the organization has the authority to set alarm parameters to "off"
  • Monitoring and responding to alarm signals
  • Check individual alarm signals for accurate settings, proper operation, and detectability.
◉ Educate appropriate staff members on the purpose and proper use of alarm systems.

Reference

1. World Health Organization (WHO). Core Medical Equipment. Geneva: WHO, 2011. Accessed Feb 20, 2018. http://apps.who.int/iris/bitstream/10665/95788/1/WHO_HSS_EHT_DIM_11.03_eng.pdf.

---

‡ Additional information on alarm safety can be found on the Association for the Advancement of Medical Instrumentation website at http://www.aami.org/PatientSafety/content.aspx?ItemNumber=1399 (accessed Feb 20, 2018). Also, the ECRI Institute has identified alarm hazards as one of the top technology hazards for 2013; more information on this hazard list can be found at http://www.ecri.org/Forms/Pages/Alarm_Safety_Resource.aspx.

RISK-ASSESSMENT TOOLBOX

1. **Download** Alternative Equipment Maintenance Checklist
2. **Download** Endoscope Reprocessing Assessment Checklist
3. **Download** Medical Equipment Assessment and Selection Decision Checklist
4. **Download** Equipment Maintenance Checklist
5. **Download** Diagnostic Imaging Compliance Checklist

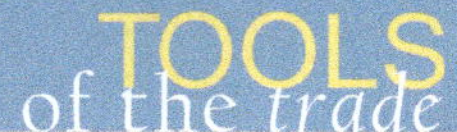

Diagnostic Imaging Compliance Checklist

Diagnostic imaging technology presents its own unique risks to health care providers and recipients. This checklist can be used with other risk-assessment tools to determine standards compliance and identify potential risk areas.

Note: *The complete checklist may be adapted and is available for internal use on the flash drive (print only) or by clicking the tool link in the Risk-Assessment Toolbox (e-book only) on page 164.*

Published in *Environment of Care Risk Assessment*, Joint Commission Resources, 2018.　　　　**File Name:** 07 05 Checklist Diagnostic Imaging

DIAGNOSTIC IMAGING COMPLIANCE CHECKLIST*

*This checklist can be used to assess various aspects of diagnostic imaging compliance. This checklist will be applicable only to organizations that use diagnostic imaging equipment. Answers to all questions should ideally be **Y** for **Yes** (unless they aren't applicable). If an answer is **N** for **No**, use the "Notes" section to document needed changes.*

ORGANIZATION: ________________________________　　DEPARTMENT/UNIT: ________________________________

DATE OF REVIEW: ________________________　　REVIEWER: ____

QUESTIONS	YES	NO	NA	NOTES
AREAS TO ASSESS APPLICABLE TO CT, MRI, NM, AND PET				
Are equipment QC and maintenance activities identified?				
Are time frames established for how often QC and maintenance activities should be performed?				
Are equipment QC and maintenance activities done?				
QC logs are complete?				
Is a performance evaluation that includes all required tests and parameters performed on each image acquisition monitor annually by a medical physicist or MRI scientist (for MRI only)?				
AREAS TO ASSESS APPLICABLE TO CT, NM, AND PET				
Are staff dosimetry results reviewed quarterly by one of the following?				
• Radiation Safety Officer				
• Medical physicist				
• Health physicist				

chapter 8

Utilities

Utilities are like the skeleton around which a health care facility is built (*see* page 169). It is very difficult, if not impossible, to provide safe, high-quality health care without reliable utility systems such as water supply, electricity, piped medical gas, and ventilation. When operating efficiently and effectively, utility systems can contribute significantly to the safe and reliable delivery of patient care in health care organizations. Because of the impact utility systems have on a health care organization, it is important to establish and maintain an effective utility risk-management program to ensure that utility systems function properly, are reliable, and do not negatively affect patients, such as through the spread of infection.

Overview of Assessing Risks

Required by Joint Commission Environment of Care (EC) Standard EC.02.05.01, the primary method of assessing utility risks is creating and maintaining an inventory. The inventory must be current and in writing, in accordance with the standard.

Inventory

Requirements for the inventory vary, depending on the setting and whether the organization uses Joint Commission accreditation for deemed status purposes. Not all settings (for example, home care) are required to maintain a utilities inventory. The following sections describe the inventory requirements for those settings that must maintain a utilities inventory (check the *Comprehensive Accreditation Manual* or E-dition to determine which settings this is applicable to).

For All Organizations That Are Required to Maintain a Utilities Inventory

Organizations must identify on their utilities inventory which devices are classified as high risk. *High-risk devices* are defined as those that pose a risk of serious harm or death to patients or staff if they were to fail, and include all life-support devices.

The inventory also must provide details on maintenance plans. This includes maintenance activities, inspections, and testing for every piece of equipment listed on the inventory. The frequency of these activities should be included as well.

STANDARDS to *know*

EC.02.05.01	EC.02.05.09
EC.02.05.03	EM.01.01.01
EC.02.05.05	EM.02.02.09
EC.02.05.07	

TERMS to *know*

high-risk equipment

medical equipment

Inventory requirements for fire safety systems

The maintenance, testing, and inspection of fire alarm and suppression systems are scored separately under the Environment of Care (EC) standards. For fire safety systems, an individualized component inventory is required for each device/equipment/system listed in each element of performance (EP). These include the following:

- Supervisory signal devices
- Water-flow devices
- Valve tamper switches
- Manual pull stations
- Duct, heat, and smoke detectors
- Electromechanical releasing devices
- Visual and audible fire alarms
- Automatic smoke-detection shutdown devices for air-handling units
- Water-storage tank alarms
- Main drains
- Fire department water supply connections
- Fire pumps, fire hoses, and their standpipe system
- Kitchen hood extinguishing systems and other special extinguishing systems
- Portable fire extinguishers
- Fire and smoke dampers
- Sliding/rolling fire doors

If a device is not listed in the EPs, such as sprinkler heads, there is no individual device inventory requirement.

Organizations That Use Joint Commission Accreditation for Deemed Status Purposes

For these organizations, all operating components of their utility systems must be included in the inventory. Certain types of equipment must be maintained, inspected, and tested according to the manufacturer's recommendations for specific activities and frequencies. These include the following:

- New operating components that do not have enough maintenance history (for example, records from the health care organization's contractors, records of the organization's own experience over time, information from nationally recognized sources) to support use of alternative maintenance strategies
- Any operating components that are subject to the US Centers for Medicare & Medicaid Services (CMS) Conditions of Participation (CoP), or other federal or state laws that establish other, more stringent maintenance requirements.

If a qualified individual determines a component can be safely maintained under an alternative equipment maintenance (AEM) program, it must be identified as such in the inventory (*see* page 171 for additional information about AEM programs for utilities management). Also, the inventory must support that decision with written details on the following:

- How the equipment is used, and the seriousness and prevalence of harm related to normal use
- Likely consequences if the equipment fails or malfunctions, including seriousness and prevalence of harm
- Availability of alternative or backup equipment in case of failure or malfunction
- Incident history of identical or similar equipment
- Maintenance requirements of the equipment

Hospitals and Critical Access Hospitals That Do Not Use Joint Commission Accreditation for Deemed Status Purposes

The inventory may include all operating components of its utility systems; or it may include selected components chosen by risk of infection, occupant needs, and systems critical to patient care (including all life-support equipment). Also, before a new type of component is put into use, the organization should evaluate it to determine whether it will be included in the inventory.

Participants in the Process

As in any other area of the environment of care, utilities risks are most effectively managed by a multidisciplinary group. Of course, facilities management staff will be a significant component of the team. It also is important to include representatives from infection control, fire/life safety, and any departments that have special utilities needs (such as radiology, intensive care units, or isolation rooms).

Identifying Risks

Utilities risks can be identified from several sources. First is through updating the inventory. Any systems that are high risk are natural targets for a risk assessment. Also, any equipment that is new or does not have much maintenance history may be a good candidate for assessment. The same is true for any piece of equipment that has experienced a failure or malfunction in the past.

Utility components also should be assessed for risks particular to their use. Water and air-handling systems, for example, can pose infection risks. This is particularly true for

Utility Systems in Health Care

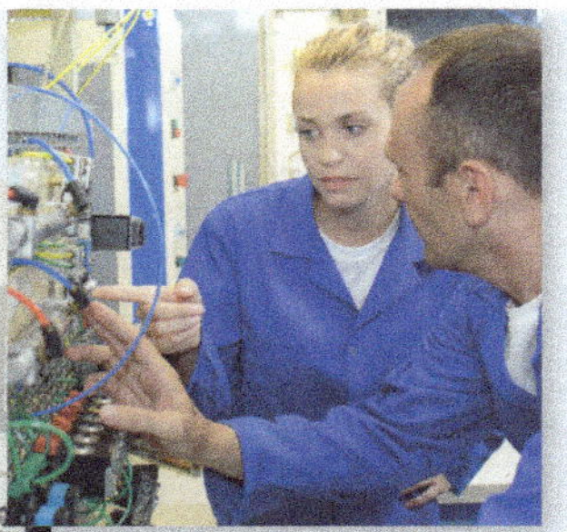

Electrical Distribution

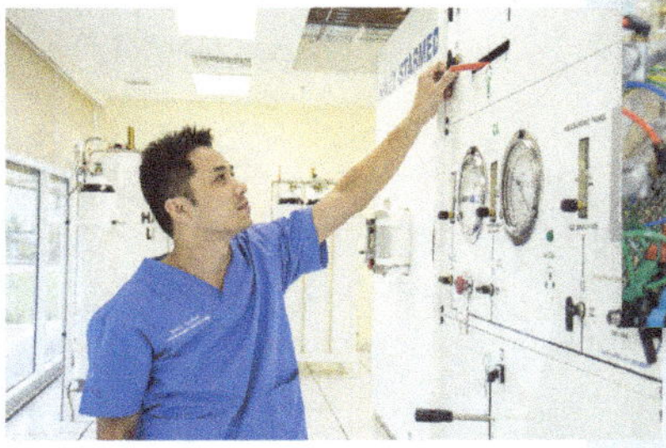

Horizontal Transport
(pneumatic tube systems
and others)

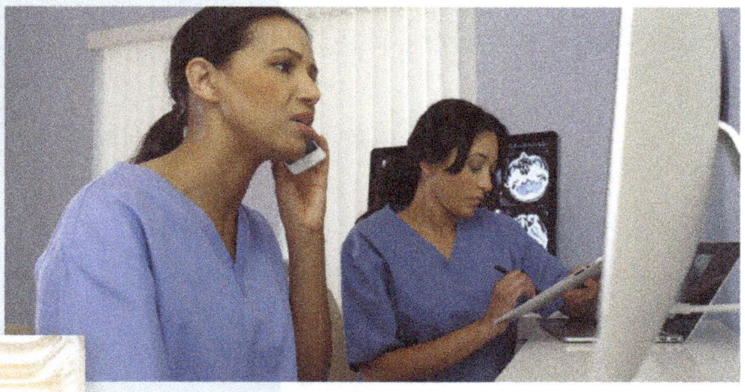

Communication Systems
(telephone, internet, public address,
nurse call system, and data exchange)

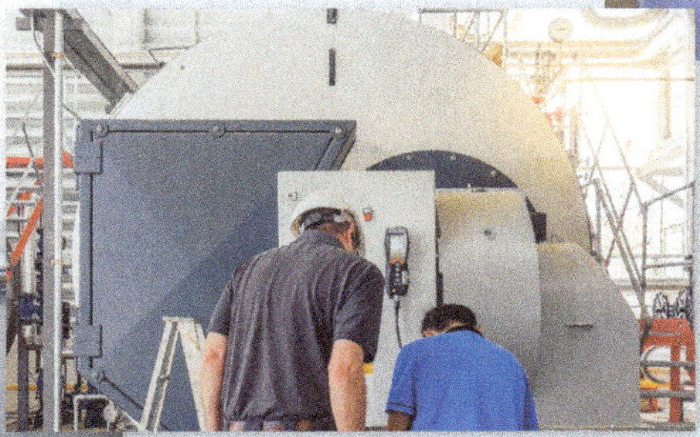

Boiler and Steam

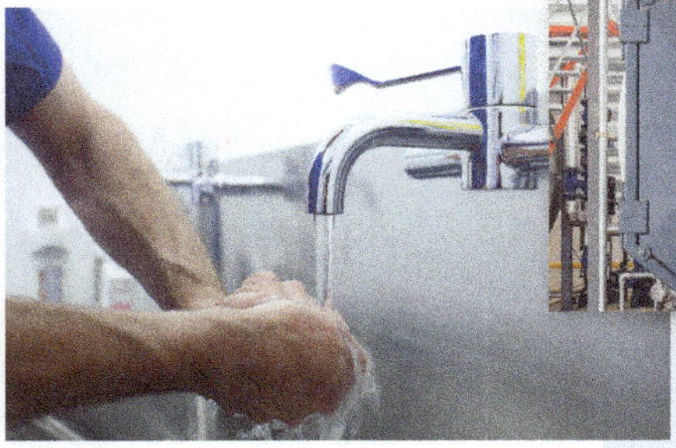

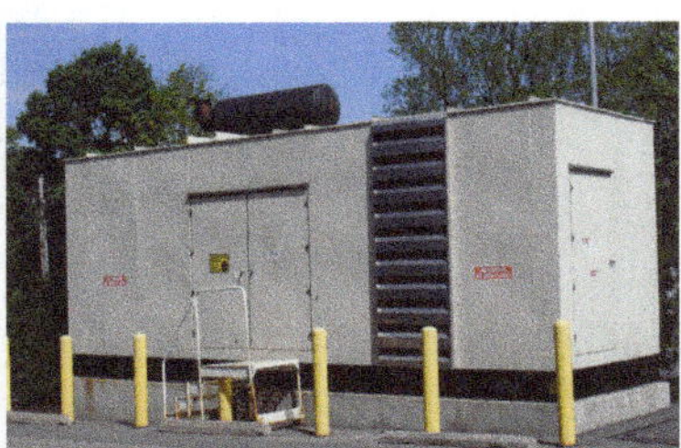

Plumbing

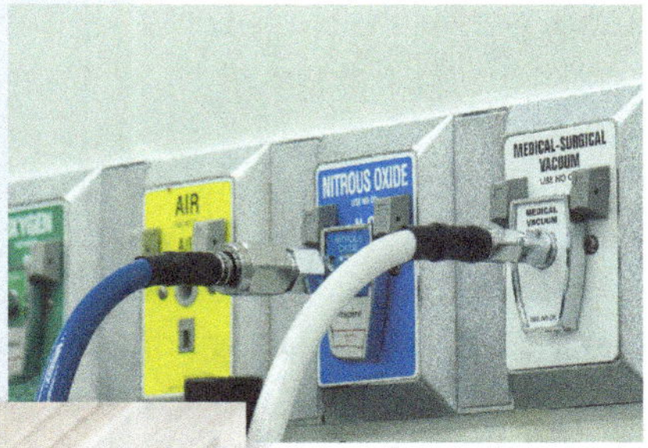

Piped Gases

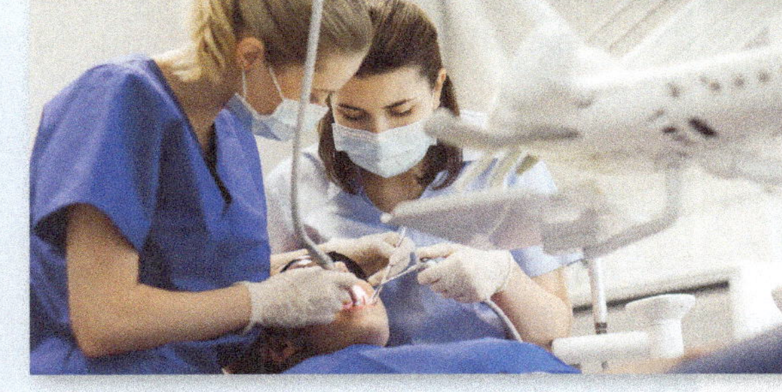

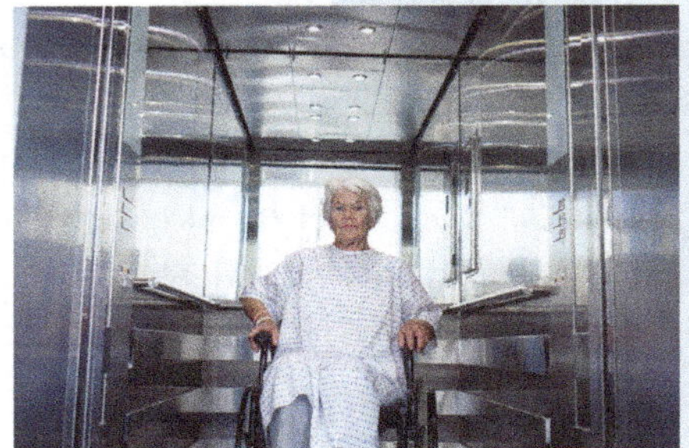

Emergency Power

Vacuum Systems

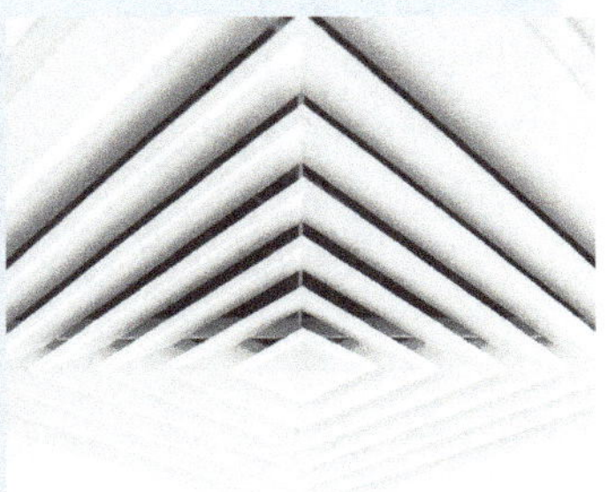

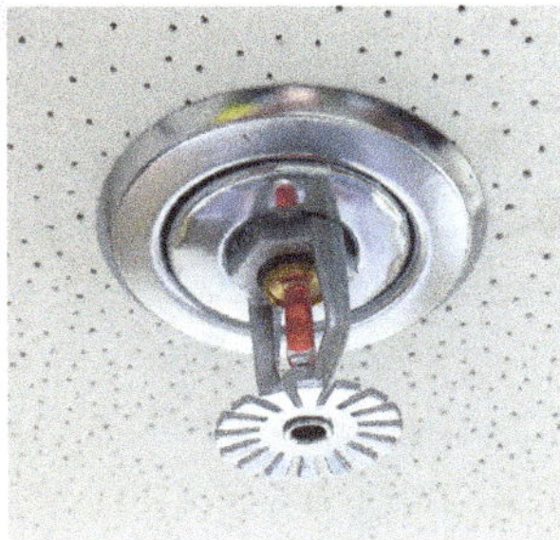

Fire Alarm
Suppression Systems

Vertical Transport (elevators)

HVAC Systems

HVAC, heating, ventilating, and air conditioning.

According to The Joint Commission, utility systems may include any of the identified systems listed
in this graphic. Some utility systems will be common to most facilities, while others may be unique
to specific settings.

special-purpose areas, such as isolation rooms, protective environments, and laboratories. For example, disinfection and sterilization devices should be assessed for infection control risks. Similarly, any device that uses a clinical alarm should be assessed for its effectiveness in the face of alarm fatigue and excessive noise levels.

Creating a Risk-Based Inventory

Most health care organizations have a full inventory of all components of the utility systems in their facilities. As with medical equipment, these components may be too numerous for effective ongoing management, given the time and resources available, or may not derive any benefit from routine preventive maintenance. Here, too, organizations have the option of creating a risk-based inventory of just those utility system components that will benefit from a systematic maintenance program (*see* page 172).

Similar to the features of fire protection, if the organization is in leased or rented space, it is not directly responsible for the operation of the utilities but is responsible for making sure that the utility systems it uses are appropriate and maintained as required. Records of utility systems' maintenance, testing, and inspection should be made available to the health care organization on request.

Maintenance Strategies

As with medical equipment, health care organizations may use any of the following inspection, testing, and maintenance inspection, testing, and strategies to ensure proper maintenance of utilities: interval-based, metered, predictive, run-to-fail, and corrective (*see* page 162 in Chapter 7 for the definitions of these strategies). Utilities-based examples for each of the five maintenance strategies include the following:

- *Interval-based maintenance* is common for such procedures as adding chemicals to cooling towers, changing filters, and lubricating parts.
- *Metered maintenance* commonly is used for compressors, which are maintained based on the number of hours run, and for the loading of variable-speed drives.
- *Predictive maintenance* is used to determine the status of electrical systems based on infrared scans, ultrasonic scans of pumps for turbulence to determine the efficiency of flow, and oil analysis for diesel generators.

- *Run-to-fail maintenance* and *corrective maintenance* are used for a variety of utility systems components that are not critical, either due to their function, the area served, or system redundancy.

Health care organizations may use any combination of these to develop an effective utilities maintenance program that enables safe, high-quality care and makes appropriate use of the time and resources of the facilities maintenance department.

Remember that manufacturers' recommendations may be overly conservative for designing maintenance strategies but should be followed at least through the warranty period for a new piece of equipment, and longer if the organization (or the field) does not have a comfortable level of professional experience with the device.

Possible Utility Failures

Assessing utility risks not only involves assessing and monitoring the operational reliability of utility systems but also minimizing the potential risks of utility system failures. Creating and exercising contingency plans, which involve backup systems that can be used in an emergency, can help minimize potential risks during a utility failure.

An Example

Consider this: It's a Sunday evening in January, and an organization is weathering the biggest snowstorm it's seen in years. It is 25°F (-4°C) outside, and the wind-chill factor makes it feel like -10°F (-23°C). The facilities manager just got off the phone with the manager of the city's steam power plant. There was a failure due to the weather, and the plant is temporarily off-line. Consequently, the health care organization is without its city-provided steam heat. The organization has a contingency plan for just this type of situation; the question is, will that plan be effective? The answer to that question may well depend on whether the organization has recently tested its steam contingency plan.

For example, say the organization's steam contingency plan involves shutting off a valve in the street behind the main facility so that steam can be diverted back into the building. But what if the valve is the same one that was installed in 1940 when the building was constructed, and the contingency

Alternative Equipment Maintenance Program

Joint Commission Environment of Care (EC) Standards EC.02.05.01 and EC.02.05.05 require health care organizations to manage risks associated with utilities. This includes proper maintenance of operating components, which generally means following manufacturers' recommendations regarding activities and associated frequencies. However, in some cases, following manufacturers' recommendations can put an unnecessary burden on a facility. The US Centers for Medicare & Medicaid Services (CMS) policy and associated Joint Commission standards now allow organizations some flexibility in their utilities maintenance program. The option of using this process, known as an alternative equipment maintenance (AEM) program, is available to hospitals and critical access hospitals that use Joint Commission accreditation for deemed status purposes.

An AEM program enables health care organizations to adopt a maintenance approach that deviates from manufacturers' requirements. The Joint Commission offers the American Society for Healthcare Engineering (ASHE) book *Maintenance Management for Health Care Facilities* as an example of guidelines for an alternative maintenance program. An AEM program must not compromise safety or put patients at increased risk, and it must be based on accepted standards of practice. The decision to use an AEM program must be based on a risk assessment performed by a qualified individual. The organization must keep documentation supporting its AEM approach and must announce its use of an AEM program at the beginning of the accreditation survey.

For hospitals and critical access hospitals that use Joint Commission accreditation for deemed status purposes, AEM programs are not permissible when any of the following conditions are present:

- Federal or state laws, or an organization's Conditions of Participation (CoPs), require adherence to manufacturers' recommendations, or otherwise establish more stringent maintenance requirements.
- New operating components do not have a sufficient amount of maintenance history to use as a basis for a risk assessment (maintenance history includes documented records provided by the organization's contractors, public information from nationally recognized sources, or records of the organization's experience over time).

In addition, certain settings (for example, ambulatory health care centers) are not allowed the use of an AEM program.

Information on AEM programs as they apply to medical equipment can be found in Chapter 7.

Utility System Components in Health Care

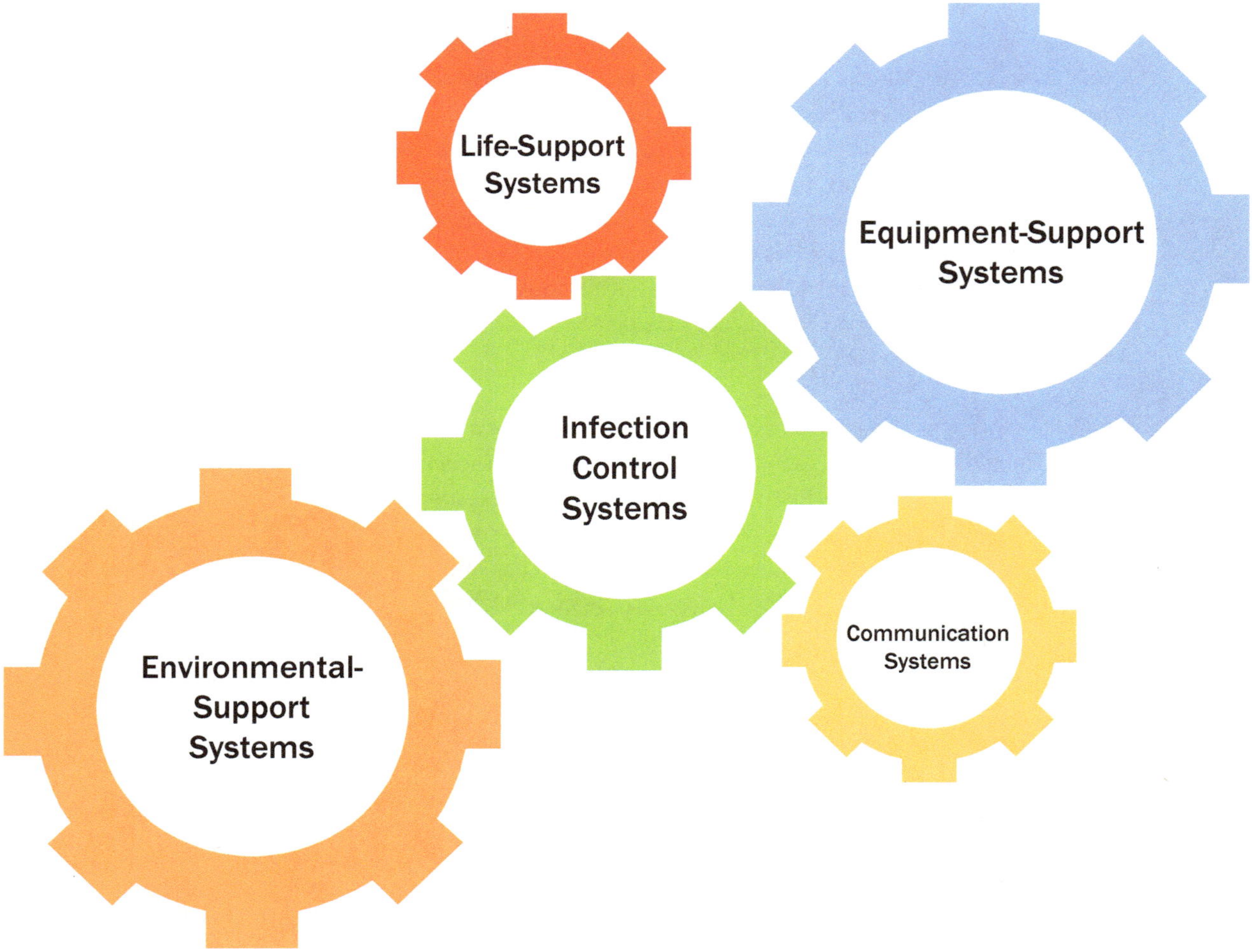

To develop a risk-based inventory for utility system components, organizations will want to consider the components' impact on the systems listed here. These systems are critical to the safety and care of the individuals served in the organization; thus, the utility system components that support or are integral to them will rank higher on a risk-based system.

plan was created by the individual who managed utilities at the time? In other words, what if the valve has never been tested? If the valve has not been tested recently, there is a good chance it will break when the facilities manager tries to shut it off. Not only would this not address the lack-of-steam problem the organization is facing, but it also might necessitate evacuating the building's occupants to another location where there is heat. What started as a utility outage would quickly transform into a crisis for the organization.

On the other hand, if the organization tested the valve last summer and it worked, the probability it will work during the crisis increases. If the valve had not worked during the test, but the organization fixed it before colder weather arrived, the crisis would have been avoided, and the organization would have ensured the continuation of steam heat during the snowstorm.

Frequent Testing as a Proactive Measure

It is important not to wait until there is a problem or an emergency before testing a contingency plan. Many organizations have contingency plans for their utilities that were created when their buildings were new, and they have not exercised them since. By frequently testing utility contingency plans, organizations can avoid crises and ensure the continuous delivery of high-quality care.

When testing contingency plans, timing is everything. Organizations should plan to conduct tests when the effects of potential failures in the utility backup systems are minimal and when the safety of patients will not be compromised. In the case of the previously mentioned steam example, an organization could consider conducting the valve test in July, when steam heat is not needed.

Emergency Operations Plan

Utility outages can be caused by several different sources. Some are planned, such as during construction. Others are unexpected, like those caused by natural disasters or terrorist situations. Improperly managed utility failures can exacerbate already heightened risks of infection, security or safety issues, equipment failure or malfunction, or other harm to patients and staff. (*See* page 175 for a utility outage mock tracer worksheet that can be used as a tool to identify risks.)

Joint Commission Emergency Management (EM) Standards EM.01.01.01 and EM.02.02.09 require health care

organizations to have an Emergency Operations Plan (EOP) that establishes procedures to manage an emergency situation. Among the issues the EOP must address is managing utilities. The EOP requires management of the following five utility systems:

1. *Electricity.* Organizations are required, according to Joint Commission Standard EC.02.05.07, to provide a reliable emergency power source for such systems and equipment as fire alarms, exit routes and signage, emergency communications, and life support. These bare minimum requirements may not be enough for most organizations. Other systems they should consider include heating, ventilating, and air-conditioning (HVAC), vertical transportation, and vital computer systems. When making decisions about emergency power beyond minimum requirements, organizations also will need to consider energy usage of these systems.

2. *Water.* Every organization uses two types of water: potable (for drinking and use in health care procedures) and nonpotable (used in cleaning systems, boilers, bathrooms, and so on). Organizations must plan for emergency provision of both types of water usage. Inability to flush toilets or provide heat will worsen an already high-risk environment.

3. *Fuel.* Organizations often focus on fuel as it applies to operating the emergency power supply, but it also is required for transportation. Ambulances, supply vehicles, and other transportation services must be available when the organization is providing service. Two solutions are stockpiling fuel at the facility and making arrangements with a local supplier (for example, a gas station). Stockpiling is not always practical, though, and gas stations might not have generators to access the fuel. These issues must be considered, and decisions must be based on the best possible solution for each organization's particular needs.

4. *Medical gas and vacuum systems.* Medical gas and vacuum systems must be connected to the emergency power system. But if they malfunction or stop working independently of power during emergency situations, these services should be restored as soon as possible. Because replacement parts may be impossible to obtain during an emergency, it is recommended that organizations keep a supply of parts on hand to fix the equipment if it does break down.

5. *Utility systems defined as essential.* This might include such systems as vertical and horizontal transport, heating and cooling systems, and steam for sterilization.

Advance planning through the EOP will ensure that all these essential utilities are provided for during emergencies.

Preparing for Utility Failure

To prepare for an unexpected utility failure, the EOP should describe how the organization will perform the following activities:

- Repair or replace components promptly.
- Provide appropriate alternative clinical care to mitigate risks to those receiving care during the outage.
- Decide when partial or total cessation of services is advisable.
- Determine when and how care recipients will be evacuated in the event of a prolonged outage.

Arranging alternative means of providing essential utilities is critical. This may entail negotiated relationships with primary suppliers, redundant or alternative equipment within the organization, or provision through a parent entity. Organizations should keep in mind that community resources may be unavailable during emergency situations, and plan accordingly.

Special Considerations

The following sections explore several important issues to consider when addressing utility system risks.

Ensuring Infection Control within Utility Systems

Health care–associated infections (HAIs) are a significant problem faced by health care organizations, despite advanced technology, cleanliness standards, and well-intentioned staff. The safety of both patients and staff is at risk because of these infections, and utility systems can either help prevent the spread of HAIs or increase the likelihood of their proliferation.

Infection prevention and control efforts in utility management require organizations to engage in monitoring and eliminating contaminants spread through the air and water.

Airborne Contaminants

Airborne contaminants could include biological agents—bacteria, viruses, and molds—as well as gases, fumes, and dust. To help prevent the spread of airborne contaminants, organizations must design, install, and maintain ventilation equipment, such as HVAC systems, to provide appropriate pressure relationships, air-exchange rates, filtration efficiencies, temperature, and relative humidity. The particulars of an organization's ventilation policies will depend on what types of procedures it performs, what types of patients it serves, and, of course, what kinds of organisms it identifies. Different areas might require different levels of temperature, humidity, velocity, and filtration.

To ensure that an effective HVAC system is designed properly, organizations should involve design professionals who are appropriately credentialed and adhere to specifications contained in state and/or local codes and in guidelines available from ASHRAE (American Society of Heating, Refrigerating, and Air-Conditioning Engineers) and the Facility Guidelines Institute.

Cleaning, inspection, and preventive maintenance schedules for the HVAC system also should be prudently established and strictly followed for such parts as fans, coils, belts, and filters. Proper fit of filters is essential to their effective functioning. A related issue is the maintenance, testing, and inspection of negative-pressure rooms for suspected or confirmed tuberculosis.

Waterborne Pathogens

Similar to airborne contaminants, waterborne pathogens can wreak havoc in a health care organization. Pathogenic biological agents—primarily, but not exclusively, *Legionella*—must be managed specifically in cooling towers, domestic hot- and cold-water systems, and aerosolizing water systems, which includes showers, humidifiers, and fountains. Although it is at their discretion to choose how to manage waterborne pathogens, organizations should use appropriate references when establishing programs. CMS also requires organizations to develop and adhere to policies and procedures that reduce the risk of microbial growth and spread of *Legionella* and other pathogens in the water systems.[1]

As with airborne contaminants, a risk assessment should be conducted to identify areas serving the individuals most susceptible to waterborne contaminants. Actually, one assessment process can be used for both kinds of contaminants. A separate assessment should be made to determine (1) if the organization has had any history of identified cases of *Legionella*, and (2) the layout and status of the domestic hot- and cold-water system. Issues to look

Utility Outage Mock Tracer Worksheet

Organizations can use this tool or create a mock tracer worksheet to focus on risks associated with utility outages.

Note: *The complete worksheet may be adapted and is available for internal use on the flash drive (print only) or by clicking the tool link in the Risk-Assessment Toolbox (e-book only) on page 177.*

Published in *Environment of Care Risk Assessment*, Joint Commission Resources, 2018.   **File Name:** 08 01 Worksheet Utility Outage Tr

UTILITY OUTAGE MOCK TRACER WORKSHEET

This tracer worksheet is filled in with questions pertinent to utility outages, but can be revised to fit a particular program sett. or health care facility. Review the relevant standards listed in the next section to determine what requirements are applicabl to specific programs and settings.

Relevant Standards for these questions include the following: EC.02.05.01, EC.02.04.01, and EM.02.02.09. Relevant standards cited are not necessarily applicable to every question. To determine applicability with a specific program/setting, check the *Comprehensive Accreditation Manual* Edition

---

for include dead ends in the plumbing system and sections of the system that have been shut off for any reason, resulting in stagnant water.

Mitigation activities for *Legionella* can include delivering water to the outlets at higher temperatures and installing thermostatic mixing valves to cool water down before use. In addition, the warm-water pipe between the valve and the shower should be self-draining. In areas where susceptible care recipients are housed, consider recirculation of the water in the system and make sure that any dead ends are short. Organizations should locate cooling towers in such a way that their drift is directed away from air intakes. They also should install drift eliminators, which need to be cleaned and treated prior to seasonal start-up and shutdown. Maintenance should be performed on a regular schedule, with the addition of an appropriate biocide. Decorative fountains also should be kept clean and undergo regular chemical treatment to control microbiological growth.

Culturing of the water systems for *Legionella* is not required by The Joint Commission, but may be required by a local authority having jurisdiction (AHJ). Those who support routine water culturing believe that it is the proactive way to address risks associated with *Legionella*. On the other hand, the US Centers for Disease Control and Prevention (CDC) does not recommend culturing because *Legionella* is indigenous to the water: If you culture for it, you will find it and then have to take action, even though—according to the CDC—not all occurrences will lead to disease. The CDC recommends maintaining a high index of suspicion for *Legionella* as a clinical diagnosis and taking action if there is a clinical reason to do so.

Regardless of where they come down on this controversial issue, all health care organizations should develop a plan of remediation for use in an outbreak of *Legionella*. Remediation methods, each of which has pros and cons, include the following:

- Chlorine dioxide
- Copper-silver ionization
- Hyperchlorination
- Monochloramine
- Superheating

Organizations should investigate the options thoroughly to determine the method most appropriate for their own use.

Ensuring the Reliability of Emergency Electrical Power

A reliable electrical power distribution system is vital to the safety of all facility occupants, particularly those who are dependent on electronic life support or other critical equipment. The complex demands placed on electrical distribution systems reflect the need for close supervision, careful risk assessment, and performance evaluation to ensure their reliability (*see* page 178 for a real-world scenario of an organization maintaining proper documentation of its testing, inspection, and maintenance of its power supply systems).

An emergency power system provides the facility with sufficient power to maintain essential functions during power failures, thereby reducing the risks associated with such failures. Emergency power systems are required for all health care organizations that intend to provide continuous service under emergency conditions.

Maintenance and Testing

Because a health care facility generally does not use its emergency power system regularly, potential problems relating to emergency power may not be immediately evident. Consequently, it is crucial that such systems be maintained and tested properly. An effective management and maintenance program for emergency power systems covers areas that should be provided with emergency power, key elements of an emergency power system, and testing procedures.

Fueling the System

An acceptable emergency power system should be powered by an on-site emergency standby generator of sufficient size to serve the connected load. The amount of on-site fuel storage should take into account past outages and anticipated delivery problems caused by shortages, weather, and geographic conditions and locations. This is determined by the individual health care organization, unless specifically dictated by an AHJ.

An emergency generator powered only by natural gas is acceptable if the documented probability of simultaneous gas and electrical failure is low. Such documentation may include written verification from the gas and electrical services, as well as a diagram of where such services enter the building.

In a residential or outpatient facility, batteries may be used instead of a generator to power the emergency electrical system. However, the amount of power provided by the batteries should conform to the degree of reliability required at the installation. Specifically, battery systems should provide power to supply corridor lighting for not less than 1½ hours, as well as to alarm systems and any equipment used in the provision of care, until regular power is restored. In addition, storage batteries are to be maintained according to the manufacturer's specifications.

Exercising Emergency Backup Generators

The EC standards require organizations to test their emergency power systems regularly.

Different types of emergency power equipment have different testing methods and frequencies, including battery-powered lights required for egress, stored emergency power supply systems (SEPSSs), non-SEPSS battery backup emergency power systems that are determined to be critical for operations during a power failure, emergency generators, diesel-powered emergency generators, and automatic transfer switches. If a system fails a test, the organization must enact measures to ensure safety until the problem can be corrected and retested.

Contingencies for Emergency Backup Failure

Similar to other utilities, organizations should have contingency plans in place should emergency backup power fail during a test. Organizations might want to consider obtaining a secondary generator unit before each four-hour generator test. Although not a requirement, proactively evaluating the need for redundant systems can be considered a best practice. The Joint Commission does not specify the interim measures that should be implemented; however, the following options outline possible interim steps that organizations could consider:

- *Communicate.* Notify clinical staff and organizational leadership that backup power is compromised.
- *Ready staff for the backup plan.* Place staff on standby to implement power failure contingency plans.
- *Restrict services.* Consider canceling elective surgeries and any other nonessential services that would put patients in danger if power failed.

Because the standards require health care organizations to provide reliable emergency electrical power at all times, an organization that experiences a generator test failure must obtain a backup generator immediately.

Organizations also may want to consider testing a utility contingency plan during an emergency management exercise. For example, if an organization is conducting an exercise that involves a loss of potable water, the organization may want to test the water valves at this time to see if they function and if an effective contingency plan is in place.

Other Backup Utility Systems

Depending on the type of organization, there may be many different utility systems present. Addressing risks and potential failures in all utility backup systems at once is not realistic due to the potential lack of resources, such as time, money, and staff. Before testing contingency plans, organizations need to make sure they are testing the most critical plans first. For example, addressing the lack of backup steam may be more critical than addressing an issue in the backup pneumatic tube system.

Organizations should consider conducting a proactive risk assessment to prioritize what needs to be addressed first. This type of assessment can help the organization determine potential utility backup system failures, identify the risks associated with those failures, prioritize issues to be fixed, determine ways to fix the priorities, and implement solutions to avoid potentially harmful situations. By conducting a risk assessment first, organizations can address the most critical issues immediately and create a timetable for addressing other issues in the future.

Testing the Contingency Plan

Before embarking on a test of a utility contingency plan, organizations should set aside resources to address whatever failures may be discovered during the test. For example, if the organization is going to test the previously mentioned valve to divert steam heat, it should have funds in place to replace that valve should it break during the test. If an organization cannot allocate sufficient funds, then plans must be made for a secondary backup to the system being tested to ensure that a loss in backup utilities will not affect the environment of care or patient safety.

When planning a test of a utility system contingency plan, EC professionals should discuss the test with the organization's multidisciplinary group that addresses EC issues. It is important that any discipline that could be affected by the test be aware of it. Also, a multidisciplinary group may help anticipate problems the EC professional might not consider. For example, if an organization is planning to test its medical gas utility backup system, everyone in the organization who would use medical gas should be aware that the test is taking place and that there is a chance the backup system could be compromised.

Organizations should schedule tests well in advance and process any requests for tests in writing to ensure that the verification and approval of the tests are documented. Before conducting a test, organizations should make sure any backup equipment or personnel are on site and ready to step in should the backup system fail.

The middle of a utility failure is not the time to discover that a contingency plan is not effective. Organizations that regularly test their contingency plans and address any problems that arise are better prepared for an emergency and increase the likelihood that patient safety and quality of care will be preserved.

Reference

1. US Centers for Medicare & Medicaid Services. Memorandum: Requirement to Reduce *Legionella* Risk in Healthcare Facility Water Systems to Prevent Cases and Outbreaks of Legionnaires' Disease (LS). Jun 2, 2017. Accessed Feb 20, 2018. https://www.cms.gov/Medicare/ Provider-Enrollment-and-Certification/Survey CertificationGenInfo/Downloads/Survey-and -Cert-Letter-17-30.pdf.

RISK-ASSESSMENT TOOLBOX

1. **Download** **Utility Outage Mock Tracer Worksheet**
2. **Download** **Emergency Power Supply System Testing Dashboard**

Proper Documentation of Testing, Inspection, and Maintenance of Emergency Power Supply Systems

Medical facilities cannot afford to be without backup power, especially during a catastrophic weather event like a hurricane or flood. One health care organization that has adopted a proactive strategy to avert a power outage emergency is University of Texas MD Anderson Cancer Center in Houston.

One of the largest cancer centers in the United States, this organization spans more than 15 million square feet across 40 structures, and three campuses; it serves hundreds of patients at any given time. University of Texas MD Anderson Cancer Center is served by an emergency power supply system (EPSS) consisting of 61 backup generators, a sophisticated fuel system that feeds 300,000 gallons of diesel to the generators, and an electrical distribution system composed of 200 automatic transfer switches, electrical switch gears, and parallel gears supported by breakers, synchronizers, and other sophisticated controls. The hospital's facilities managers and engineers make sure this complex network of backup power runs well when needed, and they're careful to comply with crucial codes and industry standards that call for regular monitoring and upkeep of the equipment as well as proper documentation.

To organize and simplify this process as well as improve the reliability of its EPSS, MD Anderson Cancer Center created a documentation protocol using customized spreadsheets designed to improve the efficiency and transparency of date logging and recordkeeping. Thanks to this protocol, the organization can now ensure high reliability of its EPSS. In addition, it can very quickly provide information requested by surveyors or auditors: Demonstrating the reliability of its EPSS now takes as little as 30 minutes.

Plugging in to a New Approach

Pouyan Layegh, PE, MBA, LEED, AP, director of Campus Services, Administrative Facilities and Campus Operations, MD Anderson Cancer Center, says the documentation protocol provides better peace of mind for everyone involved.

"Our mission here is to eliminate cancer, but we're sitting on the Gulf of Mexico, where we can get flash flooding, hurricanes, tornadoes, and power grid interruptions from extreme heat or cold," says Layegh. "Therefore, we need a robust and dependable emergency power supply system. The EPSS aspect of our operation has a direct impact on patient treatment success, as these systems support the treatment for our patients. Fortunately, our EPSS has never been compromised, but proper documentation of a system with so many parts and technical components is very challenging, especially when you're trying to remain in compliance with many industry requirements."

These requirements include the 2012 editions of the National Fire Protection Association's *Life Safety Code*®* (NFPA 101) and *Health Care Facilities Code* (NFPA 99). For example, the *Standard on Stored Electrical Energy Emergency and Standby Power Systems* (NFPA 111–2010) specifies how standby power systems and emergency generators providing power to emergency lighting systems shall be installed, tested, and maintained; NFPA 111 provides specifics regarding installation and testing of stored electrical energy systems.

The organization must also comply with Joint Commission Environment of Care (EC) Standard EC.02.05.07, which requires the testing, inspection, and maintenance of emergency power systems. Compliance with this standard has been problematic for many organizations: More than 21% of surveyed hospitals were found noncompliant with EC.02.05.07 during the first half of 2016.

Dashboard Documentation

Layegh and his team devised a dashboard that consists of a series of handy spreadsheets to enable quick and easy data logging of important testing, inspection, and maintenance results in a user-friendly single-page/screen view (*see* page 180 for a sample screen from the dashboard). The dashboard consists of a series of detailed spreadsheets that help the hospital ensure complete and accurate documentation of EPSS testing. The organization chose a project management software application for the task because it offers document collaboration flexibility among multiple personnel, who can view, access, and edit the spreadsheet data across multiple devices.

* *Life Safety Code*® is a registered trademark of the National Fire Protection Association, Quincy, MA.

"The EC.02.05.07 and NFPA 110[–2010 *Standard for Emergency and Standby Power Systems*] testing frequency—weekly, monthly, annually, and tri-annually—and technical requirements can get cumbersome and complicated," Layegh says. Thanks to the dashboard tool, he says, "We can now easily review in a summarized format all the needed information regarding the regulatory compliance of these systems."

Layegh says that the new documentation system is used by a dedicated team of electricians, generator mechanics, and instrumentation technicians. Managers check compliance and verify that all documentation is in place. This team coordination is important to guarantee that documentation is both efficient and effective.

Power Steps to Success

Layegh recommends the following tips to better ensure the reliability of your organization's EPSS and compliance with industry standards, codes, and requirements:

- **Prepare and test your EPSS for worst-case scenarios.** In accordance with code requirements, your EPSS should be up and running within less than 10 seconds of a power failure, and you should have enough fuel stored to support your facility's operation for at least 96 hours.
- **Engage the manufacturers of EPSS components and equipment.** It is important to ensure that your program covers manufacturers' minimum expectations. "MD Anderson requires proper commissioning, which includes visits to generator manufacturing sites to witness original equipment test results and to assure that design characteristics have been met," Layegh says.
- **Be proactive in your maintenance and exceed minimum recommendations/requirements.** NFPA 110 recommends that lead-acid starting batteries be replaced every 24 to 30 months. Layegh says, "We not only electronically monitor our batteries and cells around the clock and check their integrity weekly, we also replace all our batteries every two years, whether they are failing or not."

- **Explore strategies to improve your comprehensive protocol for compliance and control of your EPSS.** Consider ways to more efficiently and accurately document your related testing, inspection, and maintenance efforts.
- **Be honest and transparent in your documentation.** Documentation of tests, inspections, and maintenance of the EPSS is useful only if it is done honestly and transparently.
- **Audit your EPSS documentation system.** Auditing should be done both internally and via third-party validation.
- **Conduct consistent training, drills, and exercises.** Such tests should put your EPSS and staff to the test in mock emergencies.
- **Network and partner with area health care organizations and local authorities.** Collaboration is needed to establish the coordination and sharing of resources that will occur during an emergency that requires backup power.
- **Stay active with professional associations and industry organizations.** The American Society for Healthcare Engineering (ASHE) and other organizations recommend programs and best practices that can help your organization prepare for emergencies.

Make the Paperwork a Priority

Confirming the efficacy and reliability of your EPSS requires diligent effort, consistent supervision, and unwavering commitment from everyone involved—from administrators to maintenance technicians. Given that your EPSS is crucial to your operations and those receiving treatment within your facilities when the conventional power supply is interrupted, the constant vigilance and resources needed to certify the integrity of your system are worthwhile.

"Having the right skills, training, and resources will determine your success. In the current culture where doing more with less is often emphasized, cutting corners on testing, inspecting, and maintaining your emergency power supply system creates a slippery slope," says Layegh.

Example Dashboard—Emergency Power Supply System Testing

Pouyan Layegh and his team at the University of Texas MD Anderson Cancer Center developed this time-saving dashboard tool, consisting of a series of carefully organized spreadsheets, to more efficiently log EPSS testing procedures. Layegh encourages organizations to consider similar streamlining efforts.

Note: *This EPSS dashboard may be adapted and is available for internal use on the flash drive (print only) or by clicking the tool link in the Risk-Assessment Toolbox (e-book only) on page 177.*

Source: University of Texas MD Anderson Cancer Center, Houston, TX. Used with permission.

Published in *Environment of Care Risk Assessment*, Joint Commission Resources, 2018.

UT MD Anderson Cancer Center Standby Emergency Power Supply System Testing Summary

Generator:	XYZ	Nameplate kW Rating:	1750 kW	2188 kVA		Nameplate AMP Rating:	2631
Location:	XYZ	30% Nameplate Rating:	525 kW			30% Nameplate Rating:	789
Serves:	Building ABC	Asset Number:	XXX11			Power Factor:	0.8

Date	>20 and <40 Days Between Tests?	Techs Performing Test	Average Volts	Average Amps	Frequency (HZ)	Load Tested (kW)	% of Nameplate (Load)	Gen Test Runtime (Mins)	Exh Gas Temp (Min 685 Deg)	H₂O Temp (160–185)	Battery-Specific Gravity (>1.25)	Oil Temp	Oil PSIG (50–70)	JC Require's Met?
1/9/16	Yes	WM	478	765	60	0	0%	50	772	180	1.281	NA	72	
2/13/16	Yes	WM	477	805	60	0	0%	50	780	180	1.281	NA	73	
3/12/16	Yes	WM	479	810	60	0	0%	50	789	179	1.284	NA	72	
4/4/16	Yes	WM	478	829	60	0	0%	50	787	180	1.283	NA	72	
5/16/16	Yes	WM	477	816	60	0	0%	50	795	180	1.28	NA	72	
6/11/16	Yes	WM	477	961	60	0	0%	50	819	181	1.28	NA	73	
7/9/16	Yes	WM	477	914	60	0	0%	50	826	181	1.281	NA	71	
8/13/16	Yes	WM, VT	478	851	60	0	0%	50	811	179	1.281	NA	72	
9/10/16	Yes	WM	478	907	60	0	0%	50	834	179	1.28	NA	72	

Note: *Annual load bank is not required as it has met stack temperature for the last 12 months.*

Source: University of Texas MD Anderson Cancer Center. Used with permission. May be adapted for internal use.

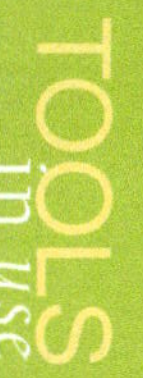

Example Dashboard—Emergency Power Supply System Testing *continued*

Published in *Environment of Care Risk Assessment*, Joint Commission Resources, 2018.

4-HOUR BUILDING LOAD TEST   DATE: 4/1/2016   WO #P1282662

	TIME	VOLTAGE			AMPS			FREQ (HZ)	KW	% OF NAME-PLATE (LOAD)	EXH GAS TEMP (MIN 550 DEG)	H₂O TEMP (160-185)	OIL TEMP	OIL PSIG (50-70)
		A-B	B-C	C-A	A	B	C							
	0:15	478	477	477	792	825	819	60	0	0%	769	176	N/A	74
	0:30	478	477	477	800	832	829	60	0	0%	770	179	N/A	73
	1:00	478	478	477	803	797	840	60	0	0%	777	179	N/A	72
	1:30	478	478	478	815	845	860	60	0	0%	790	180	N/A	72
	2:00	478	477	478	810	820	845	60	0	0%	785	180	N/A	72
	2:30	478	477	477	802	840	850	60	0	0%	786	180	N/A	72
	3:00	478	478	478	815	830	840	60	0	0%	780	180	N/A	72
	3:30	478	477	478	820	825	842	60	0	0%	785	180	N/A	72
	4:00	478	478	477	815	835	828	60	0	0%	780	180	N/A	72

4-hour building load test required by EC.02.05.07.07

2-HOUR LOAD BANK TEST   DATE: 1/9/2013   WO # P126564

DATE	TIME	VOLTAGE			AMPS			FREQ (HZ)	KW	% OF NAME-PLATE (LOAD)	EXH GAS TEMP (MIN 550 DEG)	H₂O TEMP (160-185)	OIL TEMP	OIL PSIG (50-70)
		A-B	B-C	C-A	A	B	C							
	0:00	481	481	482	690	690	691	60	500	29%	690	154	n/a	90
	0:15	481	481	481	691	690	690	60	500	29%	795	180	n/a	74
	0:30	481	481	482	691	690	691	60	500	29%	798	180	n/a	74
	0:45	481	481	481	1317	1317	1316	60	1000	57%	960	180	n/a	72
	1:00	481	481	482	1317	1316	1317	60	1000	57%	984	181	n/a	70
	1:15	481	481	481	1930	1938	1936	60	1500	86%	1149	192	n/a	66
	1:30	481	480	481	1929	1935	1935	60	1500	86%	1155	192	n/a	66
	1:45	481	481	481	1930	1932	1934	60	1500	86%	1161	192	n/a	67
	2:00	480	480	481	1931	1938	1938	60	1500	86%	1158	192	n/a	67

2-hour load bank test required by EC.02.05.07.06

Source: University of Texas MD Anderson Cancer Center. Used with permission. May be adapted for internal use.

continued

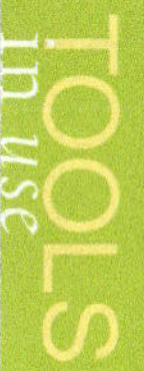

Example Dashboard—Emergency Power Supply System Testing *continued*

Published in *Environment of Care Risk Assessment*, Joint Commission Resources, 2018.

Transfer Switches Operated Monthly

DATE	BPATS-ES1	BPATS-ES2	BPATS-ES3	BPATS-ES4	BPATS-ES22	ATS-FP-1	ATS-FP-2
1/9/2016	Pass	Pass	Pass	Pass	Pass	Pass	Pass
2/13/2016	Pass	Pass	Pass	Pass	Pass	Pass	Pass
3/12/2016	Pass	Pass	Pass	Pass	Pass	Pass	Pass
4/4/2016	Pass	Pass	Pass	Pass	Pass	Pass	Pass
5/16/2016	Pass	Pass	Pass	Pass	Pass	Pass	Pass
6/11/2016	Pass	Pass	Pass	Pass	Pass	Pass	Pass
7/9/2016	Pass	Pass	Pass	Pass	Pass	Pass	Pass
8/13/2016	Pass	Pass	Pass	Pass	Pass	Pass	Pass
9/10/2016							

Battery Backup Lights Tested Monthly

DATE	Light, Battery Backup #17, T2.4100 46176	Light, Battery Backup #17, T2.4100 46177	Light, Battery Backup #17, T2.4100 46178	Light, Battery Backup #17, T2.4100 46179
1/9/2016	Pass	Pass	Pass	Pass
2/13/2016	Pass	Pass	Pass	Pass
3/12/2016	Pass	Pass	Pass	Pass
4/4/2016	Pass	Pass	Pass	Pass
5/16/2016	Pass	Pass	Fail A826376	Fail A826380
6/11/2016	Pass	Pass	Pass	Pass
7/9/2016	Pass	Pass	Pass	Pass
8/13/2016	Pass	Pass	Pass	Pass
9/10/2016				

Source: University of Texas MD Anderson Cancer Center. Used with permission. May be adapted for internal use.

chapter 9

Emergency Management

Emergencies. They happen in an instant, last for days, and oftentimes have negative ramifications for weeks, months, or years.

Recently, the topic of emergency management (EM) has been the subject of headlines across the country. The public, press, and government are all concerned that communities, and the health care organizations within those communities, are not as prepared for emergencies as they should be. Unfortunately, there is some evidence that validates these concerns. In recent years, there have been several large-scale disasters that have resulted in emergency responses in which communications broke down, resources ran out, utilities were compromised, or patient and staff safety and security were at risk.

Emergencies can happen within the health care organization or in its community; they can occur with or without warning and often take unexpected turns in scope or severity. An emergency situation can significantly affect demand for a health care organization's services, while at the same time limiting its ability to provide those services. Therefore, organizations must prepare before an emergency strikes. Comprehensive, proactive steps should identify risks, create effective response plans, train and equip staff, and practice putting those plans into effect. Because some emergencies originate in the community, health care organizations also need to collaborate with local organizations in risk assessment, preparedness, and drills whenever possible.

There are many types of emergencies:

- *Human-made threats.* Including chemical spills, airplane crashes, and train derailments
- *Terrorist events.* Including chemical, biological, radiological, nuclear, or explosive threats
- *Natural disasters.* Including hurricanes, floods, snowstorms, and earthquakes
- *Escalating events.* These occur when multiple disasters happen at once, or one right after another, thus building the complexity and scope of the emergency. For example, during Hurricane Katrina, the hurricane led to high winds, which caused levees to break, which led to flooding, which led to a loss of utilities, extensive damage to healthcare facilities, an overwhelmed public safety infrastructure, extensive emergency rescue activity, excess mortality, and civil unrest.

Health care organizations need to prepare in an all-hazards manner to protect their critical capabilities, understanding that the specifics of their response depend on the nature of

STANDARDS *to know*

EM.01.01.01	EM.02.02.07
EM.02.02.01	EM.02.02.09
EM.02.02.03	EM.02.02.11
EM.02.02.05	EM.03.01.03

TERMS *to know*

Emergency Operations Plan (EOP)

hazard vulnerability analysis (HVA)

the emergency, geographical location, community demographics, and other factors specific to each organization.

Overview of Assessing Risks

Joint Commission standards require health care organizations to review their risks, hazards, and potential emergencies annually. These are defined in the organization's hazard vulnerability analysis (HVA), a Joint Commission–required emergency risk assessment. Annual reviews also are required of the objective and scope of the Emergency Operations Plan (EOP) and of the organization's inventory of emergency resources and assets. All findings must be documented and reviewed by senior organization leadership. (The HVA process and the EOP will be discussed in greater detail later in this chapter.)

Participants in the Process

Emergency management is most effective when responsibility starts with high levels of leadership. Senior leadership plays the important role of mobilizing support for EM planning, assessment, and improvement throughout the organization. Also, leadership has the authority to allot resources and make necessary changes. Leaders should enlist support for and encourage cooperation among the emergency managers, facilities and information technology (IT) managers, clinical and administrative department heads, and other staff who will be expected to take a role in emergency planning, response, or recovery.

Hazard Vulnerability Analysis

To respond effectively to emergencies, organizations must use an approach that is planned and structured, yet flexible and scalable. A critical component of an organization's emergency preparedness program is its HVA. This is a risk-assessment process, required by Joint Commission Standard EM.01.01.01, which organizations use to help identify potential emergencies. The HVA helps organizations determine the direct and indirect impact of these emergencies. The HVA process serves as a starting point for organizations to evaluate their vulnerability to specific hazards, and it helps them get a clear picture of the risks that threaten their operation.

Using a Multidisciplinary Approach

An organization's HVA typically is conducted via a multidisciplinary process, which includes the EM staff, as well as leadership, nurses, physicians, facilities, IT, ancillary services, and others. To achieve this multidisciplinary perspective, an organization may choose to form a diverse team whose express purpose is to conduct the HVA, or it may choose to give the responsibility to the multidisciplinary environment of care (EC) or safety committee.

An emerging area of risk and opportunity for multidisciplinary effort is in the area of cyber emergencies that affect patient care. Systems for documenting, transmitting, and tracking prescriptions, laboratory reports, radiology studies, and other essential information for care can be vulnerable and must be protected from loss, tampering, intrusion, destruction, or malicious denial-of-service attacks from hackers. Effective management of cyber emergencies that affect patient care requires a similar conceptual framework as for utilities management, infection prevention and control, and emergency management in general. This framework is rooted in the following three areas:

1. Risk awareness
2. Incident detection
3. Incident response and recovery

To explore cyber risks, the organization should incorporate its IT staff in EM planning to help identify and address the following:

- To what extent are key care functions—such as the following—reliant on networked systems or internet connectivity?
  - Patient clinical information
  - Patient care, treatment, and services activities (including telemedicine)
  - Medical devices and equipment (including implantables or devices/equipment patients use in their homes
- To what extent are external vendors used to support these systems, devices, or equipment?
- What cyber risks has the organization identified that could affect its ability to provide care, treatment, and service?
- Does the organization currently use well-recognized practices to protect its IT systems from failures or intrusions (such as password protection, authentication procedures, limited use of USB devices and other

removable media, staff education on spam and phishing, and other cyber hygiene practices)?

◉ Does the organization currently manage interruptions to information processes as effectively as possible?

◉ Are there recovery (business continuity) strategies in place to restore systems after a cyber emergency has occurred?

Staff from IT, as well as staff responsible for electronic health records, facilities, biomedical engineering, nursing, telemedicine, and other areas, all have a role to play in identifying risks for potential cyber attacks or catastrophic cyber failures that could affect patient care.

Involving the Community

Health care organizations, the public health department, fire departments, police departments, and other community groups may be involved in responding to different types of emergencies; consequently, health care organizations should not plan for emergencies in isolation (*see* page 186). Standard EM.01.01.01 requires organizations to identify and prioritize potential threats with potential community response partners through the HVA process. To do this, the organization may want to have the fire chief, police chief, health department, and other emergency preparedness personnel participate on the multidisciplinary HVA team. At minimum, the organization should share its HVA with potential community response partners to share information on risks of threats from different organizations' perspectives.

In communitywide emergency response and recovery, responders and health care organizations are interdependent. For this reason, it is important that all responding agencies have an understanding of what services each can provide and what support each will need from other sources. The standards require the health care organization to communicate with its community partners about the organization's needs and how they can help meet those needs. In some cases (as, for example, with some nursing care center organizations), an organization may not have a specific role in an emergency. Nevertheless, the organization will have needs that would have to be met, and that organization might rely on the community to meet those needs (for example, evacuation support). Consequently, the organization should communicate its needs and understand if and how the community is able to assist in meeting them.

Conducting an HVA

The HVA should list all possible emergencies that could affect the health care organization and the population(s) and community it serves. To develop this list of possible emergencies, the organization may want to conduct a brainstorming session. During this session, participants should consider probable emergencies, such as power failures, floods, ice storms, multiple-casualty transportation accidents, and chemical spills. But participants also should consider more unlikely emergencies that could wreak havoc on the organization if it is not prepared for them, such as an influenza pandemic or an active shooter.

Multisite organizations may choose to create one comprehensive HVA, or separate HVAs for each location. If one HVA is used, it must accurately reflect all sites. Multiple HVAs may be appropriate when an organization encompasses sites in different communities or geographic locations, as these may face significantly different hazards.

Categorize Hazards

When identified, hazards should be categorized into areas such as natural hazards, technical hazards, human events, and hazardous materials. Then the multidisciplinary team should determine each risk's probability of occurrence, possible impact, and the organization's level of preparedness to respond to the risk. Organizations should evaluate these risk factors objectively. Just because an organization has never experienced a particular type of event does not mean there is no potential for it to occur in the future, particularly if aspects of the organization, patient population, or surrounding environment have changed.

Determine Impact

Members of the multidisciplinary team will have varying viewpoints on the possible impact and level of preparedness associated with different risks. Consider this example: One year, when an organization was updating its HVA, the EM committee assumed that an electrical power outage would be a catastrophic issue for the facility. However, the facilities manager pointed out that, due to backup power systems, a power outage would not be catastrophic, but a water outage could shut down the entire institution in a short period of time. The facilities manager's input into the HVA process helped redirect the organization's focus and shape the organization's response efforts.

Partners in the Community

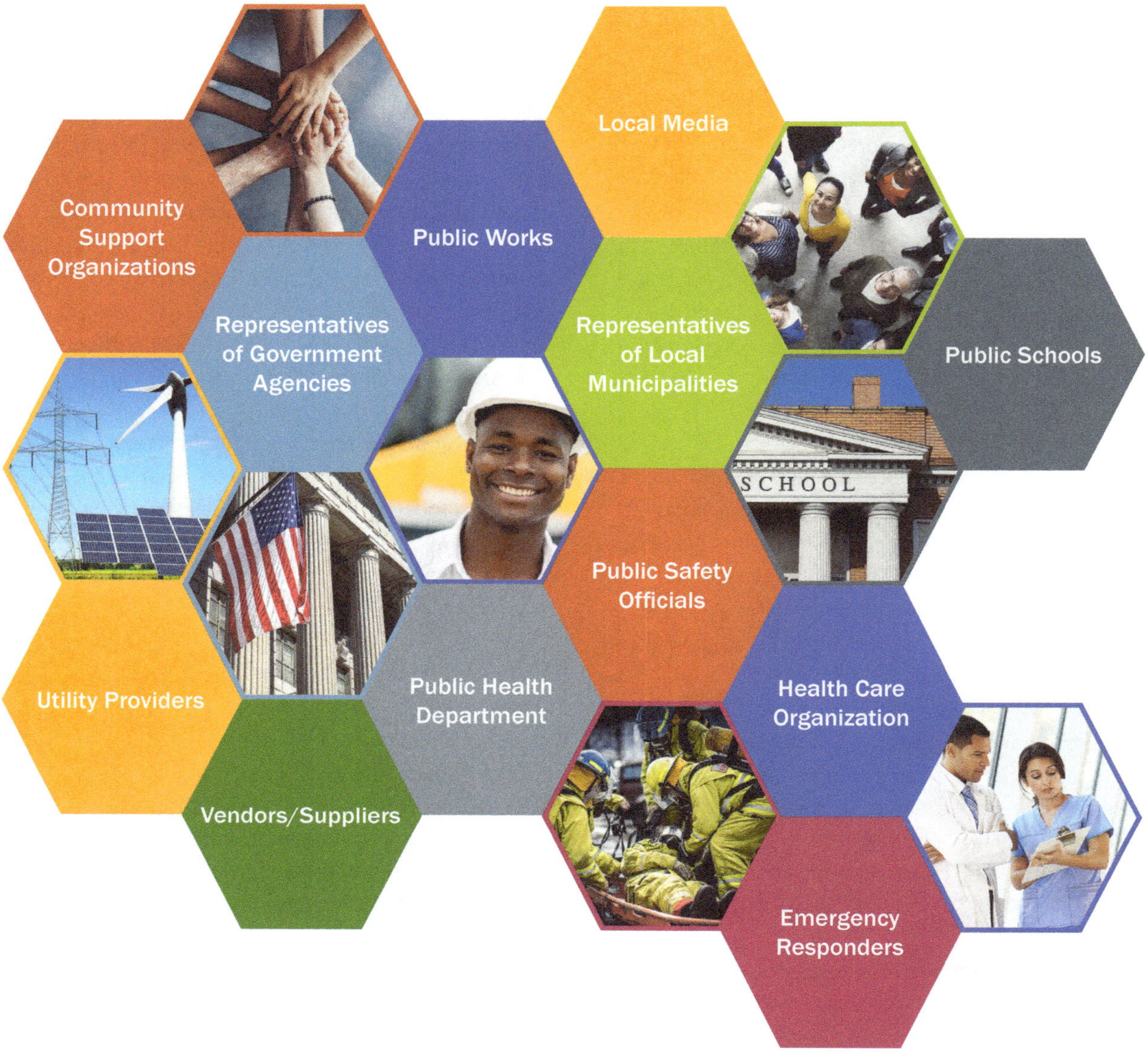

Emergencies oftentimes affect an entire community. Building strong ties between community groups and agencies will help health care organizations provide high-quality care when an emergency occurs. Organization leadership can hold periodic meetings with community leaders to demonstrate the health care organization's willingness to collaborate to support the safety of all community members. The health care organization's facilities directors and their emergency management teams should work with organization leadership to confirm that leaders are aware of key points of the Emergency Operations Plan. Finally, because collaboration with community response partners is required, the organization's accreditation professionals should be included to ensure that all Joint Commission requirements are being addressed.

for example...

Wildfires pose immediate risk to individuals in the fire zone for injuries and illness due to heat, smoke, and flames. Health care organizations have remained on high alert for surges related to these conditions, as well as the frequent evacuations that impact not only emergency department services but also availability of staff and suppliers affected by road closures, evacuation orders, and their own personal risks of danger to property and family. As individuals return to their communities to recover and rebuild, injuries associated with these clean-up and restoration efforts increase, along with visits to urgent care centers and emergency departments. Studies have begun to assess other long-term risks associated with recurring wildfires throughout the United States.

According to an article by Jia Coco Liu, et al, "The estimated increase in respiratory admissions due to future wildfire smoke highlights one of the potential human health impacts from a changing climate. Our results indicated that under climate change, increased threat of wildfire will generate smoke that can affect populations living far from wildfire centers. In addition to increasing fire suppression resources and evacuation efforts in areas directly affected by future wildfires, policy-makers also should consider improving the capacity of emergency care facilities to meet the needs of communities affected by wildfire smoke. These results, summed with other health outcomes from climate change impacts such as cardiovascular diseases, infectious diseases, heat stress, and death[22,30,31], contributed to our overall understanding of the public health burden of climate change."[1]

Health care facilities in areas prone to wildfires need to consider not only the immediate impact but also the longer-term effects as individuals seek care for injuries or illnesses that occur long after the flames have been suppressed.

Prioritize Threats

After an organization has assessed the impact of potential emergencies, the team can rank the most probable and serious threats to patient care services and organization safety. When prioritizing threats, organizations should consider not only the short-term effects of the emergency but also the long-term effects.

for example...

A fire may occur within the health care facility. The short-term effects may be the relocation and continued medical needs of the patients, residents, or individuals served. The long-term effects may be related to damage of the physical building and continuation of services provided while the repairs are being made to the affected area(s) of the facility.

To help with the HVA process, an organization may choose to create a form. This tool can be used to help with brainstorming, prioritization, ranking, and documentation. (*See* the sample HVA beginning on page 188.)

It is important to remember that an organization's hazards may change from year to year. For example, a medical center that decides to construct a landing pad for helicopters on the hospital's roof will need to revise its HVA to include the potential for a helicopter incident as a potential emergency. The Joint Commission requires organizations to reevaluate their HVAs every year to ensure a current and comprehensive risk analysis of potential emergencies and their effects.

Mitigating the Risk of Identified Threats

For each emergency identified in an HVA, an organization should implement mitigation activities designed to reduce the risk of any potential damage due to the emergency. For example, if an organization has identified an active shooter as a realistic, probable, and high-priority threat to the organization, it could mitigate the risk and impact of such an emergency by reconfiguring the reception and waiting areas, installing cameras and panic buttons, establishing patrol routes of sensitive areas by internal security staff, designating safe rooms and routes, and training and

text continued on page 193

Example Hazard Vulnerability Analysis

This sample tool shows part of an organization's required Hazard Vulnerability Analysis (HVA). This tool is used to recognize hazards that may affect demand on an organization's resources.

Note: *This assessment tool may be adapted and is available for internal use on the flash drive (print only) or by clicking the tool link in the Risk-Assessment Toolbox (e-book only) on page 199.*

Source: Kaiser Permanente, Oakland, CA. Used with permission.

Published in *Environment of Care Risk Assessment*, Joint Commission Resources, 2018.

HAZARD AND VULNERABILITY ASSESSMENT TOOL — Naturally Occurring Events

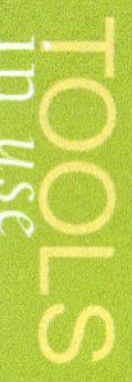

Event	Probability	Severity = (Magnitude – Mitigation)						Risk
		Human Impact	Property Imact	Business Impact	Preparedness	Internal Response	External Response	
	Likelihood this will occur	Possibility of death or injury	Physical losses and damages	Interruption of services	Preplanning	Time, effectiveness, resources	Community/ Mutual Aid staff and supplies	Relative threat*
Score	0 = N/A 1 = Low 2 = Moderate 3 = High	0 = N/A 1 = Low 2 = Moderate 3 = High	0 = N/A 1 = Low 2 = Moderate 3 = High	0 = N/A 1 = Low 2 = Moderate 3 = High	0 = N/A 1 = Low 2 = Moderate 3 = High	0 = N/A 1 = Low 2 = Moderate 3 = High	0 = N/A 1 = Low 2 = Moderate 3 = High	0 – 100%
Blizzard	0							0%
Dam Inundation	0							0%
Drought	2	1	1	1	1	2	1	26%
Earthquake	0							0%
Epidemic	0							0%
Flood, External	2							0%
Hurricane	3	2	2	2	1	1	2	56%
Ice Storm	0							0%
Landslide	0							0%
Severe Thunderstrom	3	1	1	1	2	1	1	39%
Snowfall	0							0%
Temperature Extremes	2	1	2	2	2	2	3	44%
Tidal Wave	1	3	3	2	2	1	1	22%
Tornado	1	2	2	2	2	2	1	20%
Volcano	0							0%
Wildfire	2	1	1	1	2	1	1	26%
Average Score	**1.00**	**1.57**	**1.71**	**1.57**	**1.71**	**1.43**	**1.43**	**8%**

*Threat increases with percentage.

RISK = PROBABILITY x SEVERITY		
0.08	0.33	0.23

Source: Kaiser Permanente, Oakland, CA. Used with permission.

Published in *Environment of Care Risk Assessment*, Joint Commission Resources, 2018.

HAZARD AND VULNERABILITY ASSESSMENT TOOL — Technological Events

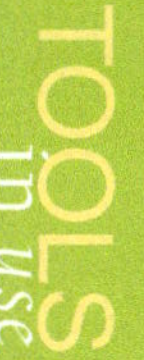

Event	Probability	Severity = (Magnitude – Mitigation)						Risk
		Human Impact	Property Impact	Business Impact	Preparedness	Internal Response	External Response	
	Likelihood this will occur	Possibility of death or injury	Physical losses and damages	Interruption of services	Preplanning	Time, effectiveness, resources	Community/ Mutual Aid staff and supplies	Relative threat*
Score	0 = N/A 1 = Low 2 = Moderate 3 = High	0 = N/A 1 = Low 2 = Moderate 3 = High	0 = N/A 1 = Low 2 = Moderate 3 = High	0 = N/A 1 = Low 2 = Moderate 3 = High	0 = N/A 1 = Low 2 = Moderate 3 = High	0 = N/A 1 = Low 2 = Moderate 3 = High	0 = N/A 1 = Low 2 = Moderate 3 = High	0 – 100%
Communications Failure	2	0	0	1	1	1	2	19%
Electrical Failure	3	1	1	2	1	1	1	39%
Fire Alarm Failure	1	2	3	3	1	1	1	20%
Fire, Internal	1	1	3	3	1	1	1	19%
Flood, Internal	2	0	2	2	1	1	1	26%
Fuel Shortage	1	0	0	1	2	2	1	11%
Generator Failure	2	1	1	2	1	1	1	26%
Hazmat Exposure, Internal	3	2	1	1	1	1	1	39%
HVAC Failure	2	0	2	1	1	1	1	22%
Information Systems Failure	2	0	1	3	2	2	2	37%
Medical Gas Failure	2	2	1	1	1	1	2	30%
Medical Vacuum Failure	1	1	0	1	2	1	1	11%
Natural Gas Failure	1	0	0	1	2	2	1	11%
Sewer Failure	1	0	0	1	2	2	1	11%
Steam Failure	1	0	0	1	2	2	2	13%
Structural Damage	1	1	3	3	2	2	1	22%
Supply Shortage	2	1	1	1	2	1	1	26%
Transportation Failure	1	0	0	2	2	1	1	11%
Water Failure	2	0	0	1	1	1	1	15%
Average Score	**1.63**	**0.63**	**1.00**	**1.63**	**1.47**	**1.32**	**1.21**	**22%**

*Threat increases with percentage.

RISK = PROBABILITY x SEVERITY		
0.22	0.54	0.40

Source: Kaiser Permanente, Oakland, CA. Used with permission.

continued

Example Hazard Vulnerability Analysis *continued*

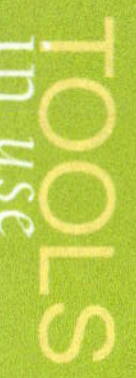

HAZARD AND VULNERABILITY ASSESSMENT TOOL — Human-Related Events

KAISER PERMANENTE.

Event	Probability	Severity = (Magnitude – Mitigation)						Risk
		Human Impact	Property Impact	Business Impact	Preparedness	Internal Response	External Response	
	Likelihood this will occur	Possibility of death or injury	Physical losses and damages	Interruption of services	Preplanning	Time, effectiveness, resources	Community/ Mutual Aid staff and supplies	Relative threat*
Score	0 = N/A 1 = Low 2 = Moderate 3 = High	0 = N/A 1 = Low 2 = Moderate 3 = High	0 = N/A 1 = Low 2 = Moderate 3 = High	0 = N/A 1 = Low 2 = Moderate 3 = High	0 = N/A 1 = Low 2 = Moderate 3 = High	0 = N/A 1 = Low 2 = Moderate 3 = High	0 = N/A 1 = Low 2 = Moderate 3 = High	0 – 100%
Chemical Exposure, External	2	0	0	1	1	1	1	15%
Large Internal Spill	1	0	0	0	1	1	1	6%
Mass Causalty Hazmat Incident (from historic events at your MC with ≥ 5 victims)	2	0	0	2	2	1	1	22%
Radiologic Exposure, External	1	1	0	0	1	1	1	7%
Radiologic Exposure, Internal	1	1	0	1	1	1	1	9%
Small Casualty Hazmat Incident (from historic events at your MC with ≥ 5 victims)	2	0	0	1	2	1	1	19%
Small- to Medium-Sized Internal Spill	3	0	0	0	1	1	1	17%
Terrorism, Chemical	1	2	1	1	1	1	1	13%
Terrorism, Radiologic	1	1	0	0	1	1	1	7%
Average Score	**1.56**	**0.56**	**0.11**	**0.67**	**1.22**	**1.00**	**1.00**	**13%**

*Threat increases with percentage.

RISK = PROBABILITY x SEVERITY		
0.13	0.52	0.25

Source: Kaiser Permanente, Oakland, CA. Used with permission.

Published in *Environment of Care Risk Assessment*, Joint Commission Resources, 2018.

HAZARD AND VULNERABILITY ASSESSMENT TOOL — Human-Related Events

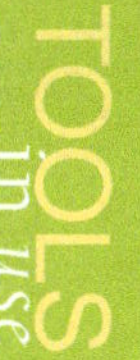

Event	Probability	Severity = (Magnitude – Mitigation)						Risk
		Human Impact	Property Impact	Business Impact	Preparedness	Internal Response	External Response	
	Likelihood this will occur	Possibility of death or injury	Physical losses and damages	Interruption of services	Preplanning	Time, effectiveness, resources	Community/ Mutual Aid staff and supplies	Relative threat*
Score	0 = N/A 1 = Low 2 = Moderate 3 = High	0 = N/A 1 = Low 2 = Moderate 3 = High	0 = N/A 1 = Low 2 = Moderate 3 = High	0 = N/A 1 = Low 2 = Moderate 3 = High	0 = N/A 1 = Low 2 = Moderate 3 = High	0 = N/A 1 = Low 2 = Moderate 3 = High	0 = N/A 1 = Low 2 = Moderate 3 = High	0 – 100%
Chemical Exposure, External	2	0	0	1	1	1	1	15%
Large Internal Spill	1	0	0	0	1	1	1	6%
Mass Causalty Hazmat Incident (from historic events at your MC with ≥ 5 victims)	2	0	0	2	2	1	1	22%
Radiologic Exposure, External	1	1	0	0	1	1	1	7%
Radiologic Exposure, Internal	1	1	0	1	1	1	1	9%
Small Casualty Hazmat Incident (from historic events at your MC with ≥ 5 victims)	2	0	0	1	2	1	1	19%
Small- to Medium-Sized Internal Spill	3	0	0	0	1	1	1	17%
Terrorism, Chemical	1	2	1	1	1	1	1	13%
Terrorism, Radiologic	1	1	0	0	1	1	1	7%
Average Score	**1.56**	**0.56**	**0.11**	**0.67**	**1.22**	**1.00**	**1.00**	**13%**

*Threat increases with percentage.

RISK = PROBABILITY x SEVERITY		
0.13	0.52	0.25

Source: Kaiser Permanente, Oakland, CA. Used with permission.

continued

Example Hazard Vulnerability Analysis *continued*

Published in *Environment of Care Risk Assessment*, Joint Commission Resources, 2018.

KAISER PERMANENTE.

Summary of Medical Center Hazards Analysis

	Natural	Technological	Human	Hazmat	Total for Facility
Probability	0.33	0.54	0.60	0.52	0.49
Severity	0.23	0.40	0.47	0.25	0.34
Hazard-Specific Relative Risk	0.08	0.22	0.28	0.13	0.17

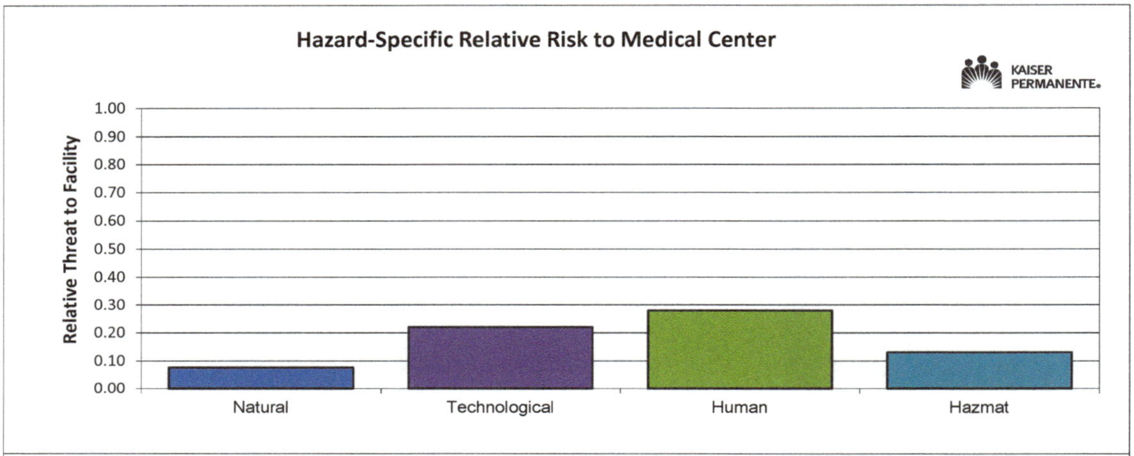

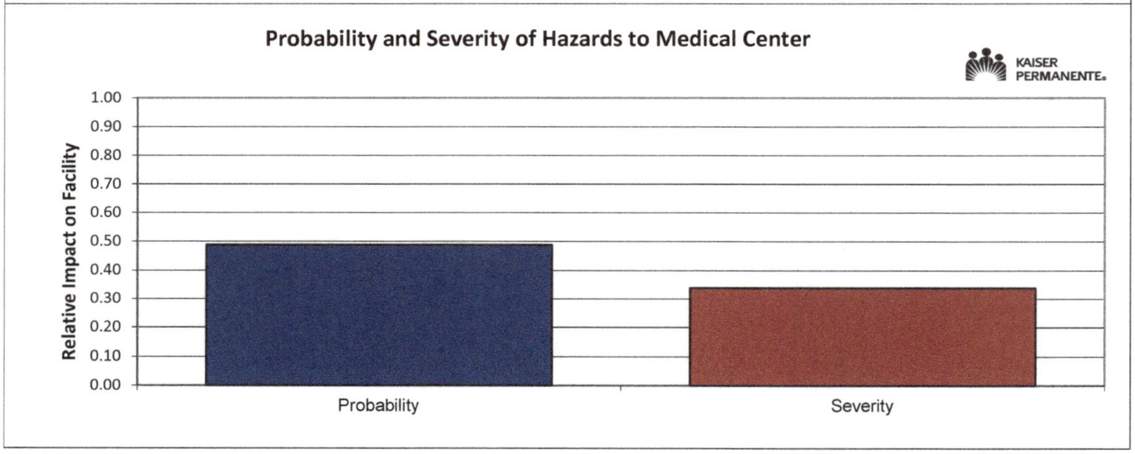

Hazard-Specific Relative Risk to Medical Center

KAISER PERMANENTE.

Probability and Severity of Hazards to Medical Center

KAISER PERMANENTE.

This document is a sample Hazard Vulnerability Analysis tool. It is not asubstitute for a comprehensive emergency preparedness program.

Individuals or organizations using this tool are solely responsible for any hazard assessment and compliance with applicable laws and regulations.

drilling staff in evasive and defensive strategies. Another organization located near a large chemical plant may choose to build a decontamination room outside of its emergency department to address its identified risk of a hazardous materials spill or release.

Emergency Operations Plan

The HVA can give the organization a good indication of where to focus its preparedness efforts. The organization's EOP is an all-hazards plan in terms of protecting key capabilities regardless of the emergency, but it must be linked to priorities identified in the HVA so that resources, training, and other plan components effectively support preparedness response and resilience.

The EOP is a document the organization creates to help guide its emergency response and recovery efforts (*see* page 198 for a breakdown of the contents in an EOP plan). The Joint Commission standards require organizations to create such a plan, and it should include a description of the organization's incident command system (ICS). The ICS helps the organization identify who is in charge during an emergency and who will carry out the decisions of those in charge. It does not need to be rigid, but everyone in an organization should understand the basic principles of the ICS and how it applies during emergency response and recovery.

Over many years, The Joint Commission has studied the response of health care organizations to various disasters by going on-site and conducting debrief conference calls, gathering their lessons learned, and discussing the issues they faced. By analyzing information from this process and consulting with national and international experts in disaster preparedness, The Joint Commission identified six areas that are critical to effective emergency management. According to the EM standards, organizations must address the six areas within their EOPs:

1. Communications
2. Resources and assets
3. Safety and security
4. Staff responsibilities
5. Utilities management
6. Patient clinical and support activities

These areas are discussed in more detail in the following sections.

Communications

In the event that community infrastructure is damaged and/or an organization's power, IT systems, or facilities are disabled, communication pathways—whether dependent on fiber-optic cables, electricity, satellite, Internet, or other conduits—can be at risk. In accordance with Standard EM.02.02.01, the organization must develop a plan to maintain communication pathways both within the organization and to critical community resources.

The standard also encourages organizations to strive for standardized communication both internally and externally. Organizations that receive federal EM funding should align with the Federal Emergency Management Agency's National Incident Management System (NIMS) and other federal guidance related to communication structures and processes (*see* page 194 for more information about NIMS).

Resources and Assets

A solid understanding of the type and availability of an organization's resources and assets is arguably more important during an emergency than during times of normal operation. Medical and nonmedical supplies, pharmaceuticals, and personal protective equipment are some of the essential resources that organizations must know how to access in times of crisis in order to sustain patient care, treatment, and services during response and recovery.

Standard EM.02.02.03 requires organizations to create inventories of on-site assets and resources that would be needed during an emergency. Organizations also must actively monitor those assets and resources during an emergency using their supply chain management and incident command reporting tools to support situational awareness and timely decision making. Organizations should take the opportunity during emergency planning to tighten relationships with suppliers and make sure they can deliver supplies during an emergency. This includes discussing with suppliers how they will get supplies to the health care facility, and how many other health care organizations they have agreed to supply.

Contingency Planning

One important aspect of emergency response addressed in the EM standards is monitoring the evolving incident and ongoing resource utilization to ensure that the organization can function effectively throughout the emergency. Organizations must understand how they will continue operations

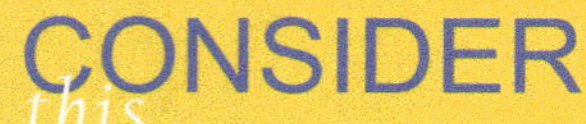

National Incident Management System

The National Incident Management System (NIMS) was created by the US Federal Emergency Management Agency (FEMA) to be a systematic, proactive system of managing emergency incidents of all sizes and complexity. It is designed to be used to coordinate efforts of departments and agencies at all levels of government, nongovernmental organizations, and private-sector organizations to reduce loss of life and property and minimize harm to the environment.

NIMS is a standardized—yet flexible—set of practices that is built on existing structures, such as the Incident Command System (ICS). It focuses on five components:

1. Preparedness
2. Communications and Information Management
3. Resource Management
4. Command and Management
5. Ongoing Management and Maintenance

More information on NIMS is available on the FEMA website at https://www.fema.gov/national-incident-management-system.

even when the community cannot support them. The EOP should describe the organization's response plans and decision criteria (which may include curtailing services, conserving resources, and other measures) to support functioning for up to 96 hours if the organization could not be supported by its local community. The organization is not required to stockpile 96 hours of supplies; it is required to maintain situational awareness and inventory management so that should essential patient care resources (staff, supplies, space, and so on) be projected to run out in less than 96 hours, the organization can implement contingency plans that will allow them to continue to provide the standard of care, or plan for partial or full evacuation. (*See* page 195 for a 96-hour operational chart.)

It is important for the community to understand what health care services may be affected by a disaster in the community. The organization should coordinate public information between its own ICS and the community's ICS so that the public is informed in a timely way about what services will continue to be provided, and where they may go for other services that will not be available from their usual source of care.

Safety and Security

The safety and security of patients is the prime responsibility of the organization during an emergency. Beyond daily safety and security measures, the organization's safety and security plans and strategies will involve many components, depending upon the type of emergency it is planning for, including the following examples:

- *Mass vaccination during a disease outbreak.* Considerations include vehicle access control; guided movement of community members to designated vaccination tents in the health care organization's parking lot; and identification arm bands to distinguish clinical volunteers.
- *Bomb threat.* Considerations include targeted evacuation and search coordinated with local and federal law enforcement; additional security patrols on the organization's campus and at points of entry and exit; and coordination of staff interview and evidence collection.
- *Presidential inauguration.* Considerations include designation of primary VIP organization; clearance and coordination with Secret Service and other federal agencies; and rapid response plans to clear ambulance bay and redirect internal movement of visitors, patients, and nondesignated staff from sensitive areas.

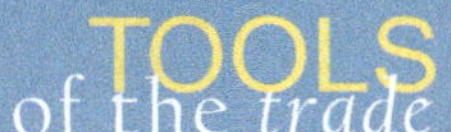

96-Hour Operational Impact Chart

This chart may help organizations keep track of supplies during 96 hours of operation or during emergency exercises that rehearse and plan strategies for times when support from the local community is not possible. Note that the Emergency Operations Plan does not require organizations to conduct an emergency exercise lasting 96 hours, nor are organizations required to stockpile supplies to last for 96 hours of operation.

Note: *The complete chart may be adapted and is available for internal use on the flash drive (print only) or by clicking the tool link in the Risk-Assessment Toolbox (e-book only) on page 199.*
Source: Mercy Health Partners, Cincinnati, OH. Used with permission.

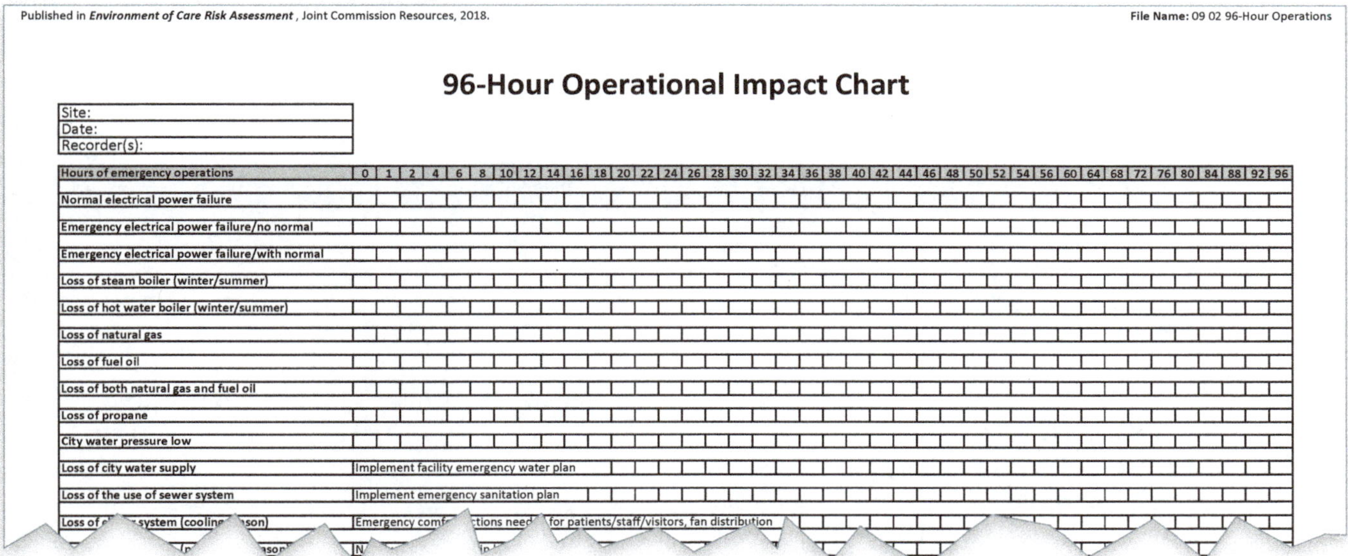

Published in *Environment of Care Risk Assessment*, Joint Commission Resources, 2018.　　　　File Name: 09 02 96-Hour Operations

96-Hour Operational Impact Chart

Site:
Date:
Recorder(s):

Hours of emergency operations	0	1	2	4	6	8	10	12	14	16	18	20	22	24	26	28	30	32	34	36	38	40	42	44	46	48	50	52	54	56	60	64	68	72	76	80	84	88	92	96
Normal electrical power failure																																								
Emergency electrical power failure/no normal																																								
Emergency electrical power failure/with normal																																								
Loss of steam boiler (winter/summer)																																								
Loss of hot water boiler (winter/summer)																																								
Loss of natural gas																																								
Loss of fuel oil																																								
Loss of both natural gas and fuel oil																																								
Loss of propane																																								
City water pressure low																																								
Loss of city water supply	Implement facility emergency water plan																																							
Loss of the use of sewer system	Implement emergency sanitation plan																																							
Loss of … system (cooling season)	Emergency comfort … ctions need … for patients/staff/visitors, fan distribution																																							

Staff Responsibilities

During an emergency, staff may be challenged to perform their usual jobs under dynamically changing conditions, with limitations in supplies or space, with different team members or response partners or equipment, or for different patient populations. The EOP defines the emergency functions to be performed by staff; the organization trains staff in these roles and facilitates drills and exercises so that staff can become familiar with any changes in their roles or procedures that may be required under an emergency situation. Even the most comprehensive EOP cannot anticipate all possible emergency scenarios, but regular training in their expected emergency procedures prepares staff to respond quickly at the start of an emergency and to communicate and coordinate effectively as the emergency situation evolves (*see* page 196 for an emergency response staff training checklist).

Utilities Management

An organization is dependent on the uninterrupted function of its utilities during an emergency. The supply of key utilities, such as electrical power, water, ventilation, and fuel, must not be disrupted or the ability of the organization to provide patient care reliably and in a safe environment will be compromised. Organizations must plan for hardening the infrastructure that supports these systems, rapid detection of failures or degradation (which may require automatic sensors, staff rounding, or other methods), rapid repair capability, transfer to backup systems, and alternative external sources of these utilities in the event of total disruption or failure.

Many of the systems that operate the utilities that support patient care are run by or monitored through Internet connections, often with vendor support. In addition, with reliance on Internet-connected medical devices, automated dispensing machines, telemedicine, and other networked capabilities, IT is as fundamental as electricity in providing health care in most organizations. IT must be included in consideration of utilities management when addressing EM planning, response, and recovery.

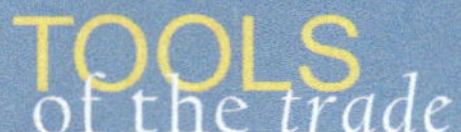

Emergency Response Staff Training Checklist

Organizations can use this tool to assess the completeness of its emergency response staff training.

Note: *The complete checklist may be adapted and is available for internal use on the flash drive (print only) or by clicking the tool link in the Risk-Assessment Toolbox (e-book only) on page 199.*

Published in *Environment of Care Risk Assessment*, Joint Commission Resources, 2018.　　　**File Name:** 09 03 Checklist Emergency Response Train

EMERGENCY RESPONSE STAFF TRAINING CHECKLIST

*This checklist can be used to identify potential gaps in emergency response staff training. Answers to all questions should ideally be Y for **Yes** (unless they aren't applicable). If an answer is N for **No**, use the "Notes" section to document needed changes. Unless otherwise noted, this checklist is applicable to all program settings.*

ORGANIZATION: ____

DATE OF REVIEW: _________________________　　REVIEWER: _______________________________

QUESTIONS	YES	NO	NA	NOTES
Does the organization have an emergency response training program?				

Patient Clinical and Support Activities

The clinical needs of patients during an emergency are of prime importance. The EOP must address patient scheduling, triage, assessment, treatment, admission, transfer, and discharge; any of these processes may be affected, either for patients already in the facility during an emergency or patients arriving at the facility because of an emergency in the community. Organizations should pay special attention to the needs of their high-risk patients. These could include patient groups in which an emergency could cause negative health effects, such as pediatric patients, geriatric patients, immunocompromised patients, and surgical patients. Particular kinds of emergencies give rise to particular patient care issues that need to be addressed in the EOP, including the following examples:

- An outbreak of infectious disease, including novel and emerging diseases, will require the organization to use isolation space, trained and/or dedicated staff, and safe disposal procedures for contaminated supplies and equipment.
- An industrial explosion with mass casualties will require the organization to activate decontamination procedures, consult with clinical or environmental specialists within the organization or outside of the organization (regional medical center, state health department, US Centers for Disease Control and Prevention [CDC], US Occupational Safety and Health Administration [OSHA], and so on), and provide psychological first aid for patients, their families, and staff.
- A facility damaged by a hurricane or other short-notice event will need to plan for evacuation; for example, by having evacuation sleds on each floor, establishing decision criteria for which groups of patients will be evacuated in what order, and preparing clinical record summaries to accompany each evacuated patient.

Patients with Access and Functional Needs

During community emergencies, vulnerable populations that seek care at a hospital when their typical sources of care are not available may create surge situations for hospitals. These situations may include the following examples:

- Home care patients who lose power at home after a tornado and arrive at the hospital in need of electricity for their oxygen machines.
- Elderly low-English–proficiency patients whose clinics have closed due to civil unrest and who urgently need medications for complications due to diabetes.
- An explosion in an industrial park that requires decontamination and trauma care for individuals at a nearby factory that employs people who rely on assistive devices (for example, visual and hearing aids, wheelchairs).

- Individuals in behavioral health crisis during a natural disaster who cannot locate a provider in the community and are boarded in designated spaces in the emergency department while referral and transport are arranged.
- Residents from a nearby homeless shelter arriving at the emergency department during a flu pandemic with upper respiratory infections and acute symptoms from untreated serious chronic conditions.

Some access and functional needs can be anticipated and addressed in advance with patients and/or community partners. The American College of Emergency Physicians provides resources on its "EMS and Disaster Preparedness" portal that address management of patient needs, including a Disaster Planning Toolkit for the Elderly and Special Needs Persons and links to resources developed by the Substance Abuse and Mental Health Services Administration (SAMHSA). For additional resources, *see* https://www.acep.org/Clinical---Practice-Management/EMS-and-Disaster-Preparedness/.

Changes to Emergency Management in Health Care Facilities

Organizations should note that the US Centers for Medicare & Medicaid Services (CMS) final rule for emergency preparedness became effective November 15, 2016, with all health care organizations expected to comply by November 15, 2017. The Joint Commission has deemed status designation from CMS to survey five specific settings addressed in the CMS EM final rule:

1. Hospitals
2. Critical access hospitals
3. Ambulatory surgical centers
4. Hospices
5. Home health agencies

Commencing with the CMS implementation date (November 15, 2017), the Joint Commission onsite survey of these five settings will include additional requirements that meet the CMS EM final rule requirements (*see* page 200 for additional information about this ruling).

Emergency Response Exercises

EOPs are only as good as the staff's ability to carry them out. Testing, exercising, and evaluating the plans are all essential steps in helping organizations to prepare for potential emergencies. Joint Commission Standard EM.03.01.03 requires organizations to conduct two exercises every year that test and stress the EOP. (If an organization experiences an actual emergency, it can serve in place of the exercise.) Although tabletop exercises can be excellent for training and evaluating focused components of the EOP, exercises must be actual activities that deploy the organization's staff, supplies, and equipment required for emergency response. (*See* pages 202 and 203, respectively, for an EM exercise planning guide and an after-action review report.)

The exercise must be designed based on a specific scenario, with defined exercise objectives that will be revisited during the evaluation of the exercise. Examples and tools to aid in exercise design and evaluation are available from several medical centers, consortia, and centers of excellence, including the Emergency Preparedness Research, Evaluation & Practice (EPREP) program at the Harvard T.H. Chan School of Public Health (for additional information, visit https://www.hsph.harvard.edu/preparedness/drills-exercises/).

Escalating Events

Choosing to exercise the scenarios identified in the HVA can help organizations prepare for the most likely threats. However, to truly test response plans and organization preparedness, organizations need to integrate escalating events into their emergency response exercises.

As previously mentioned, escalating events involve incidents that build on each other to create a large-scale emergency that significantly disables the organization's capabilities, creates an overwhelming influx of patients in terms of number or type, and/or affects the entire community. For example, organizations should consider not just exercising a tornado but a tornado that hits the organization, takes out the power, damages the emergency room, and knocks out electronic communication systems. Not only is the organization facing the aftermath of a tornado, it also

Contents of an Emergency Operations Plan

If starting from scratch or fully revising an Emergency Operations Plan (EOP), this outline can serve as a guide.

Note: *The complete EOP contents list may be adapted and is available for internal use on the flash drive (print only) or by clicking the tool link in the Risk-Assessment Toolbox (e-book only) on page 199.*

Source: University of Toledo Medical Center, Toledo, OH. Used with permission.

Published in *Environment of Care Risk Assessment*, Joint Commission Resources, 2018.　　　　**File Name:** 09 04 EOP Contents

CONTENTS OF AN EMERGENCY OPERATIONS PLAN

INTRODUCTION

Objectives and Background ....

Scope ....

Framework and Planning..

HVA...

---

is contending with a power outage, communication failure, and a lack of facility space for triage and emergency services.

Other Requirements

Depending on its role in the community and the services it offers, an organization may need to conduct specific types of emergency response exercises. For example, each site that offers emergency services or is a community-designated disaster receiving station must include an escalating event for one of its two yearly exercises. These sites also must incorporate an influx of simulated patients into one of its two yearly exercises. In addition, if an organization plays a role in its community's response plan, one of its two annual exercises should include participation in a communitywide exercise.

When designing exercises, organizations also should consider the needs of their most vulnerable populations. Depending on the organization, these may include immuno-compromised patients, pediatric patients, geriatric patients, rehabilitation patients, and patients with physical or mental disabilities. Vulnerable populations may have specific needs during an emergency that should be considered ahead of time to ensure that they are addressed appropriately. For example, pediatric patients are not small adults—equipment and supplies used in their examination and treatment must be appropriately sized, medication dosages must be adjusted, and additional care and comfort appropriate to their age and maturity level must be provided. People who use assistive devices and supports (including wheelchairs and service animals) due to vision, hearing, speech, or mobility challenges benefit physically and psychologically from using their devices and supports throughout emergency response activities, including evacuations. Exercises should be designed to test, evaluate, and improve the ability of the organization to meet the special needs of its vulnerable populations. *See* page 204 for examples of state requirements and best practices for managing vulnerable populations in emergency situations.

Evaluate the Exercises

The fundamental purpose of conducting an emergency response exercise is to determine the effectiveness of the EOP. In other words, does the plan effectively guide staff in procedures for providing care safely under emergency conditions? Has the organization invested in the space, supplies, and staffing required to carry out the plan? The evaluation should be documented to inform decisions on improvements that will strengthen the organization's preparedness, response, and recovery efforts, and guide any needed revisions to the EOP.

There are several factors to consider when evaluating an emergency response exercise. These include the following:

- *Scope.* Did the exercise test the six critical areas as relevant to the incident—communications, resources and assets, safety and security, staff responsibilities, utilities, and patient clinical and support activities? There may be gaps in the EOP that come to light only when put into action. During the exercise, any gaps or deficiencies should be noted and documented.

- *Staff participation.* Did the exercise activate staff from throughout the organization to test knowledge of emergency processes? Participation must go beyond clinical services to include leadership and management; support functions, such as patient registration, transportation, and housekeeping; night and weekend shifts; satellite locations that can supplement staff or patient care and support activities of the main site, and so on. Emergency response exercises should encompass all staff assets relevant to the incident, and staff should understand their critical role in emergency preparedness.
- *Collaboration.* Was communication and collaboration with other health care entities and community response partners (emergency medical service [EMS], health department, police, fire, and so on) well coordinated or were there gaps or mistakes that created additional risk?
- *Relevance.* Was the exercise conducted in a way that reflects the "on-the-ground" reality of the organization? Did it contain procedures that added burden or complexity that was not useful in providing patient care or protection during the emergency scenario?

For example, an evaluation for a surge exercise would document the performance of key tasks and tactics under each of these plan processes as follows:

- Receiving and acting on initial incident information
- Assessing and identifying strategies for information flow, coordinating messages, and communication
- Assessing and identifying resources needs during the emergency
- Meeting and responding to the surge event
- Maximizing space within the facility
- Recovering from the incident

The exercise evaluation documentation should be reviewed by the EM staff, the EC committee, senior leadership, and the performance improvement team. Any deficiencies or gaps in the EOP should be prioritized for improvement before the next emergency exercise.

Improving the EOP may require significant modifications (construction projects, for example) that take a long time to implement. If these cannot be completed before the next emergency response exercise, the organization must use interim measures to maintain readiness until the final modifications are completed.

To Sum Up

The very nature of emergencies is unpredictable, stressful, and resource-consuming. Those organizations that have experienced wildfires, widespread flooding, civil disturbances, shooting or other violence in the workplace, or other natural and man-made emergencies, certainly can attest to that. Risk assessment, planning, training, and exercises are essential in preparing an organization to respond to and recover from an emergency. Without such measures, an emergency can become a catastrophe, and an organization can feel the effects on its operations, staff, and clinical services for months, and sometimes years, to come.

Reference

1. Liu JC, et al. Future respiratory hospital admissions from wildfire smoke under climate change in the Western US. *Environ Res Lett.* 2016 Dec 8;11(12).

RISK-ASSESSMENT TOOLBOX

1. **Download** Hazard Vulnerability Analysis
2. **Download** 96-Hour Operational Impact Chart
3. **Download** Emergency Response Staff Training Checklist
4. **Download** Emergency Operations Plan Contents
5. **Download** After-Action Review

CMS Emergency Preparedness Final Rule

The US Centers for Medicare & Medicaid Services (CMS) published its final rule for emergency management (EM) late in 2016. As previously discussed, healthcare organizations are expected to comply with the ruling by November 15, 2017. The Joint Commission also released newly revised EM standards and elements of performance that align with this final rule, and the following is a breakdown of what is expected from healthcare organizations.

Four Required Sections

The CMS emergency preparedness final rule requirements are divided into four major sections:

1. Emergency Plan
2. Policies and Procedures
3. Communication Plan
4. Training and Testing

In addition, there are sections related to integrated healthcare systems and transplant hospitals that will apply depending on the structure of and services provided by the organization. Key elements of the four major sections are outlined as follows:

- Develop a plan that includes the following:
  - Facility and community-based risk assessment
  - Strategies to address identified events
  - Address patients, including those at risk
  - Cooperation and collaboration
- Develop specific procedures based on the plan addressing the following:
  - Subsistence needs
  - Food, water, medical supplies
  - Alternative sources of energy
  - Temperature and humidity for health and safety
  - Emergency lighting
  - Fire detection, extinguishment, alarm systems
  - Sewage and waste disposal
  - Location of staff and patients during and post event
  - Evacuation
  - Shelter in place for staff, patients, volunteers
  - Manage patient information
  - Use of volunteers
  - Arrangements with other hospitals and providers
  - Role in accordance with a waiver under Section 1135 of the Social Security Act, for care and treatment at alternate care sites, when the president declares a disaster or emergency under the Stafford Act or the National Emergencies Act
- Develop a communications plan as part of the emergency plan that includes the following:
  - Name and contact information
  - Staff and other service provider entities
  - Physicians
  - Other hospitals
  - Volunteers

- Contact information
- Federal, state, tribal, regional, and local emergency preparedness staff
- Primary and alternate means of communication to reach staff, federal, state, tribal, regional, and local emergency management agencies
- Method to share information about patients
- Method to release patient information if evacuating
- Develop a training program that includes the following:
  - Review at least annually
  - Specific to expected roles
- Testing through exercises*
  - Community or facility exercise
  - Evaluation
  - Improve plan based on exercise
- Emergency and standby power systems
  - Generator location in accordance with NFPA 99–2012, 101–2012, and 110–2010
  - Testing in accordance with NFPA 110–2010
  - Emergency generator fuel

* Please note that although the CMS EM final rule permits tabletop exercises, The Joint Commission will not allow tabletop exercises to be used to meet the annual exercise requirements for hospitals, critical access hospitals, and ambulatory surgical centers. For these settings, the current exercise requirements for accreditation purposes continue to apply. Home care settings are already permitted to use tabletop exercises for accreditation purposes.

NFPA, National Fire Protection Association.

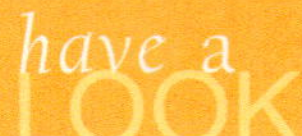

Emergency Management Exercise Planning Guide

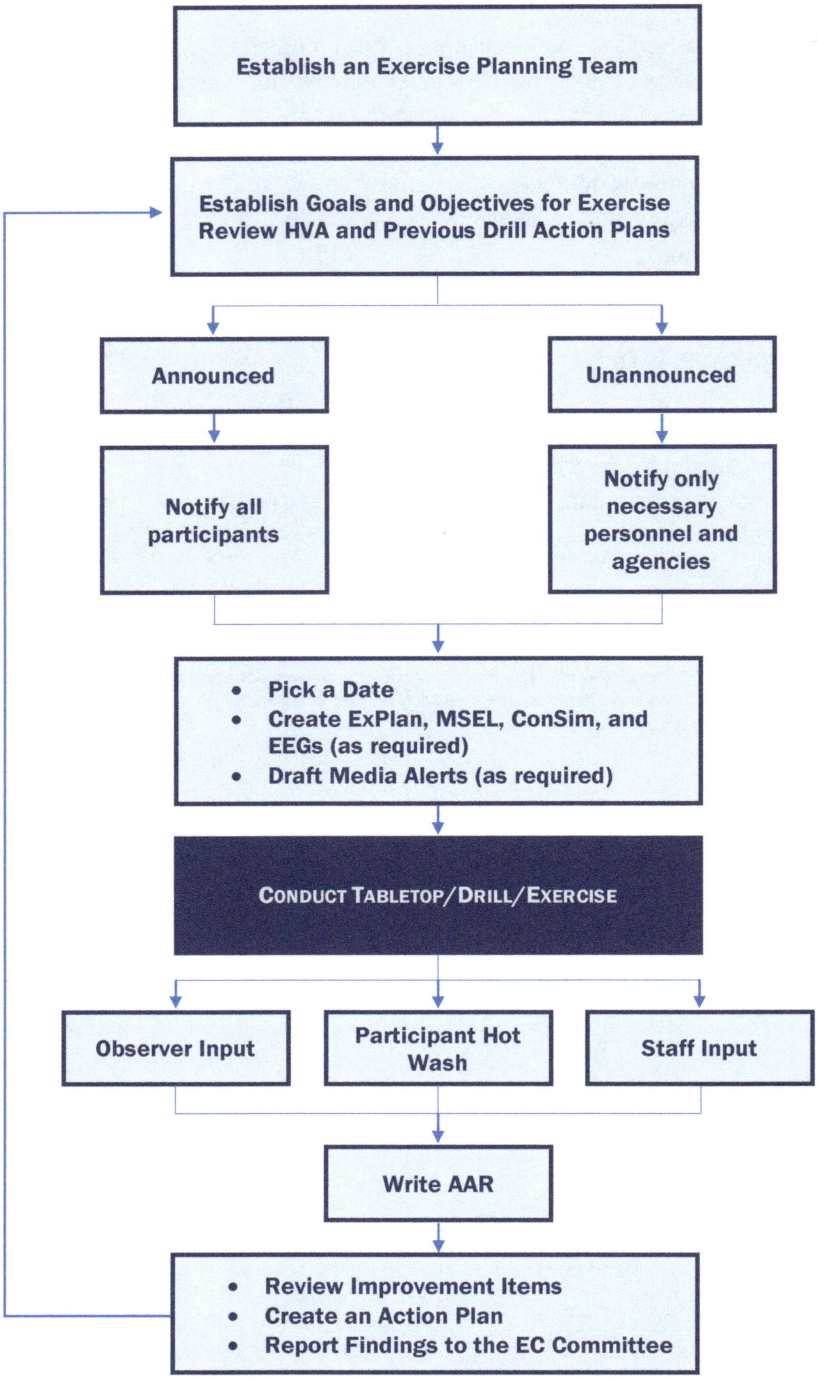

HVA, hazard vulnerability analysis; ExPlan, Exercise Plan; MSEL, Master Scenario Event List; ConSim, Control Simulator; EEG, exercise evaluation guide; AAR, After Action Report; EC, environment of care.

Source: Adapted from Tangredi E. Emergency Management: Exercise Planning Guide. White Plains Hospital, White Plains, NY. Used with permission.

Organizations can use a process flow map, such as the one illustrated here, to plan its emergency exercises.

After-Action Review Report

After-action reviews are a critical step to ensure all participants and observers can relay information about the effectiveness or areas of weakness seen during an emergency response exercise. Once compiled, after-action report data can be used to drive performance improvement efforts for areas that the organization did not meet the desired standard of performance.

Note: *The complete report may be adapted and is available for internal use on the flash drive (print only) or by clicking the tool link in the Risk-Assessment Toolbox (e-book only) on page 199.*

Source: Niemer P. Children's Hospital Colorado, Aurora, CO. Used with permission.

Published in *Environment of Care Risk Assessment*, Joint Commission Resources, 2018.   **File Name:** 09 05 After-Action Review Report

AFTER-ACTION REVIEW REPORT

DATE OF EVENT: _________________   TYPE OF DISASTER: COMMUNITY ☐   INTERNAL ☐   OTHER ☐

PLANNED EVENT   ☐   DATE REVIEWED BY EMERGENCY MANAGEMENT COMMITTEE OR MANAGER:

ACTUAL EVENT   ☐

PERSON(S) RESPONSIBLE FOR COMPLETING   ____
THE SUMMARY OF INFORMATION:

AUDITORS	AREAS OR ACTIVITIES MONITORED

TYPE OF EXERCISE: ____

SCENARIO: ____

MEASURABLE PERFORMANCE EXPECTATIONS FOR THE SIX CRITICAL FUNCTIONS: ____

1. Communications	SATISFACTORY ☐	UNSATISFACTORY ☐	NA ☐
Items to consider ✓ Activation of emergency management all-hazards command structure ✓ Notification of appropriate members of peri-operative, surgical and anesthesia services ✓ Communication with the media, suppliers, patient families ✓ Internal communications	Comments from staff debriefing and auditors:		

2. Resources and Assets	SATISFACTORY ☐	UNSATISFACTORY ☐	NA ☐
Items to consider ✓ Additional resources located and addressed before receiving patients (stocking up)	Comments from staff debriefing and auditors:		

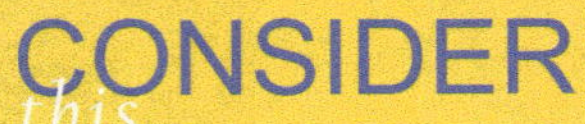

Best Practices for When the Worst Strikes

Proactive planning with community partners is an integral part of sustaining various services when disaster strikes. Solid emergency planning coupled with strong partnerships in the community help facilitate the recovery and restoration of health care services. The following examples provide real-world experiences of best practices for emergency planning for different health care settings.

- The state of Maryland requires all dialysis centers to have emergency management plans. Best practices from these plans include notification to patients, families, and other facilities regarding provision of services; triaging the most vulnerable patients and rescheduling high-priority patients; self-care messaging to patients; emergency power hookup and utility return-of-service prioritization; and participation in regional planning efforts and drills.[1]

- Home care organizations rose to the challenge during Hurricane Sandy, working closely with the Home Care Association (HCA) of New York State and other key partners to coordinate response and recovery activities. According to the communications director of the HCA, "The intimate, day-to-day connection between patients and their home care aides, therapists, nurses, and social workers makes these front-line caregivers a valuable asset before, during, and after a crisis. They know which patients have life-limiting disabilities that require transportation assistance, or which patients are technology-dependent and need immediate triage before the power is knocked out."[2]

- The university medical center that received trauma cases during the San Bernardino terrorist shooting rapidly activated its trauma team and the trauma chief pulled in extra staff. Additional surgeons from the local Veteran's Administration (VA) medical center came in; it was an informal process, but the VA surgeons were already privileged. The university medical center had good working relationships with other hospitals, and received many offers for staffing help from other triage physicians and nursing from other locations, and from some out-of-state medical centers.

- A chemical spill in a local river contaminated the water supply for several communities in West Virginia, including the supply used by hospitals, clinics, and most other health care providers in the area. An ambulatory dialysis company was notified of the incident at 6 P.M. and immediately contacted its biomedical engineer and regional director, and the command center serving the four-hospital system it supported. The biomedical engineer confirmed that city water could not be used; through their national contract, the ambulatory dialysis company received a 6,000-gallon tanker truck within four hours to one of the hospitals that had no water available for patient care purposes. The company set up a distribution center, which it had done previously at ambulatory sites, but this was its first time setting up at a hospital. The hospital building engineers set up a delivery system to the floors, but it was difficult to maintain sufficient pressure to operate all the medical equipment. The local fire department worked with the dialysis tanker to pressurize the system so that water for patient care could flow continuously without interruption.

References

1. Kidney Community Emergency Response. Scenarios and Best Practices for Emergency Management of End Stage Renal Disease Patients. Ingram K, et al. 2013. Accessed Feb 20, 2018. http://www .kcercoalition.com/en/resources/patient-resources/emergency-preparedness/.
2. Noyes RL. Home care emergency response: Hurricane Sandy lessons learned and actions taken. *Caring.* 2013 Jun;32(5):10–14.

Source: The Joint Commission. Building resilience with vulnerable populations. *Environment of Care® News.* 2014 Jul;17(7):1, 3–4, 10.

chapter 10

Construction

Construction and renovation are messy, and when these activities occur in a health care organization, they can significantly compromise patient and staff safety in the environment of care (EC). Construction activities can create or spread contaminants, produce noise and/or vibration, and disrupt essential services. Construction often entails the temporary shutdown of utilities, such as electrical power or water. The risk of health care–associated infections increases when construction activity disrupts and disperses airborne or waterborne microorganisms. Construction work also can interfere with fire safety measures by blocking egress or perforating fire and smoke compartments.

Overview of Assessing Risks

In accordance with Standard EC.02.06.05, the Joint Commission requires organizations to manage safety risks during any construction, renovation, or demolition project. This is done through a required preconstruction risk assessment (PCRA) (*see* the focus areas of a PCRA on page 206), which identifies potential risks, and plans ways to mitigate them before the first hammer is swung (*see* page 207 for a PCRA tool).

Infection prevention and control (IC) and life safety (LS) risks have their own required assessment processes according to Standards IC.01.03.01 and LS.01.02.01, respectively. The infection control risk assessment (ICRA) will be described later in this chapter. LS risks are identified and addressed through the interim life safety measures (ILSM) assessment (*see* Chapter 6).

Participants in the Process

Because construction projects affect every aspect of the environment of care, the team that assesses the risks should reflect those aspects. The makeup of the team may vary depending on the type and scope of the planned construction activity, but should include representatives from the EC, risk management, and facilities management committees, as well as leadership from the department(s) where the activity will take place. Also, the team should include individuals with expertise in the following areas:

- Safety
- Infection prevention and control
- Ventilation
- Facility design

Preconstruction Risk Assessment Focus Areas

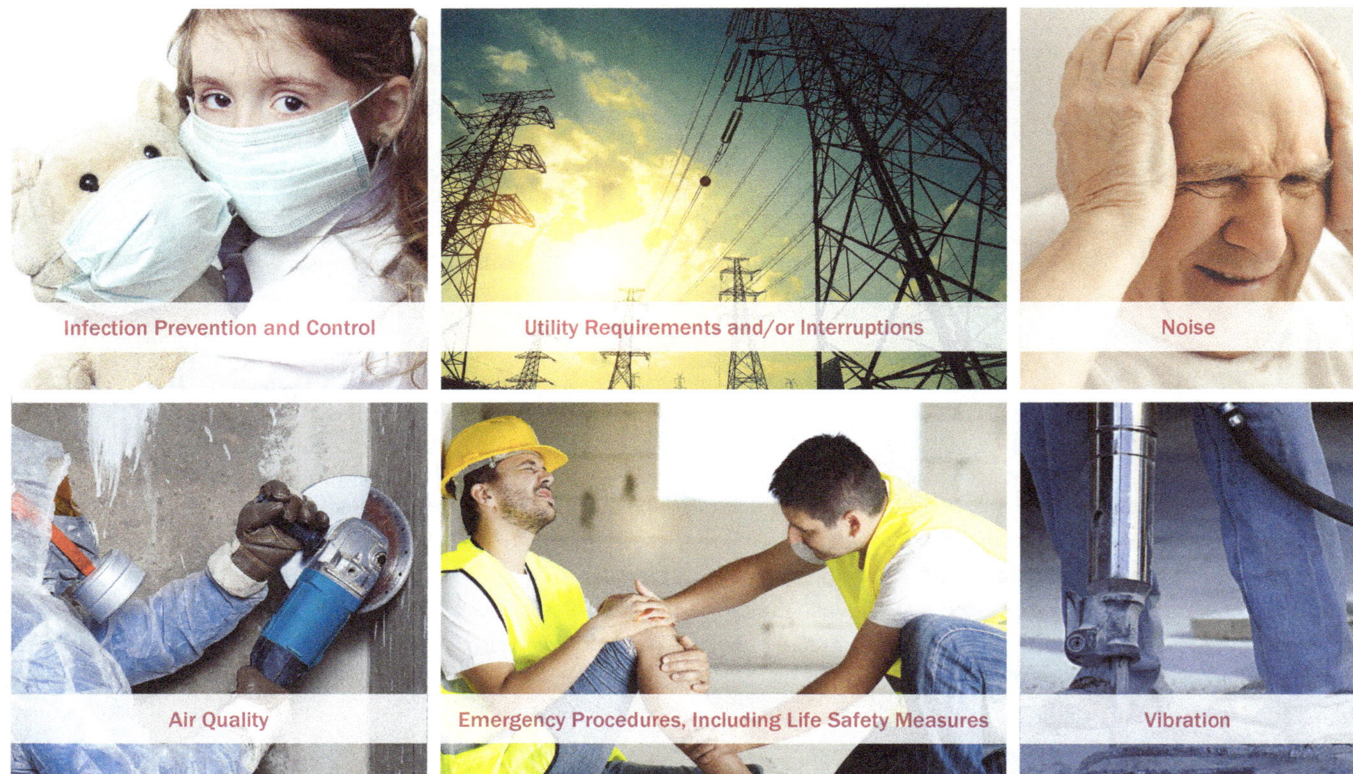

Before a construction project beings, the preconstruction risk assessment tool is used to determine the affect the construction will have on these identified areas.

Building engineers and the project's contractor should be included in risk-assessment activities as well. *See* page 209 for a construction-based mock tracer worksheet.

Frequency

Construction risks should be assessed early in the planning process. As the planning and design phases progress, risks should be assessed and reassessed frequently. Frequent assessment serves the following purposes:

- Ensures that the risk-management activities are effective
- Allows the team to adapt those activities as plans change
- Helps the team identify new risks that may arise due to changes in the design or other factors

Many PCRA teams meet weekly to evaluate the current status of the project and discuss updates on the risk-management activities. These meetings generally continue throughout the life of the project—including planning, design, and active construction phases (*see* page 209 for a daily project safety inspection checklist).

Identifying Risks

As previously described, the PCRA should assess risks related to infection prevention and control, air quality, utilities, noise, vibration, and emergency procedures. The specific risks and the severity of their potential impact will vary depending on the size, type, and location of the project.

for example...

When conducting a preconstruction risk assessment, the patient population within, next to, above, or below the area of construction must be taken into consideration, such as the following:

- Construction noise will be a significant concern to a neonatal intensive care unit, since hearing is still developing for these infants.
- Appropriate ventilation will be a priority in areas where immunocompromised patients receive care.

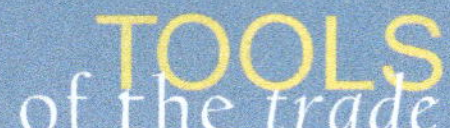

Preconstruction Risk Assessment

Construction—in its very nature—is fraught with risks. The environmental risks construction brings to a health care facility can have long-lasting negative effects if precautions are not taken. Prior to beginning a project, health care organizations must complete a preconstruction risk assessment (PCRA), using a tool such as this example, to identify the varying risks to the health care environment.

Note: *The complete assessment may be adapted and is available for internal use on the flash drive (print only) or by clicking the tool link in the Risk-Assessment Toolbox (e-book only) on page 214.*

Source: Charleston Area Medical Center, Charleston, WV. Used with permission.

Published in *Environment of Care Risk Assessment*, Joint Commission Resources, 2018.   **File Name:** 10 01 PCRA

PRECONSTRUCTION RISK ASSESSMENT

LOCATION OF CONSTRUCTION: _______________________   PROJECT START DATE: _______________

PROJECT COORDINATOR: _______________________   ESTIMATED DURATION: _______________

CONTRACTOR PERFORMING WORK: _______________________   PERMIT EXPIRATION DATE: _______________

It is important **not** to overlook the potential risks involved with small projects. Even the smallest project will affect the environment of care, and small projects often are more complicated than they may originally seem. Therefore, a PCRA should be conducted for every construction, renovation, or demolition project.

Conducting a PCRA should cover the most common areas that will affect the care, treatment, and services of a health care facility. However, there are some specific construction-related risks to look for, including the following:

- *Mercury.* In earlier decades, mercury was commonly used in temperature gauges and switches. Today it still can be found in fluorescent lamps and, sometimes, in research laboratories.
- *Lead.* Still present in many health care facilities, lead can be found in paint, roof flashings, plumbing, and shielding in imaging departments. Special care should be taken when removing or installing lead shielding in these areas.
- *Asbestos.* Typically a concern in older buildings, removing asbestos must be done under very specific conditions to prevent the fibers from becoming airborne and spreading through the facility.
- *Radiation.* Whenever construction will house equipment that produces ionizing radiation or in which radioactive material will be used and/or stored, a qualified medical physicist or health physicist should be consulted. For computed tomography, positron emission tomography, or nuclear medicine, a medical physicist or health physicist must conduct a structural shielding design assessment to specify required radiation shielding. After construction and prior to clinical use of the area, a medical physicist or health physicist must conduct a radiation protection survey to verify the adequacy of installed shielding.

The Infection Control Risk Assessment

Construction projects create an environment that increases the risk of creating and spreading infection. Opening walls can expose infectious particles such as fungi or mold, causing those particles to become airborne. Work on boilers, cooling towers, or plumbing can disturb biofilm and spread waterborne infections such as *Legionella*. For these reasons, The Joint Commission–required PCRA includes an ICRA component so organizations can determine construction-related infection risks.

Although there is no single method available to conduct an effective ICRA, the widely used matrix on page 211 consists of a multistep process, as follows:

- *Step 1.* The risk-assessment team must identify the type of construction activity, which ranges from inspection and noninvasive activities, such as minor plumbing and painting, to major demolition or construction, including new construction.

- *Step 2.* Using the table provided, the team identifies the risk groups that will be affected. Groups are listed on the matrix from low to high risk. One example of a low-risk group would be office staff; the highest-risk groups might include patients in a burn unit or immunocompromised patients. If more than one group will be affected, such as a remodeling project that affects both the radiology and oncology departments, the higher-risk group should be selected.
- *Step 3.* The information gleaned from the first two steps is used to determine the level of IC activities needed. The infection control precautions are delineated in a matrix from Class I to Class IV. The matrix then prescribes the precautions to use during construction and at the end of construction.
- *Steps 4 through 7.* After the infection control precautions have been determined, the team will identify specific activities and issues related to the project.
- *Steps 8 through 13.* These steps require the team to assess and consider how the construction project will affect the organization.
- *Step 14.* The team will discuss with the project team the containment issues and the schedule and timing for identified issues.

This template, including the risk groups, precautions, and a sample infection control construction permit, is provided as an example only. Each organization should use an ICRA process that reflects its individual situation, and should use precautions that meet its particular needs.

Review Guidelines from Outside Organizations

The Joint Commission is not the only organization that requires an assessment of the risks of construction. The *Guidelines for Design and Construction of Health Care Facilities* from the Facility Guidelines Institute (FGI) also requires organizations to consider these risks, and provide an ICRA during the programming phase of a construction project[1] to determine the potential risk of transmission of various agents in the facility.

FGI. According to the FGI *Guidelines*, an ICRA should be a continuous process that begins during planning and continues throughout design and construction. An ICRA should be conducted by a panel with expertise in infection prevention and control, risk management, facility

design, construction ventilation, safety, and epidemiology. The panel should provide updated documentation of the risk assessment through planning, design, and construction. The ICRA should address only building areas anticipated to be affected by construction.

Construction issues to assess in the ICRA may include, but are not limited to, the following:
- Disruption of essential services
- Relocation or placement of patients
- Barrier placements to control airborne contaminants
- Debris cleanup and removal
- Traffic flow

American Institute of Architects (AIA). AIA also requires organizations to consider noise and vibration that result from construction activities.

Association for Professionals in Infection Control and Epidemiology (APIC). After a risk-assessment team is selected, APIC recommends that an authority should be assigned to coordinate the process. APIC notes that contractor accountability for attention to IC issues should be written into the contract documents. Furthermore, APIC reminds organizations to focus not only on patients but also on the risks to health care workers, volunteers, and the contractors themselves.[2]

US Centers for Disease Control and Prevention (CDC). The concept of an ICRA also is supported by the CDC's *Guidelines for Environmental Infection Control in Health-Care Facilities*, 2003 edition, which lists three major preliminary considerations[3]:
1. Design and function of the new structure or area
2. Assessment of environmental risks for airborne disease and opportunities for prevention
3. Measures to contain dust and moisture during construction or repairs

The CDC also recommends that consideration be given to construction projects that occur outside the health care facility's walls and perhaps even outside the property lines. Adjacent construction, whether undertaken by the health care facility or others, can affect patients within the facility if dust and airborne contaminants are permitted to enter the building via air intakes or other openings.[3]

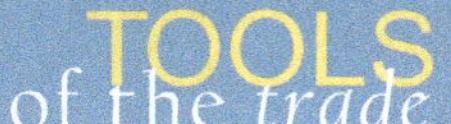

Construction Mock Tracer Worksheet

This worksheet can be used for construction-related mock tracers. Answers to these questions or questions added to the tool can provide insight about risks construction projects present to the health care organization.

Note: *The complete worksheet may be adapted and is available for internal use on the flash drive (print only) or by clicking the tool link in the Risk-Assessment Toolbox (e-book only) on page 214.*

Published in *Environment of Care Risk Assessment*, Joint Commission Resources, 2018. **File Name:** 10 02 Worksheet Construction Tracer

CONSTRUCTION MOCK TRACER WORKSHEET

This tracer worksheet is filled in with questions pertinent to construction, but can be revised to fit a particular program setting or health care facility. Review the relevant standards listed in the next section to determine what requirements are applicable to specific programs and settings.

Relevant Standards for these questions include the following: EC.02.06.05, LS.01.01.01, LS.01.02.01, and LS.02.01.10. Relevant standards cited are not necessarily applicable to every question. To determine applicability with a specific program/setting, check the *Comprehensive Accreditation Manual* or E-dition.

Organization		Department/Unit	
ate o... ...r	Time of ...er	Trac... ...op...	Constructio...

Construction Daily Project Safety Inspection Checklist

Health care organizations can complete this form daily. When complete, the form should be delivered to the project manager or another identified individual weekly. If a hazardous condition that cannot be fixed is observed, staff should contact the project manager or call the emergency operator to report the emergency situation.

Note: *The complete checklist may be adapted and is available for internal use on the flash drive (print only) or by clicking the tool link in the Risk-Assessment Toolbox (e-book only) on page 214.*

Source: Edwards Hospital & Health Services, Naperville, IL. Used with permission.

Published in *Environment of Care Risk Assessment*, Joint Commission Resources, 2018. **File Name:** 10 03 Checklist Daily Construction Safety

CONSTRUCTION DAILY PROJECT SAFETY INSPECTION

*This checklist can be used daily to identify safety issues that may develop over the course of a project. The "Corrective Action" section allows users to document the corrective actions taken, as well as the completion dates. Answers to all questions should ideally be Y for **Yes** (unless they aren't applicable). If an answer is N for **No**, use the "Notes" section to document needed changes. Unless otherwise noted, this checklist is applicable to all program settings.*

INSPECTOR: ______________________________   DATE: ______________________________

PROJECT NAME: ______________________________   LOCATION: ______________________________

QUESTIONS	YES	NO	NA	CORRECTIVE ACTION	DATE COMPLETED
1. Do all exits provide free and un...structed ...ress?					

Assess the IC Risks

Health care facilities have many potential IC risks from day-to-day tasks. Construction or renovation projects add another level of potential IC risks that could negatively affect the individuals served by a facility. The following are considered the common construction-related IC risks:

Dust and Fumes

These can compromise patient safety, even in small-scale projects. Dust can have severe effects on patients with compromised respiratory systems, including chronic obstructive pulmonary disease and asthma. Volatile organic compounds (VOCs), which are chemicals typically contained in cleaners, paint, adhesives, and the off-gas of new carpeting and upholstered furniture, also can cause adverse health effects.

Mold

Mold occurs on a construction site when materials get wet. This could be due to a burst pipe, water leak, or rain intrusion—all common construction scenarios. Mold can be hazardous to patients with compromised immune systems and others.

The CDC offers specific guidelines on how to handle materials that come in contact with moisture. Organizations must dry the materials completely before use or remove them within 72 hours. Some organizations choose to use a conservative approach to mold prevention and ban the use of materials that have become wet in construction projects.

Fungi

When renovating an older building, construction teams have to deal with fungi, such as *Aspergillus*. Sources of fungi include outdoor air; previously water-damaged ceilings, plaster, or drywall; construction dust; excavation; wet areas in the heating, ventilating, and air-conditioning (HVAC) system; living plants; and bird and bat droppings. Fungal spores easily become airborne when disturbed, and care must be taken to wet any affected material carefully before its removal so that spores do not become airborne.

Construction presents a risk for opportunistic airborne fungal infections in immunocompromised patients because normal ventilation may be disrupted, possibly releasing hazardous airborne spores into the environment. The phases of construction that usually create the greatest risk include demolition, window or wall removal, ventilation and utility outages, application of volatile chemicals, and placement of combustion engines.

Water Contaminants

During construction projects, bacteria can enter the water system, thus contaminating it. Many existing water systems already contain contaminants such as *Legionella* in the biofilm. This does not pose a threat if left undisturbed. However, during construction, vibration can shake this loose, releasing *Legionella* into the water supply.

Utility Disruption

During the course of construction, the organization may be required to shut off main power, heat, water, or air conditioning. Organizations must consider the impact of these shutdowns on a system and patient level. For example, if the water is shut off for two hours, how will patients be affected? How will staff be affected? How will equipment be affected? What is the most appropriate time for the shutdown that will have the least impact?

Hand Hygiene

Frequent hand washing helps prevent the spread of infection. This is critical in an area as fraught with IC risks as a construction site. Organizations must keep in mind locations for hand-washing stations or hand-sanitizer dispensers within a construction site to ensure that everyone on the job site has access to a convenient location for hand hygiene.

Storage

Oftentimes contractors will need to store tools and raw materials during the project. Organizations should plan for appropriate storage areas that prevent further creation of dust and mold and are out of the way of patient and staff traffic areas.

Debris Removal

Construction projects generate a lot of debris. Managing the removal of debris is essential to maintaining infection prevention and control during construction. Care should be taken to ensure that it is removed promptly. Use of covered containers, tacky mats, and other precautions ensure that debris and associated dust and contaminants do not spread beyond the construction site.

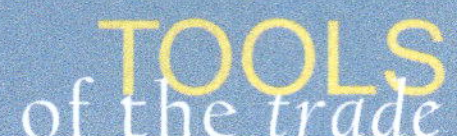

Infection Control Risk-Assessment Matrix of Precautions for Construction and Renovation

Health care facilities work to keep individuals healthy. When an organization begins a construction, renovation, or demolition project, it needs to assess the risks to its infection prevention and control (IC) efforts. This infection control risk-assessment matrix can help organizations identify what steps need to be taken to ensure the health of the individuals served.

Note: *The complete matrix may be adapted and is available for internal use on the flash drive (print only) or by clicking the tool link in the Risk-Assessment Toolbox (e-book only) on page 214.*

Source: Adapted from Judene Bartley, Epidemiology Consulting Services, Inc. Beverly Hills, MI. © 2002. Updated 2017.

Published in *Environment of Care Risk Assessment*, Joint Commission Resources, 2018.　　　　**File Name:** 10 04 ICRA

INFECTION CONTROL RISK-ASSESSMENT MATRIX OF PRECAUTIONS FOR CONSTRUCTION AND RENOVATION

STEP 1.	Using the following table, identify the type of construction project activity (Types A–D).
TYPE A	**Inspection and noninvasive activities** Includes, but is not limited to, the following: • Removal of ceiling tiles for visual inspection only (e.g., limited to one tile per 50 square feet) • Painting (but not sanding) • Wall covering, electrical trim work, minor plumbing, and activities that do not generate dust or require cutting of walls or access to ceilings other than for visual inspection
TYPE	**Small-scale, short-duration activities that create minimal dust** Includes, but is not limited to, the following: • Installation of telephone and computer cabling

---

Respond to the Risks

After IC risks have been assessed, the team should determine the appropriate responses for the risks and patients involved. These could include the following:

Project Isolation

Construction projects should be isolated from the rest of the facility. Large-scale projects, such as constructing a new wing or renovating an old one, might be easier to isolate than small-scale projects, such as painting a few rooms or repairing ceiling tiles. In accordance with the 2012 edition of the *Life Safety Code*®† the National Fire Protection Association's (NFPA) standard requires a minimum one-hour fire-rated separation from slab to slab in order to separate any construction areas from the rest of the building.

Work Methods

Organizations should consider all types of work methods that could reduce the likelihood of future patient safety problems.

---

† *Life Safety Code*® is a registered trademark of the National Fire Protection Association, Quincy, MA.

Using high-efficiency particulate air (HEPA)–filtered fan units and vacuums to minimize dust, working off-hours or on weekends to reduce patient and staff impact, wetting down materials with a fine spray to prevent the spread of dust and fungi, as appropriate, and other strategies could help address risks.

Effective HVAC System

Because virtually all buildings have some degree of recirculation in their ventilation systems, requiring both a supply and a return, careful preconstruction planning helps prevent buildingwide contamination during construction. This could include contamination from dust, fumes, or other airborne particles.

To prevent contamination from the construction site, the organization must ensure that air flows from clean to dirty. The facility's HVAC engineer must determine how to isolate the system. This may include sealing vents, adding additional filters, or using other means to prevent contamination. Elevator shafts require special consideration because of their tendency to function like a chimney, drawing odors, dust, and fumes up through the shaft onto other floors. This is known as the stack effect.

Negative-Pressure Areas

No matter how well an area is sealed up with plastic sheeting or rigid barrier walls, air leaks can occur. The use of negative pressure can prevent seepage into adjacent areas and can draw air containing dust, fumes, and other particles back into the construction area. Recirculation of air is prevented. Exhaust from the construction area should be filtered and directed outside to a predetermined area.

Negative-air machines, capable of drawing in and filtering not more than 2,000 cubic feet per minute of air, can be used. Although these units once were expensive, their cost has dropped and they work extremely well. HEPA–filtered units are capable of filtering out 99.97% of particulate matter. One downside to negative-pressure machines is that they can be noisy. Organizations will need to address this noise during the PCRA process. Organizations also should assess how much negative pressure will be needed at the construction site, where the exhaust will go, how the pressure will be monitored, and whether to use existing equipment.

Negative pressure also can be used with small-scale projects. For example, if workers need to run wires above a ceiling, they can contain just the area they are working in by building a plastic cube around the work area and putting the cube under negative pressure with a small negative air unit or a HEPA–filtered vacuum cleaner. With proper exhausting outside the cube, dust and fumes can be kept from migrating to occupied areas.

Clean and Dirty Anterooms

Just outside the construction site, organizations may wish to set up clean and dirty rooms. This will help construction workers remove particles, such as dust, fungi, and bacteria, from their persons before leaving the project area. This can minimize the transfer of particles outside of the construction zone.

Tacky Mats

Placing these at the entrance to and exit from the construction site can minimize the spread of dust and debris throughout the facility.

Covered Containers for Waste Removal

This can prevent the spread of odors, dust, and other particles that can cause patient harm. Waste should be removed every day. In addition, containers of paints and adhesives should be kept closed when not in use, which reduces the off-gassing of VOCs.

Air and Water Testing

The CDC does not recommend routine sampling of air and water, noting that "Conducting quality-assurance sampling on an extended basis, especially in the absence of an adverse outcome, is usually unjustified."[3(p. 89)] But in some specific situations, such as evaluating the effects of a change in IC practice, or ensuring that equipment or systems perform according to specification and expected outcomes (situations that may arise during a construction project), the CDC indicates that sampling may be advised.

A common measurement is an ongoing sampling of air quality during construction to determine breaks in environmental IC measures. In addition, sampling is recommended during the commissioning of newly constructed space, such as operating suites, immunosuppressed units, or areas for other vulnerable populations.

Monitoring Immunocompromised Patients

Careful monitoring of immunocompromised patients is particularly important during a construction or renovation project to detect any airborne contaminants as early as possible. The monitoring is not environmental sampling but a close watch on any type of unexpected infections in patients.

Protective Clothing

Workers at the construction site should be provided with appropriate clothing to protect them from potential infection and harm. This may include coveralls, masks or eye shields, respirators, gloves, or other types of clothing. These items must be managed effectively, particularly with regard to donning and doffing procedures, and disposal or reprocessing of the items.

Barriers

Barriers can help seal off the construction site. As part of the risk assessment, organizations should determine where to place barriers, with what materials to make barriers, and the LS considerations associated with those barriers.

Cleaning

This could include wiping down work services with disinfectant, daily vacuuming with HEPA–filtered vacuums, or ensuring that all trash is removed from the construction site on a regular basis.

Implementing the PCRA

It is up to the organization to implement appropriate recommendations to reduce and/or control the risks inherent in the project. Furthermore, the controls instituted as a result of the assessment must be enforced. Organizations should revisit the assessment throughout the construction process to ensure that all risks are being addressed appropriately.

Interim Life Safety Measures

Periods of construction or renovation are the most common times when an organization may be unable to comply with the *Life Safety Code®*. Organizations are required to have a policy in place that describes how they will assess *Life Safety Code* compliance and respond to deficiencies that occur during construction (*see* page 140 in Chapter 6 for a sample ILSM policy). Those responses are known as interim life safety measures, and they are identified through an ILSM risk assessment. Both ILSM and ILSM risk assessments are discussed in detail in Chapter 6.

Some organizations use the same team to conduct the PCRA and the construction-related ILSM risk assessment. This method ensures that both assessments are coordinated and that no critical areas are overlooked. It is important to remember that ILSM are intended to be temporary—they should be used only while the compliance lapse exists. As work progresses and the situation changes, ILSM should be removed or added, as determined by frequent reassessment of the LS risks in a construction area (*see* page 209 for a construction daily project safety inspection checklist).

Other PCRA Issues

Not all PCRA risks are related to infection prevention and control or life safety. Other issues to consider include the following:

Low-Emitting Materials

By using low-emitting materials during construction, organizations can prevent off-gassing of VOCs and carcinogens into the air. This can help preserve the environment, as well as the safety of construction staff, health care organization staff, patients, and visitors.

Traffic Control

Preconstruction planning defines how workers will enter and exit the building and the route they will take to the construction area. Separation of patient/visitor/staff traffic from construction traffic is highly desirable, if possible. Signs should direct patients, staff, and visitors away from the construction area.

In larger buildings, it might be appropriate to designate use of freight elevators for construction traffic. These are designed for heavier use and rarely are used by patients. If this is not feasible, one or more elevators can be keyed off, allowing use only by construction staff. Organizations should consider how to protect non-freight elevators because they can be damaged quickly during construction.

Placement of the construction office for large projects requires planning as well. An office trailer should not get in the way of entering or exiting patients, visitors, and staff.

Communications

Effective communication is an essential—and perhaps the most important—activity in a health care organization's efforts to minimize construction-related problems. The key to the successful implementation of a plan to manage such issues as noise, vibration, dust, and utility interruptions during a construction project is ensuring that everyone who may be affected by this work is aware of what is happening and why it is happening. Good communication not only minimizes the impact on operations but also helps to identify potential problems or issues that otherwise may have been overlooked.

Emergency Procedures

Construction projects can dramatically affect an organization's emergency response procedures by moving entrances and exits, rerouting traffic, and disabling alarm systems. An organization must consider how it would respond to an emergency during construction, including how to defend in place and, if necessary, evacuate.

Construction workers play a major role in emergency procedures during the project. It is important that an organization consider the impact these additional workers, who may number in the thousands, will have on their emergency planning efforts.

The organization also should consider revising its hazard vulnerability analysis (HVA) to reflect the construction activities. For example, if a tower crane is being brought on-site, does the HVA consider what would happen if this were to tip and block access to the facility or injure a large number of people in the area?

Finally, it is important to train the construction workers on how to respond to an emergency (for example, fire, earthquake, storm event). This is a critical part of emergency planning, and the organization needs to provide appropriate training when necessary.

Documenting the Process

It is essential that the PCRA process be documented. The organization is ultimately responsible for conducting the assessment and implementing recommendations. But responsibilities for specifications and implementation also lie with the contractor on the project, and these responsibilities should be outlined clearly in the contract. It is recommended that the PCRA (including the ICRA) and ILSM documentation be included in contract documents to clarify which entities are responsible for which activities.

References

1. Facility Guidelines Institute. *Guidelines for Design and Construction of Health Care Facilities*. Chicago: American Society for Healthcare Engineering, 2010.
2. Bartley JM. APIC State-of-the-Art Report: The role of infection control during construction of health care facilities. *Am J Infect Control*. 2000 Apr;28(2):156–169.
3. US Centers for Disease Control and Prevention. *Guidelines for Environmental Infection Control in Health-Care Facilities: Recommendations of the CDC and the Healthcare Infection Control Practices Advisory Committee (HICPAC)*. 2003. (Updated: Feb 15, 2017.) Accessed Feb 20, 2018. https://www.cdc.gov/infection control/pdf/guidelines/environmental-guidelines.pdf.

RISK-ASSESSMENT TOOLBOX

1. [Download] Preconstruction Risk Assessment
2. [Download] Construction Mock Tracer Worksheet
3. [Download] Construction Daily Project Safety Inspection Checklist
4. [Download] Infection Control Risk-Assessment Matrix of Precautions for Construction and Renovation

Notes:

Glossary

access control The management of admission to areas within a facility based on permission levels assigned to users. Access control often includes authentication of the identity of the user.

active shooter An individual actively engaged in killing or attempting to kill people in a confined and populated area; in most cases, active shooters use firearms, and there's no pattern or method to their selection of victims.

adverse event A patient safety event that resulted in harm to a patient.

alternative equipment maintenance (AEM) program A program that enables hospitals to adopt a medical equipment maintenance approach that deviates from manufacturers' requirements. The Joint Commission offers the American National Standards Institute/Association for the Advancement of Medical Instrumentation document ANSI/AAMI EQ56–2013, *Recommended Practice for a Medical Equipment Management Program*, as an example of standards for an AEM program. An AEM program must not compromise safety or put patients at increased risk. The decision to use an AEM program must be based on a risk assessment performed by a qualified individual. The organization must keep documentation supporting its AEM approach, and must announce its use of an AEM program at the beginning of the accreditation survey.

ambulatory health care occupancy An occupancy used to provide services or treatment to four or more patients (or one or more patients in an ambulatory surgical center that elects to use The Joint Commission deemed status option) at the same time that either (1) renders them incapable of providing their own means of self-preservation in an emergency or (2) provides outpatient surgical treatment requiring general anesthesia.

annual evaluation A review every 12 months of environment of care (EC) management plans to make sure the plans are still relevant, applicable, and effective, and reflect any changes at the organization.

annually One year from the date of the last event, plus or minus 30 days. Synonymous with every 12 months, once a year, or every year.

authority having jurisdiction (AHJ) The organization, office, or individual responsible for approving equipment, materials, an installation, or a procedure.

automatic transfer switch (ATS) Switchgears that transfer the power from the utility to the emergency generator in the event of an electrical outage. Upon the loss of power, the transfer switch signals the generator to start. When the generator gets up to speed and produces the proper voltage and frequency, the transfer switch transfers the load to the generator.

barrier A separation made up of walls, doors, windows, and so on, intended to prevent the spread of fire or smoke.

Basic Building Information (BBI) One of four parts within the Statement of Conditions™ (SOC) tool. This is a summary of patient care facilities that are defined by the *Life Safety Code®* as health care, ambulatory, or residential occupancies, as applicable. Although The Joint Commission does not require patient care facilities defined as business occupancies to be managed in the SOC, it is still recommended. Sites are populated based on an organization's Electronic Application for Accreditation (E-App), while buildings for each site are created and managed by the organization. Although no longer mandatory, a BBI is required to manage other parts of the SOC.

best practices Clinical, scientific, or professional practices that are recognized by a majority of professionals in a particular field as being exemplary. These practices are typically evidence-based and consensus driven.

building assessment An established process to assess compliance with the *Life Safety Code* and self-identify deficiencies in the built environment, as well as establishing corrective action measures. The Joint Commission requires each organization to conduct a building assessment at a time frame established by the organization; however, annually is recommended.

Building Maintenance Program (BMP) A method for tracking, managing, and correcting deficiencies through maintenance activities. The program can consist of written strategies to manage items covered in the program, a documented schedule for the frequency of inspecting the items, and processes for evaluating the effectiveness of the program.

business occupancy An occupancy used to provide outpatient care, treatment, day treatment, or other services that does not meet the criteria in the ambulatory health care occupancy definition (for example, three or fewer individuals at the same time who are either rendered incapable of self-preservation in an emergency or are undergoing general anesthesia). For ambulatory surgical centers that elect to use The Joint Commission deemed status option, treatment of one or more incapacitated patients renders the area an ambulatory health care occupancy.

clinical alarm A component of some medical devices that is designed to notify caregivers of an important change in a patient's physiologic status. A clinical alarm typically provides audible and/or visible notification of the changed patient status.

close call A patient safety event that did not reach the patient; also called near miss or good catch.

commissioning A series of activities before taking ownership of a building, project, or renovation, in which an organization makes sure that all specifications are met and that all systems, components, equipment, and such are fully operational.

culture of safety An environment in which safety is the top priority. In a culture of safety, not only are processes designed for optimal safety but employees feel safe in reporting unsafe situations. Also referred to as a *safety culture*.

decontamination Removing or neutralizing dangerous materials and/or substances.

deemed status, deeming Approval given by the US Centers for Medicare & Medicaid Services (CMS) to an organization like The Joint Commission that uses standards and survey processes equivalent to those used by Medicare or other federal programs to "deem" a health care organization as meeting such requirements. Those accredited organizations do not then have to go through the CMS survey and certification process; they are said to have "deemed status." Seeking deemed status through accreditation is generally an option, not a requirement. Deemed status is available for Joint Commission–accredited ambulatory surgical centers, clinical laboratories, critical access hospitals, home health agencies, hospice organizations, hospitals, and psychiatric hospitals.

defend in place An emergency fire strategy for health care occupancy in which occupants remain within the health care facility rather than be evacuated. This is accomplished by limiting the development and spread of a fire emergency to the room of fire origin and reducing the need for occupant evacuation, except from the room of fire origin.

disaster A type of emergency that, due to its complexity, scope, or duration, threatens an organization's capabilities and requires outside assistance to sustain care, safety, or security.

drills Emergency exercises designed to test individual facets of an organization's response capabilities so that emergency planners can evaluate individual parts of the Emergency Operations Plan.

E-App An electronic form used for collecting information pertaining to the applicant organization. Information collected on this form will be used to determine the accreditation requirements applicable to the organization, the types of surveyors needed, the length of survey, and the survey fee.

element of performance (EP) Specific action(s), process(es), or structure(s) that must be implemented to achieve the goal of a standard. The scoring of EP compliance determines an organization's overall compliance with a standard.

elopement When a patient wanders away or leaves a health care facility unsupervised and/or without permission.

emergency An unexpected or sudden event that significantly disrupts the organization's ability to provide care, treatment, or services or the environment of care itself, or that results in a sudden, significantly changed or increased demand for the organization's services. Emergencies can be either human-made or natural (such as an electrical system failure or a tornado), or a combination of both, and they exist on a continuum of severity.

emergency management The overarching discipline that ensures that organizations are building and testing plans using the four phases of emergency management:
1. Mitigation
2. Preparedness
3. Response
4. Recovery

Emergency Operations Plan (EOP) An organization's written document that describes the process it would implement for managing emergencies that could disrupt the organization's ability to provide care, treatment, and services. (For behavioral health care, this document is called an *Emergency Management Plan*.)

emergency power supply system (EPSS) and stored emergency power supply system (SEPSS) Systems that automatically supply emergency illumination or power to critical areas and equipment essential for safety to human life. An SEPSS has a stored energy source (battery) as part of the system. An organization may have both an EPSS and an SEPSS for a specific utility or type of equipment; in case the EPSS fails, the SEPSS is a backup system. Or an organization may have only one or the other for a specific utility or type of equipment.

environment of care (EC) The physical environment of a health care organization, which includes the building itself and its grounds, utilities, medical equipment, and more. Some organizations refer to this as the EOC; however, The Joint Commission refers to this by the acronym "EC."

environment of care (EC) management plans One or more written plans that provide an overview of an organization's approach to the environment of care and how that approach complies with Joint Commission Environment of Care (EC) standards.

environment of care (EC) risk assessment A proactive examination of functions and processes in the physical environment used to assess actual and potential risks. Results from the assessment are then prioritized to identify improvement opportunities. Joint Commission standards require risk assessments in each of the seven functional areas of the environment of care:
1. Safety
2. Security
3. Fire and life safety
4. Hazardous materials and waste
5. Medical equipment
6. Utilities
7. Preconstruction

environment of care (EC) rounds A daily walk-through of an area in which staff look for basic environment of care (EC) issues that can be corrected right away, rather than waiting until the more in-depth environmental tour. This type of monitoring is not required under Joint Commission standards.

environment of care (EC) tour A proactive multidisciplinary comprehensive facility tour used to evaluate the physical environment and the effectiveness of current policies and procedures used to manage environmental safety risks. An EC tour also is used to determine staff knowledge and evaluate compliance with Joint Commission standards, codes, regulations, and laws. This tour is not required by The Joint Commission, but organizations who elect to conduct them set the frequency of the tour. Also called an environmental tour.

environment of care (EC) tracer A multidisciplinary assessment method used by surveyors on site to assess a health care organization's compliance with Joint Commission standards by following an entire system or process as it relates to the environment of care, emergency management, and fire protection and life safety.

equipment management Activities selected and implemented by the organization to assess and control the clinical and physical risks of fixed and portable equipment used for diagnosis, treatment, monitoring, and care.

equivalency A Joint Commission–approved alternate approach to a known *Life Safety Code*® deficiency that is mitigated by other building features so that the noncompliant condition is no longer identified as deficient. The Joint Commission has two types of equivalencies, a traditional equivalency and a Fire Safety Evaluation System (FSES) equivalency. The traditional equivalency requires field validation by a registered architect, a fire safety professional, or a fire marshal responsible for community fire safety. The FSES is a formula-based approach that evaluates the entire building and deducts deficient conditions. If the net score is 0 or better, the building is considered "equalized." Both types of equivalencies require submittal to and review by The Joint Commission. When The Joint Commission completes its analysis, the request is forwarded to the appropriate US Centers for Medicare & Medicaid Services (CMS) regional office for final disposition.

evacuation Removing individuals from a dangerous situation. An evacuation could be partial (at the site of an incident, affect certain groups of patients or areas within the facility, horizontally move individuals beyond corridor fire doors and/or smoke zones on the same floor, vertically move individuals from one floor[s] to the floor[s] above or below) or be complete and encompass the entire organization.

Evidence of Standards Compliance (ESC) A report submitted by a surveyed organization, which details the action(s) that it took to bring itself into compliance with an accreditation requirement or clarifies why the organization believes that it was in compliance with the accreditation requirement for which it received a Requirement for Improvement. An ESC report must address compliance at the element of performance level.

exercise An activity conducted by an organization to practice, train, and/or drill for emergency events using mock scenarios intended to gauge the effectiveness of the organization's Emergency Operations Plan (EOP).

failure Lack of success, nonperformance, nonoccurrence, breaking down, or ceasing to function. In most instances, and certainly within the context of this book, failure is what is to be avoided. It takes place when a system or part of a system performs in a way that is not intended or desirable.

failure mode and effects analysis (FMEA) A systematic way of examining a design prospectively for possible ways in which failure can occur. It assumes that no matter how knowledgeable or careful people are, errors will occur in some situations and may even be likely to occur. Synonym: failure mode, effects, and criticality analysis (FMECA).

fire barrier A continuous membrane or a membrane with discontinuities created by protected openings with a specified fire protection rating, where such membrane is designed and constructed with a specified fire resistance rating to limit the spread of fire, that also restricts the movement of smoke.*

fire door The door component of a fire door assembly.*

fire safety The minimum requirements for protecting against injury to life as a result of smoke, fire, and combustion, dependent on human intervention. This includes fire drills, use of fire safety equipment, and maintenance of alarm and sprinkler systems.

---

* **Source:** NFPA Glossary of Terms, June 2012, National Fire Protection Association, Quincy, MA.

fire watch The assignment of a person or persons to an area for the express purpose of protecting occupants from fire or similar emergencies. Examples of this protection include the following:
- ➤ Notifying the fire department, the building occupants, or both of an emergency
- ➤ Preventing a fire from occurring
- ➤ Extinguishing small fires

fire-resistance rating The time, in minutes or hours, that materials or assemblies have withstood a fire exposure (as determined by the tests, or methods based on tests, prescribed by the *Life Safety Code*®). Normally used to describe a fire wall or fire barrier wall.*

Focused Standards Assessment (FSA) A requirement of the accreditation process whereby an organization reviews its compliance with a selected subset of applicable Joint Commission accreditation requirements (including the applicable National Patient Safety Goals, a subset of direct and indirect impact standards, a selection of standards that address accreditation program–specific high-risk areas, and the organization's Requirements for Improvement [RFIs] from its last triennial survey); completes and submits to The Joint Commission a Plan of Action (POA) for any accreditation requirement with which it is not in full compliance; and chooses whether to engage in a telephone discussion with a member of the Standards Interpretation Group staff to determine the acceptability of the POA or discuss any other area of concern. Alternatives for a Full FSA submission include FSA Option 1 (attestation that an FSA was completed, but not submitted to The Joint Commission), Option 2 (on-site survey with documented findings), and Option 3 (on-site survey without documented findings). The FSA encourages organizations to be in continuous compliance with Joint Commission accreditation requirements and helps them to identify and manage risk. The organization retains the option to complete self-assessment with all applicable accreditation standards in the FSA tool, available on the organization's *Joint Commission Connect*™ extranet site. *See also* Intracycle Monitoring (ICM).

hazard vulnerability analysis (HVA) A process for identifying potential emergencies and the direct and indirect effects these emergencies may have on the organization's operations and the demand for its services.

---

* **Source:** NFPA Glossary of Terms, June 2012, National Fire Protection Association, Quincy, MA.

hazardous condition A circumstance (other than a patient's own disease process or condition) that increases the probability of an adverse event.

hazardous materials Dangerous materials (radioactive, flammable, explosive, or poisonous) that would be harmful to people or to the environment if released without taking necessary precautions, in accordance with local, state, and/or federal laws or regulations.

hazardous waste A term with a specific legal meaning, as determined by the US Environmental Protection Agency (EPA) and the US Department of Transportation (DOT), that applies to certain materials that have been generated as wastes from processes applied to hazardous materials.

health care occupancy An occupancy used for purposes such as medical or other treatment or care of persons suffering from physical or mental illness, disease, or infirmity; and for the care of infants, convalescents, or infirm aged persons. Health care occupancies provide sleeping facilities for four or more occupants and are occupied by persons who are mostly incapable of self-preservation because of age, physical or mental disability, or security measures not under the occupant's control. Health care occupancies include hospitals, critical access hospitals, skilled nursing homes, and limited care facilities.

health care–associated infection (HAI) An infection acquired concomitantly by an individual who is receiving or who has received care, treatment, or services from a health care organization. The infection may or may not have resulted from the care, treatment, or services.

health information Any information, oral or recorded, in any form or medium, that is created by a health care provider, health plan, public health authority, employer, life insurer, school or university, or health care clearinghouse that relates to past, present, or future physical or mental health or condition; the provision of health care; or payment for the provision of health care to an individual.

high-risk equipment Any medical equipment or operating components of utility systems that may result in serious injury or death to patients or staff if it fails. High-risk medical equipment includes life-support equipment. The term is equivalent to the US Centers for Medicare & Medicaid Services (CMS) term *critical equipment*.

high-risk process A process that, if not planned and/or implemented correctly, has a significant potential for affecting the safety of a patient or an individual served.

human factors The study of how individuals interact with each other, products, equipment, procedures, and the environment (including considerations of known human behavior, abilities, limitations, and other characteristics), applied to ensure safer, more reliable outcomes.

Immediate Threat to Health or Safety A situation that poses an immediate risk of serious adverse effects on the health or safety of a patient. This is identified on-site by a surveyor during survey. Also known as *immediate threat to life (ITL)* .

incident command system (ICS) The combination of personnel, procedures, communications, equipment, and facilities, operating within a common organizational structure, designed to aid in incident management activities. ICS is used for a broad spectrum of emergencies, from small to complex incidents, both natural and human-made, including acts of catastrophic terrorism.

incident report (occurrence report) A written report, usually completed by a nurse and forwarded to risk management personnel that describes and provides documentation for any unusual problem, incident, or other situation that is likely to lead to undesirable effects or that varies from established policies and procedures.

individual served An individual who receives care, treatment, or service; the individual can be a child, a youth, or an adult. When required for the well-being or age of the individual served, a legally responsible individual is also involved in the care, treatment, or service of the individual served.

infection control risk assessment (ICRA) A determination of the potential risks of transmission of various airborne and waterborne biological contaminants in the facility.

influx *See* surge event.

interim life safety measures (ILSM) A series of 11 administrative actions intended to temporarily compensate for significant hazards posed by existing National Fire Protection

Association 101–2012, *Life Safety Code*®, deficiencies, or construction activities.

Intracycle Monitoring (ICM) A process that helps accredited organizations maintain continuous compliance through a self-assessment of high-risk areas and related standards. It involves use of the organization's ICM Profile available on the organization's *Joint Commission Connect*™extranet site.

leader An individual who sets expectations, develops plans, and institutes procedures to assess and improve the quality of the organization's governance, management, and clinical and support functions and processes. At a minimum, leaders include members of the governing body and medical or clinical staff, the chief executive officer and other senior managers, the nurse executive, clinical leaders, and staff members in leadership positions within the organization.

life safety The minimum requirements for protecting against injury to life as a result of smoke, fire, and combustion, dependent on building features. This includes alarm and sprinkler systems, building construction and design, maintaining means of egress, and fire protection hardware issues.

Life Safety Code® Requirements for building construction intended to protect occupants during fires, developed by the National Fire Protection Association (NFPA) and adopted by The Joint Commission. *Life Safety Code*® is a registered trademark of the National Fire Protection Association, Quincy, Massachusetts.

life safety drawings Accurate and current maps included in an organization's Statement of Conditions™ (SOC) that show sprinklered areas of the organization's buildings, barrier locations, suite boundaries, and other fire and life safety features, as well as approved equivalencies and waivers in accordance with Joint Commission requirements.

life-support equipment Any medical equipment with the purpose of sustaining life. If it fails to perform its primary function (when used according to the manufacturer's instructions and clinical protocol), that failure will lead to patient death unless there's immediate intervention.

maintenance There are five types of maintenance— predictive, metered, corrective, interval-based, and reliability-centered—defined as follows:

1. **predictive maintenance**—A type of maintenance strategy that provides the means to achieve reliability levels that exceed the performance of a piece of equipment or system. This strategy is designed to measure and track data significant to the piece of equipment or system. It confirms possible faults with the equipment, and specific repairs are completed before the equipment fails. Predictive analysis can be performed using advanced monitoring instruments and predictive software that collects data and performs an analysis. The data collected are analyzed, and corrective maintenance is performed when the equipment is performing outside the desired operating parameters.
2. **metered maintenance**—A maintenance strategy based on the hours of run time or the number of times the equipment is used (for example, number of images processed).
3. **corrective maintenance**—A maintenance strategy that restores a piece of equipment to operational status after equipment failure.
4. **interval-based maintenance**—A maintenance done according to specific intervals (for example, calendar time, running hours). A number of periodic inspections or restoration tasks are completed, based on information/data obtained from the last equipment check.
5. **reliability-centered maintenance**—A type of maintenance that begins with a failure mode and effects analysis to identify the critical equipment failure modes in a systematic and structured manner. The process then requires the examination of each critical failure mode to determine the optimum maintenance policy to reduce the severity of each failure. The chosen type of maintenance strategy must take into account cost, safety, and environmental and operational consequences.

means of egress A continuous and unobstructed way of travel from any point in a building or other structure to a public way consisting of three separate and distinct parts:
1. Exit access
2. Exit
3. Exit discharge

medical device An instrument, apparatus, implement, machine, contrivance, implant, in vitro reagent, or another similar or related article, including a component part or accessory that is:
➤ Recognized in the official National Formulary or the US Pharmacopeia or any supplement to them;

➤ Intended for use in the diagnosis of disease or other conditions or in the cure, mitigation, treatment, or prevention of disease in humans or other animals; or
➤ Intended to affect the structure or any function of the body of humans or other animals and that does not achieve any of its primary intended purposes through chemical action within or on the body of humans or other animals and that is not dependent on being metabolized for the achievement of any of its primary intended purposes.

medical equipment Fixed and portable equipment used for the diagnosis, treatment, monitoring, and direct care of individuals.

mitigation Actions taken in attempting to reduce the probability, severity, and/or impact of a potential emergency; first of the four phases of emergency management.

mitigation, emergency Those activities an organization undertakes in attempting to reduce the severity and impact of a potential emergency. *See also* emergency.

mixed occupancy Areas of a building, within some facilities classified as health care occupancies that may have uses other than the housing or treatment of patients who are incapable of self-preservation. For example, there may be a wing that is used strictly for administrative offices or an area that is only for outpatient services that do not render individuals incapable of self-preservation. These areas may be classified as other occupancies, provided they are separated from the health care occupancy by a minimum two-hour fire-resistance-rated assembly. There are some advantages to doing this.

multidisciplinary team A group of staff members composed of representatives from a range of professions, disciplines, or service areas.

National Incident Management System (NIMS) A nationwide framework created by the US government that provides an all-hazards approach to emergency management and coordinates the responsibilities of organizations and jurisdictions.

near miss A patient safety event that did not reach the patient; also called a close call or a good catch. *See* close call.

occupancy In life safety, the purpose for which a building or portion of a building is used or meant to be used. Depending on the organization, occupancies may include ambulatory health care occupancy, business occupancy, health care occupancy, and residential occupancy.

occurrence report *See* incident report.

operations The activities involved in running a health care organization.

outbreak The occurrence of more than the expected number of cases of disease, injury, or other health conditions among a specific group during a specified time frame.

outcome The result of the performance (or nonperformance) of a function(s) or process(es).

patient An individual who receives care, treatment, or services. Synonyms used by various health care fields include resident, patient and family unit, individual served, consumer, health care consumer, customer, and beneficiary.

patient safety event An event, incident, or condition that could have resulted or did result in harm to a patient. *See also* adverse event, near miss, sentinel event.

performance improvement The systematic process of identifying performance problems, developing, and implementing solutions through interventions (actions), determining their success, and sustaining the improvement.

personal protective equipment (PPE) Clothing and other equipment worn to minimize exposure to serious workplace injuries and illnesses that may result from contact with chemical, radiological, physical, electrical, mechanical, or other workplace hazards. PPE may include gloves, safety glasses, shoes, earplugs or muffs, hard hats, respirators, coveralls, vests, and full-body suits.

piped medical gas and vacuum systems Networks of pipes that distribute medical gases or vacuum from central sources, such as tanks, throughout a facility to terminal units for access.

Plan for Improvement (PFI) For purposes of Joint Commission accreditation, an organization's written statement that details the procedures to be taken and time frames to correct existing *Life Safety Code*® deficiencies. *See also Life Safety Code*®, Statement of Conditions™ (SOC).

Plan of Action (POA) A plan detailing the action(s) that an organization will take in order to come into compliance with a Joint Commission accreditation requirement. A POA must be completed for each element of performance associated with a noncompliant accreditation requirement.

policy A principle or method that is developed for the purpose of guiding decisions and activities related to governance, management, care, treatment, and services. A policy is developed by organization leadership, approved by the governing body of the organization, and maintained in writing.

preconstruction risk assessment (PCRA) A risk assessment required before construction projects that addresses the impact of construction on patient care and occupant safety in a facility during construction.

preparedness Actions taken to build capacity and identify resources that may be used if an emergency occurs; second of the four phases of emergency management.

preventive maintenance (PM) The care and servicing of equipment and utilities to help prevent failure from occurring.

quarterly Every three months, plus or minus 10 days.

reassessment Ongoing data collection, which begins on initial assessment, comparing the most recent data with the data collected at earlier assessments.

recovery Actions taken to restore services after an emergency; last of the four phases of emergency management.

renovation The replacement in kind, strengthening, or upgrading of building elements, materials, equipment, or fixtures that does not result in a reconfiguration of the building or spaces within.*

---

* **Source:** NFPA Glossary of Terms, June 2012, National Fire Protection Association, Quincy, MA.

repair The patching, restoration, or painting of materials, elements, equipment, or fixtures for the purpose of maintaining such materials, elements, equipment, or fixtures in good or sound condition.*

Requirement for Improvement (RFI) A recommendation that is required to be addressed in an organization's Evidence of Standards Compliance (ESC) in order for the organization to retain its accreditation. Failure to adequately address an RFI after two opportunities may result in a recommendation to place the organization in Accreditation with Follow-up Survey.

resident A recipient of care in a nursing care center or an assisted living community.

residential occupancy A lodging and rooming house occupancy used for facilities that provide sleeping accommodations for 16 or fewer occupants who are capable of self-preservation. Similarly, hotel and dormitory occupancies provide sleeping accommodations for 17 or more occupants who are capable of self-preservation. Both types of residential occupancies are used for residential treatment facilities, which are often accredited as behavioral health care facilities. As designated by the local authority having jurisdiction (AHJ), assisted living facilities also may be classified as one of these types of residential occupancies.

response Actions taken when an emergency occurs; third of the four phases of emergency management.

risk The probability that a disease, injury, condition, death, or related occurrence may occur for a person or population or that serious damage could occur to necessary equipment, the building, or property.

risk assessment An examination of a function or process to determine the actual and potential risks and to prioritize areas for improvement. *See also* environment of care (EC) risk assessment.

root cause A fundamental reason for the failure or inefficiency of a process.

safety The degree to which an intervention in the health care environment is free of risk for a patient and other persons, including workers. Safety risks may arise from the performance of tasks, from the structure of the physical environment, or from situations beyond the organization's control (such as weather).

safety data sheet (SDS) A sheet provided by the manufacturer that includes details about a substance's hazards. Employers must make sure that SDSs (formerly known as material safety data sheets) are readily accessible to employees.

safety management Activities selected and implemented by the organization to assess and control the impact of environmental risk and to improve general environmental safety.

safety officer A person who manages environmental risks and who also may be the person with authority to intervene when situations threaten people or property.

security Protection of people and property against harm or loss (for example, workplace violence, theft, access to medications). Security incidents may be caused by persons from outside or inside the organization.

security-sensitive areas Zones in a health care facility that require increased levels of defense to protect patients, staff, and visitors as well as dangerous materials and confidential or important data and information.

sentinel event A patient safety event (not primarily related to the natural course of the patient's illness or underlying condition) that reaches a patient and results in death, permanent harm, or severe temporary harm. *See* the "Sentinel Event" chapter of the *Comprehensive Accreditation Manual* or E-dition for a list of sentinel events, including those related to the environment of care.

smoke barrier A continuous membrane, or a membrane with discontinuities created by protected openings, where such membrane is designed and constructed to restrict the movement of smoke.*

---

* **Source:** NFPA Glossary of Terms, June 2012, National Fire Protection Association, Quincy, MA.

smoke compartment A space within a building enclosed by smoke barriers on all sides, including the top and bottom.

staff As appropriate to their roles and responsibilities, all people who provide care, treatment, and services in the organization, including those receiving pay (for example, permanent, temporary, and part-time personnel, as well as contract employees), volunteers, and health profession students. The definition of *staff* does not include licensed independent practitioners who are not paid staff or who are not contract employees.

Statement of Conditions™ (SOC) A proactive tool that helps an organization conduct a critical self-assessment of its environment of care, fire safety risks, and current level of compliance with the *Life Safety Code®*. The Statement of Conditions™ (SOC) also helps organizations manage deficiencies identified during self-assessment. An organization can access its SOC through its *Joint Commission Connect™* extranet website. The SOC tool is made up of four parts:
1. Basic Building Information (BBI)
2. Plan for Improvement (PFI)
3. Survey-Related Plan for Improvement (SPFI)
4. Time-Limited Waiver (TLW)/Equivalency

surge event An unexpected influx of patients that has the potential to or has overwhelmed organizational resources (for example, mass casualty, epidemic, flu).

survey A key component in the accreditation process, whereby a surveyor(s) conducts an on-site evaluation of an organization's compliance with Joint Commission or Joint Commission International accreditation requirements.

Survey Analysis for Evaluating Risk™ (SAFER™) Matrix The Survey Analysis for Evaluating Risk™ (SAFER™) Matrix gives a visual representation of the risk level of each Requirement for Improvement (RFI). Each observation reported by a surveyor is plotted on the SAFER Matrix according to the risk level of the finding. The risk level is determined according to two factors:
1. The likelihood of the finding to cause harm to patient(s), staff, and/or visitors
2. The scope at which the finding was observed

surveyor For purposes of Joint Commission accreditation, a health care professional who meets The Joint Commission's surveyor selection criteria, evaluates compliance with accreditation requirements, and provides education and consultation regarding compliance with accreditation requirements to surveyed organizations or systems. The type of surveyor(s) assigned is determined by the accreditation program and its services. A surveyor may be, but is not limited to, a licensed physician, surgeon, podiatrist, dentist, nurse, physician assistant, administrator, social worker, psychologist, or behavioral health care professional.

Survey-Related Plan for Improvement (SPFI) A structural environment of care or life safety deficiency that resulted in a Requirement for Improvement (RFI), but cannot be resolved within the required 60 days for completion of an Evidence of Standards Compliance (ESC). The SPFI documents the deficiency and manages the resolution with the Statement of Conditions™ (SOC).

tabletop exercise An exercise that involves key personnel discussing simulated scenarios and is used to assess plans, policies, and procedures. It is a discussion-based exercise that familiarizes participants with current plans, policies, agreements, and procedures, or may also be used to develop new plans, policies, agreements, and procedures.

Time-Limited Waiver (TLW) One of four parts within the Statement of Conditions™ (SOC) tool, this is a formal request for additional time to address an environment of care or life safety Request for Improvement that will take longer than the allowed 60 days provided in the Evidence of Standards Compliance (ESC).

tracer *See* environment of care (EC) tracer.

utility systems Building systems that provide support to the environment of care, including electrical distribution and emergency power; vertical and horizontal transport; heating, ventilating, and air-conditioning (HVAC); plumbing, boiler, and steam; piped gases; vacuum systems; and communication systems, including data exchange systems.

vulnerable population A group of individuals who may have particular needs that set them apart from a more general patient population in their ability to anticipate, cope with, resist, and recover from the impacts of disasters. These populations may include children and adolescents, mental health patients, and the elderly.

weekly Once every seven days, plus or minus two days.

workarounds Alternative, informally designed, and inconsistently applied work processes that expedite work flow but sometimes subvert specific safeguards designed to prevent risk.

workplace violence Any physical assault, threatening behavior, or verbal abuse occurring in the workplace setting.

Index

C

D

E

S

W